T0234278

A Guide to Alternative Medicine AND THE Digestive System

A Guide to Alternative Medicine ᴬᴺᴰ THE Digestive System

Anil Minocha, MD, FACP, FACG, AGAF, CPNSS
Professor of Medicine
LSU Health Sciences Center and OB-VAMC
Shreveport, Louisiana

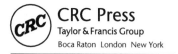

CRC Press
Taylor & Francis Group
Boca Raton London New York

CRC Press is an imprint of the
Taylor & Francis Group, an **informa** business

First published 2013 by SLACK Incorporated

Published 2024 by CRC Press
2385 NW Executive Center Drive, Suite 320, Boca Raton FL 33431

and by CRC Press
4 Park Square, Milton Park, Abingdon, Oxon, OX14 4RN

CRC Press is an imprint of Taylor & Francis Group, LLC

© 2013 Taylor & Francis Group, LLC

Dr. Anil Minocha has no financial or proprietary interest in the materials presented herein.

Library of Congress Cataloging-in-Publication Data

Minocha, Anil.

  A guide to alternative medicine and the digestive system / Anil Minocha.
    p. ; cm.
  Includes bibliographical references and index.
  ISBN 978-1-55642-863-0 (alk. paper)
  I. Title.
  [DNLM: 1. Digestive System Diseases--therapy. 2. Complementary Therapies. 3. Digestive System Physiological Phenomena. WI 140]

616.3--dc23

                          2012025043

ISBN: 9781556428630 (pbk)
ISBN: 9781003524427 (ebk)

DOI: 10.1201/9781003524427

DEDICATION

With pride and love, I dedicate this book to my daughter Geeta, the light of my life; to my loving parents for their constant encouragement and dedication that shaped my life; and to Kamal, Vimal, and Rina for their patience, love, understanding, and unconditional support— without which this book could not have been written.

CONTENTS

ACKNOWLEDGMENTS

This mammoth "solo" project would not have been possible without the teachings, assistance, and cooperation of many friends, senior colleagues, teachers, and thought leaders with whom I have interacted throughout my career and who have selflessly shared their knowledge and wisdom that carries me through to this day.

I owe a deep sense of gratitude to the anonymous peer-reviewers for their exceptionally thorough and constructive criticism, as well as helpful suggestions that exponentially enhanced the quality of this book. They are the unsung heroes!

Doug Larson once said, "A true friend is one who overlooks your failures and tolerates your success." Mike Owens fits this description to the hilt and I am grateful to him for his constant help and encouragement, even during some of the worst times of my life.

Just like any good movie, it is the people behind the scenes that make the show what it is. I am greatly indebted to my publisher, John Bond, and Acquisitions Editor, Carrie Kotlar, for providing me with this unique opportunity to contribute to my passion for learning, teaching, and healing. The team of project editors—April Billick, Dani Malady, and Jessica White—successfully transformed this bland manuscript into a book that readers can easily read, assimilate, and enjoy. I appreciate Marketing Communications Director Michelle Gatt's efforts to ensure that the book gets the exposure it needs. This exceptionally gifted "behind the scenes" cast has done wonders in their quest to make me—and my book—look good.

ABOUT THE AUTHOR

Anil Minocha, MD, FACP, FACG, AGAF, CPNSS is a nationally known physician with board certification in gastroenterology, internal medicine, and nutrition. He is also fellowship trained in clinical pharmacology and medical toxicology.

He grew up in India and received his medical school training at PostGraduate Institute of Medical Sciences in Rohtak, India. He underwent further education and training in various medical institutions in the United States, including Baylor College of Medicine in Houston, Texas, University of Virginia in Charlottesville, and Michigan State University in Lansing.

Dr. Minocha has served in various capacities at different institutions including Director, Division of Digestive Diseases at 2 different medical schools in the United States. In addition to 6 books, he has authored or co-authored over 100 publications in peer-reviewed journals.

Dr. Minocha believes in the old adage, "We are what we eat" and that our digestive system is intimately involved with the health or sickness of systems throughout the human body. What we put into our gut, which is a micro-universe of trillions of bacteria, and how we live with respect to our surrounding environment goes a long way in determining our healthy state versus sickness.

In addition to lectures to physicians across the United States, Dr. Minocha has been interviewed and/or quoted on a variety of topics in different media on numerous occasions including TV, radio, and magazines such as *Ladies Home Journal*, *GQ*, *Good Housekeeping*, and *Natural Health*.

Dr. Minocha currently holds the rank of Professor of Medicine at the Louisiana State University Health Sciences Center and OBVAMC in Shreveport, Louisiana.

PREFACE

There is no such thing as alternative medicine. There is only medicine that works and medicine that doesn't.

Richard Dawkins, *A Devil's Chaplain:*
Reflections on Hope, Lies, Science, and Love, 2004.

Consider the following real-life scenarios:

○ A pregnant woman with nausea and vomiting, who refuses all allopathic medications, asks you about the possible benefits of ginger and/or vitamin B_6. She wants to try them if you think it might help, and asks how should she take it—fresh, powder, or capsules?

○ Your hospital administrator's wife has heard that yogurt with its bacteria is good for health, but she is confused about what kind/brand of yogurt to buy. Are all yogurts created equal?

○ A young medical student with ulcerative colitis asks you if taking turmeric would be helpful. Is it helpful in acute disease, for maintaining remission, or neither?

○ Your boss's father has had 6 recurrences of *Clostridium difficile*-associated diarrhea. He wants to try probiotics and wonders which probiotic/brand he should use and how. He also asks about fecal bacterio-therapy. What are the prerequisites and potential strategies and protocols?

A Guide to Alternative Medicine and the Digestive System is one source that provides answers to the questions above and many more. The *raison d'être* for this peer-reviewed book is my conviction that there is a conspicuous need for a systematic approach to tackle questions like those outlined above. The goal is to inform so that the reader may make informed decisions. The constructive criticism and suggestions of the anonymous peer-reviewers have been a great help to me in accomplishing my goal.

As a practicing gastroenterologist and nutritionist who is also involved in training future physicians, I have frequently been frustrated and saddened by the lack of knowledge (or desire to learn) among health care providers about the vast variety of "medicines" used by patients. As a physician scientist, I have been intrigued by the demand for a much higher level of evidence from complementary and alternative medicine therapies than we demand from mainstream allopathic medicine prior to accepting its use. A comparison of studies related to mainstream allopathic medicine and complementary and alternative medicine therapies has consistently demonstrated that there is no significant difference between the average quality of the studies related to the two. Let it not be forgotten that physicians use mainstream medications for unapproved uses about half the time! The majority of the expensive devices and procedures go into mainstream practice long before controlled trials have demonstrated any benefit.

I do not profess to have covered everything. To state otherwise would be a profound exercise in ignorance and arrogance. This book represents a select portion of the knowledge base available. The carefully selected citations are meant to whet the appetite of the readers and motivate them to expand their horizons beyond what is taught in traditional medical school.

I sincerely hope that readers will find this book helpful and informative, ultimately leading to reducing suffering and bettering health care for patients. As for myself, the 5 years of research and writing have been a labor of love and a lot of fun. Cheers!

Anil Minocha, MD, FACP, FACG, AGAF, CPNSS

INTRODUCTION

Chapter

1 *Why Patients Are Frustrated*

KEY POINTS

○ Digestive illness is widespread.

○ Diagnostic and therapeutic frustrations abound, pushing patients to seek answers from Eastern systems of medicine.[1]

DIAGNOSTIC FRUSTRATIONS

Despite advances in medicine, less than a quarter of patients with dyspeptic symptoms can be documented to have peptic ulcer disease and gastroparesis. Similarly, the lower gastrointestinal problems may not consistently yield a precise diagnosis.

Most of the patients have normal results upon routine investigation and get labeled with such waste basket diagnoses as dyspepsia, gastritis, spastic colon, irritable bowel syndrome (IBS), etc. We are usually unable to offer a precise diagnosis—much less an effective, reliable treatment plan—to such patients. Despite the lack of diagnosis in many of the patients, they are treated with not only drugs like proton pump inhibitors, but even perhaps antidepressants, despite conflicting evidence of clinical efficacy.

Almost half of the patients complaining of heartburn and diagnosed with gastroesophageal reflux disease (GERD) have normal endoscopy, esophageal motility, and esophageal pH profile but still

1

Minocha A. *A Guide to Alternative Medicine and the Digestive System* (pp 1-6).
© 2013 Taylor & Francis Group.

continue to be treated with high-dose proton pump inhibitors. The majority of patients with GERD have to continue taking their anti-GERD medications long after the antireflux surgery.

For a while, especially in the 1990s, many diverse ailments were attributed to *Helicobacter pylori.* It was not unusual for experts to show slides announcing, "The only good *H pylori* is dead *H pylori.*"[2] We still do not understand *H pylori* fully, since it appears to be related to dyspepsia in only a small fraction of patients; however, its presence has been shown to be helpful against GERD. Yet we keep looking for it and killing it in many cases, even without peptic ulcer disease or malignancy. This is all done without fully understanding the ramifications of such treatments, as well as possible future effects of the absence of *H pylori* on the body.

Beyond functional dyspepsia, we do not yet have a full and clear understanding of the pathogenesis of peptic ulcer disease. Oxidative stress, *H pylori* infection, use of nonsteroidal anti-inflammatory drugs, and inadequate gastric mucosal defense are some of the mechanisms involved. As many as half of the patients continue to have epigastric pain long after healing of the ulcer. Dyspeptic symptoms improve in less than 15% of patients after eradicating *H pylori.*

We should at the same time be alert to the critical differences between functional and organic disorders. A classic example is IBS; while the endoscopic exam is normal, biochemical, physiological, and histopathological changes can be found in many patients. The diagnostic criteria are clinical and keep changing every few years (eg, Rome I, Rome II, and Rome III, all based on "expert consensus"), while the patient continues to suffer.[3] However, given the economic environment and how physicians are paid, physicians often spend more time doing procedures that carry higher reimbursement and avoid spending adequate time with their patients.

THERAPEUTIC FRUSTRATIONS

Disease states associated with chronic pain form a major component of this category.[4] Why is it that patients do not always get better using modern medicine? The answer probably lies, at least in part, in the fact that most of the modern-day ailments are multifactorial in pathogenesis and involve a multitude of interactions between the human biological systems (including the central nervous system) with the environmental factors. Modern medicines frequently rely on a single specific molecule, or a combination of few discreet molecules, to cure a disease. Countering one component of the dysfunctional biological system only allows for another component to take over. In many instances, the treatment response is no more than 10% to 25% above the placebo.

Disaster-related environmental exposures like 9/11 have been shown to contribute to the development of gastroesophageal reflux symptoms.[5] These may be potentiated by concomitant asthma and post-traumatic stress disorder. How can a prescription of a proton pump inhibitor help target the cause of the problem in such cases?

It is no wonder then, that many chemically defined treatments frequently gain limited superiority over a placebo. At the same time, the power of modern medicine cannot be underestimated. An ideal situation is a combination of the best of everything, including all of the conventional and complementary medicine that is available.

REFERENCES

1. London F. Take the frustration out of patient education. *Home Health Nurse.* 2001;19(3):158-163.

2. Fennerty MB. Is the only good *H. pylori* a dead *H. pylori*? *Gastroenterology.* 1996;111(6):1773-1774.

3. Whitehead WE, Drossman DA. Validation of symptom-based diagnostic criteria for irritable bowel syndrome: a critical review. *Am J Gastroenterol.* 2010;105(4):814-820.

4. Wang CK, Myunghae Hah J, Carroll I. Factors contributing to pain chronicity. *Curr Pain Headache Rep.* 2009;13(1):7-11.

5. Li J, Brackbill RM, Stellman SD, et al. Gastroesophageal reflux symptoms and comorbid asthma and posttraumatic stress disorder following the 9/11 terrorist attacks on World Trade Center in New York City. *Am J Gastroenterol.* 2011;106(11):1933-1941.

Chapter
2

Popularity and Status of Complementary and Alternative Medicine

KEY POINTS

○ Complementary and alternative medicine (CAM) therapies are becoming increasingly popular.

○ There is concern/criticism about the safety of complementary and alternative therapeutic formulations available in the market.

CAM has been growing in popularity in Western countries[1] and has gathered increasing recognition in recent years with regard to both treatment options and health hazards. Access to such systems is somewhat limited, and a variety of strategies have been advocated to counter that obstacle.[2] The variety of systems presents a wide range of therapeutic approaches, including diet, herbs, metals, minerals, and precious stones, as well as nondrug therapies.[3]

Many of the traditional remedies have been passed through families for generations. The patient's familiarity with the system breeds more trust, especially when modern medicine is failing him or her.

Ayurveda is the oldest system of medicine in the world and is most commonly practiced in India.[4] The written documentation of the diagnostic and healing acumen of Ayurveda predates the advent of modern medicine by thousands of years.

WHY DO PATIENTS FLOCK TO COMPLEMENTARY AND ALTERNATIVE MEDICINE?

In general, patients are more interested in relief and less in what may be causing the problem. The diagnosis may be an ulcer, gastritis, or "functional dyspepsia" based on modern medicine; or a disharmony of the body systems of Vata, Pita, or Kappa in Ayurveda. Regardless, the patient's goal remains the same. Modern medicine rarely shies away from making a diagnosis—even when there may not be enough scientific knowledge to support what that diagnosis precisely is and what can be done for a cure. The treatment, whether it is for IBS or functional dyspepsia, continues to be based on hit-or-miss trials and empiric data, despite all of the medical advances.

Criticism of Complementary and Alternative Medicine

Due to the increasing use of natural and nonmedicinal therapies (as well as herbal products) and the rapid growth of natural health foods, the herbal product industry is being viewed with increasing concern at several levels:

○ Potential for complications
○ Use of possible contraindicated treatments
○ Potential delays in getting proven and potentially more effective treatment

○ Wasting precious time and money trying possibly ineffective treatments for serious illnesses like cancer, and losing both with perhaps no reward

○ Suboptimal regulatory environment

○ Telling lies in order to achieve a placebo effect

There is and likely always will be an inherent conflict between the CAM practitioners and the purists demanding evidence for safety and efficacy. Ultimately, there is only one medicine—the medicine that works. The need of the current times is for the practitioners to work together to optimize the best possible benefit for the ailing patient.

STATUS OF COMPLEMENTARY AND ALTERNATIVE MEDICINE

There is a dire need to look at the active principles of the phytobotanicals, as well the mechanisms involved in using nonherbal therapies as potential chemotherapeutic agents. While there are only limited head-to-head comparisons with conventional chemically defined medications, the combination of extracts with various gastrointestinal active ingredients appears to be advantageous for heterogeneous conditions such as functional dyspepsia, IBS, and inflammatory bowel disease. However, the proof shall only be in the pudding!

REFERENCES

1. van der Riet P. Complementary therapies in health care. *Nurs Health Sci.* 2011;13(1):4-8.

2. Rogers J. Personal health budgets: a new way of accessing complementary therapies? *Complement Ther Clin Pract.* 2011;17(2):76-80.

3. Kiefer D, Pitluk J, Klunk K. An overview of CAM: components and clinical uses. *Nutr Clin Pract.* 2009;24(5):549-559.

4. Patwardhan B, Bodeker G. Ayurvedic genomics: establishing a genetic basis for mind-body typologies. *J Altern Complement Med.* 2008;14(5):571-576.

DIGESTIVE SYSTEM AND COMPLEMENTARY AND ALTERNATIVE MEDICINE

Chapter

3

Pivotal Role of the Digestive System in Health

KEY POINTS

- ○ Damage to the gastrointestinal system has the potential to cause illness throughout the body.
- ○ The gut offers an attractive therapeutic chance to heal multisystem disorders (eg, the use of probiotics for hepatic encephalopathy).

"Man is a food-dependent creature; if you don't feed him he will die. If you feed him improperly, part of him will die."

– Emanuel Cheraskin, MD, DMD[1]

Over hundreds of years, many complex changes have occurred in our lifestyle, nutrition, as well as in our environment. Modern agriculture and animal husbandry supplanted the jungle and then country life. Migration to large cities with fast-paced life placed heavy emphasis on industrialization and the use of processed food. Our current nutritional intake bears no semblance to the past. There is overindulgence with high glycemic load, high-fat foods with changes in macronutrient composition, micronutrient density, acid-base balance, sodium-potassium ratio, and fiber content.[2]

Minocha A. *A Guide to Alternative Medicine and the Digestive System* (pp 7-10). © 2013 Taylor & Francis Group.

Healthy Digestive System

A healthy digestive system allows optimal processing of ingested food matter and efficient absorption of nutrients, while ignoring unneeded and/or fighting off potentially noxious substances and microbes, and eliminating waste matter efficiently and rather effortlessly. The very complex intestinal barriers, including the mucin,[3,4] are evolutionarily conserved but not impervious.

One simple example is celiac sprue, where the net effect is not just malnutrition but also a variety of systemic disorders, including increased incidence of skin diseases and cancers.[5]

In genetically predisposed subjects in the setting of the "right" environmental milieu, a dyshomeostasis state is unable to repair imbalances, leading to disease. This has the potential to result in variable manifestations in different parts of the body that are seemingly unrelated to the digestive system itself.

Future of Nutrition in Health

The role of interactions between gut luminal contents (including food) and genetic predispositions in optimal health, and vice versa, that lead to the development of disease is being increasingly recognized. This has led to the new science of nutrigenomic or nutrigenetic approaches to individualizing nutrition, with the goal of disease prevention and health maintenance, as well as enhancing repair mechanisms for healing during sickness.

Understanding how our diet and nutritional status influence the composition and dynamic operations of our gut microbial communities, and the innate and adaptive arms of our immune system, represents an area of scientific need, opportunity, and challenge.[6]

References

1.   The Hummingbird's Foundation for M.E. Web site. Available at: http://www.hfme.org/healthquotes.htm. Accessed August 12, 2012.
2.   Cordain L, Eaton SB, Sebastian A, et al. Origins and evolution of the Western diet: health implications for the 21st century. *Am J Clin Nutr.* 2005;81(2):341-354.
3.   McGuckin MA, Lindén SK, Sutton P, Florin TH. Mucin dynamics and enteric pathogens. *Nat Rev Microbial.* 2011;9(4):265-278.

4. Liévin-Le Moal V, Servin AL. The front line of enteric host defense against unwelcome intrusion of harmful microorganisms: mucins, antimicrobial peptides, and microbiota. *Clin Microbiol Rev.* 2006;19(2):315-337.

5. Goh VL, Werlin SL. Discovery of gluten as the injurious component in celiac disease. *Nutr Clin Pract.* 2011;26(2):160-162.

6. Kau AL, Ahern PP, Griffin NW, Goodman AL, Gordon JI. Human nutrition, the gut microbiome and the immune system. *Nature.* 2011;474(7351):327-336.

HUMANS ARE SUPERORGANISMS

Chapter

4 *A Bacterial Universe Within Our Body*

KEY POINTS

- ○ A single layer of epithelium separates the human body from trillions of bacteria.
- ○ Trillions of microbes inside of us and in direct constant contact with us have the potential to affect our health.[1]
- ○ The human body, combined with its microbiota, represents a composite superorganism.

WHY DO WE NEED TO KNOW?

While we are always aware of the "outside" influences affecting our body, we seldom think of the even bigger universe inside our gut (technically outside the body) that may be affecting us, even while asleep.

This realization has led to a proliferation of bacterial/yeast products, also known as probiotics, all around the world. It can be different kinds of yogurt brands (healthy and otherwise), in capsules, as well as in enteral nutrition formula.[2]

11

Minocha A. *A Guide to Alternative Medicine and the Digestive System* (pp 11-46). © 2013 Taylor & Francis Group.

Mammals are superorganisms, being a composite of mammalian and microbial cells existing in symbiosis.[3] The gastrointestinal (GI) wall is in constant contact with trillions (10^{14}) of bacteria composed of over 1000 different species.[4]

GUT BACTERIA

The microbiota is critical for a normal state of health. Intestinal bacteria play a vital role in the evolution of the body's adaptive immune system.[5] Interactions between commensal and intestinal epithelial cells (IECs) are vital for the maturation of our immune system. The interplay among the gut, the mucosa-associated immune system, and microbiota has a vital role in gut homeostasis and protection against a variety of diseases.[6]

Epidemiological data implicate changes in the intestinal flora over decades as a link between a modern lifestyle and increased prevalence of certain immune-allergic diseases. Microbial restoration may occur as a result of natural processes or bacteriotherapies.[7]

Human Microbiota Fingerprint

A single layer of epithelium separates the human body from trillions of bacteria. Most of the bacteria are from about 40 to 50 species. This represents that individual's unique bacterial fingerprint, which can be disrupted as a result of infection, medication (including antibiotics), etc, leading to the potential for chronic disease in the long term.[8-10]

Individual patterns of microflora in any individual are specific and stable, and this uniqueness is controlled by physiological, and even logical, distinctive patterns.

FACTORS AFFECTING HUMAN MICROBIOTA

The gut bacteria does change with time until it is established. Numerous factors play a role (Table 4-1).

Gut Flora During Sickness/Stress[9]

The gut flora is also altered during stress and disease. When patients are admitted to an intensive care unit with severe sickness, they lose their lactic acid bacteria after a short stay. Astronauts, when they return from space, are found to have absent or reduced *lactobacilli* and overgrowth of pathogens. The imbalance between the human

---

Table 4-1. Factors Affecting Gut Flora

❖ Type of birth: Vaginal versus Cesarean

❖ Location of birth: Home versus hospital

❖ Domicile: Developed versus developing country, rural versus urban

❖ Breastfed versus formula-fed infants

❖ Maternal diet when breastfeeding

❖ Family and household size: Large versus small

❖ Antibiotic use, especially during early life

❖ Nonsteroidal anti-inflammatory drugs

❖ Emotional stress

❖ Diet: Vegetarian versus nonvegetarian

❖ Diet: Low versus high fiber; use of frozen foods, canned foods, etc

❖ Use of food additives/preservatives

❖ Type of cooking (eg, predominantly fried versus predominantly boiled foods)

---

and the intestinal bacteria predisposes the host not just to enteric infections, but to development of chronic inflammatory-allergic disorders.

FORGET THE MYTHS, HERE ARE THE FACTS ABOUT OUR MICROFLORA

○ A mere detection in feces does not mean they are inhabitant. Food-associated *Lactobacillus* species may just pass through the body and cannot be characterized as permanent inhabitants.

○ The bacteria in feces may or may not represent the bacteria actually in contact with the gut wall in contrast to the lumen.

○ A mismatch, as a result of fewer beneficial bacteria or a higher number of pathogenic bacteria in the colon, allows the pathogenic bacteria to assert their negative influence and cause disease.

○ The gut has a mind of its own, literally, via the enteric nervous system. Brain-gut axis interactions are intimately involved. There is the potential that it affects neuropsychiatric disorders as well.[1]

REFERENCES

1. Cerf-Bensussan N, Gaboriau-Routhiau V. The immune system and the gut microbiota: friends or foes? *Nat Rev Immunol.* 2010;10(10):735-744.

2. Khan SH, Ansari FA. Probiotics—the friendly bacteria with market potential in global market. *Pak J Pharm Sci.* 2007;20(1):76-82.

3. Mandel MJ. Models and approaches to dissect host-symbiont specificity. *Trends Microbiol.* 2010;18(11):504-511.

4. Fujimura KE, Slusher NA, Cabana MD, Lynch SV. Role of the gut microbiota in defining human health. *Expert Rev Anti Infect Ther.* 2010;8(4):435-454.

5. Lee YK, Mazmanian SK. Has the microbiota played a critical role in the evolution of the adaptive immune system? *Science.* 2010;330(6012):1768-1773.

6. Sekirov I, Russell SL, Antunes LCM, Finlay BB. Gut microbiota in health and disease. *Physiol Rev.* 2010;90(3):859-904.

7. Reid G, Younes JA, Van der Mei HC, Gloor GB, Knight R, Busscher HJ. Microbiota restoration: natural and supplemented recovery of human microbial communities. *Nat Rev Microbiol.* 2011;9(1):27-38.

8. Dominguez-Bello MG, Costello EK, Contreras M, et al. Delivery mode shapes the acquisition and structure of the initial microbiota across multiple body habitats in newborns. *Proc Natl Acad Sci USA.* 2010;107(26):11971-11975.

9. Cryan JF, O'Mahony SM. The microbiome-gut-brain axis: from bowel to behavior. *Neurogastroenterol Motil.* 2011;23(3):187-192.

10. Raison CL, Lowry CA, Rook GA. Inflammation, sanitation, and consternation: loss of contact with coevolved, tolerogenic microorganisms and the pathophysiology and treatment of major depression. *Arch Gen Psychiatry.* 2010;67(12):1211-1224.

Chapter

5 *Bacteria May Actually Help: The Science Behind It*

KEY POINTS

○ Gut flora is not only involved in digestive processes, but also in host defenses.

○ The intestinal flora imprint the immunological and physiological systems at or shortly after birth, and then affect systems throughout life.[1]

PROTECTOR ROLE OF BACTERIA

The intestinal surface in a human body reflects the largest surface area of the body that comes into contact with the external environment. It limits host contact with the massive load of luminal antigens that have the potential to bring pathogens into the body.

○ Microbial sensors[2] in the gut represent the tip of the spear—protection against assault by invading pathogens. Microbial sensors allow the gut mucosa to not just sense but also allow distinction between pathogens and nonpathogenic commensal microbes (based on their molecular patterns).

○ The commensal bacteria help in the development of immunity and prevent colonization by pathogens.[3] The intestinally derived bacterial signals that are incorporated into white blood cells and transported to the lactating breast potentiate the neonatal immune system.

Specific patterns of gut bacteria are responsible for the induction of specific immune cells.

GASTROINTESTINAL BACTERIA USUALLY DO NOT CAUSE INFLAMMATION

There is a critical need for homeostatic balance between tolerance[4] and immunity. Any perturbation of a key pathway involved in inflammation or repair results in disorder of the normal homeostatic mechanisms, leading to a chronic uncontrolled inflammation.

Host-Based Dendritic Cells[5]

Mature dendritic cells are usually involved in activation of the immune system. Tolerogenic dendritic cells do the opposite (ie, suppress immune system activity):

○ They serve as the sentinels that capture antigens in the periphery, process them into peptides, and present these to lymphocytes in lymph nodes.

○ They adapt their responses and discriminate between virulent microbes and innocuous bacteria.

These seemingly disparate actions are highly organized. A breakdown in any of the mechanisms results in chronic intestinal inflammation.

Intestinal Epithelial Cells, Immune System, Bacteria, and Inflammation

IECs[6] facilitate receptor-mediated recognition, as well as different bacteria and host-derived feedback mechanisms. Toll-like receptors (TLRs) and nod-like receptors play a key role in controlling mucosal immunity.[7,8]

Differentiating Pathogens From Commensals

In contrast to the pathogens, commensals from the healthy gut develop a variety of different chemical signals for a totally opposite response that maintains homeostasis. Commensal bacteria secrete TLR ligands,[9] which correlate with surface TLRs in the normal gut. These signals, the patterns of which have been conserved during the course of evolution, are released by the commensals. This allows commensals to be recognized as nonthreatening and turn down the pathogenic cascade of events.

Mice deficient in key TLR pathways do not have TLR signaling mechanisms. This results in an exaggerated response to intestinal injury. Similarly, depleting normal mice of intestinal microflora induces an exaggerated injury response. Thus, exposure of the intestinal surface to commensal-derived TLR ligands is key to positive health.

> The gut epithelium and its immune cells do not just sit there disregarding the commensals. These nonpathogenic bacteria play an important role in epithelial development and differentiation.

How Commensal-Intestinal Dysregulation Occurs

Numerous communicating signals are constantly exchanged in the regulation of inflammatory responses at the level of IEC. These delicately balanced interactions are complex and susceptible to dysregulation. The predominant response of the IEC to the bacteria is activated by pattern recognition receptors. Pattern recognition receptors include TLRs.

Evolutionary preserved pattern recognition receptors[10] are needed for recognition and differentiation between nonpathogenic and pathogenic bacteria. Gut commensal bacteria signals utilize the same pattern recognition receptor pathways as the pathogenic bacteria. These interactions at the GI mucosal surface are critical for driving both the protective and pathological immune responses.[11]

REFERENCES

1. Cerf-Bensussan N, Gaboriau-Routhiau V. The immune system and the gut microbiota: friends or foes? *Nat Rev Immunol.* 2010;10(10):735-744.

2. Ronald PC, Beutler B. Plant and animal sensors of conserved microbial signatures. *Science.* 2010;330(6007):1061-1064.

3. Hajishengallis G, Lambris JD. Microbial manipulation of receptor crosstalk in innate immunity. *Nat Rev Immunol.* 2011;11(3):187-200.

4. Bluestone JA, Auchincloss H, Nepom GT, Rotrosen D, St Clair EW, Turka LA. The Immune Tolerance Network at 10 years: tolerance research at the bedside. *Nat Rev Immunol.* 2010;10(11):797-803.

5. Tuettenberg A, Becker C, Correll A, Steinbrink K, Jonuleit H. Immune regulation by dendritic cells and T cells--basic science, diagnostic, and clinical application. *Clin Lab.* 2011;57(1-2):1-12.

6. Maldonado-Contreras AL, McCormick BA. Intestinal epithelial cells and their role in innate mucosal immunity. *Cell Tissue Res.* 2011;343(1):5-12.

7. Khoo JJ, Forster S, Mansell A. Toll-like receptors as interferon-regulated genes and their role in disease. *J Interferon Cytokine Res.* 2011;31(1):13-25.

8. Dagenais M, Dupaul-Chicoine J, Saleh M. Function of nod-like receptors in immunity and disease. *Curr Opin Investing Drugs.* 2010;11(11):1246-1255.

9. Oberg HH, Juricke M, Kabelitz D, Wesch D. Regulation of T cell activation by TLR ligands. *Eur J Cell Biol.* 2011;90(6-7):582-592.

10. Kumagai Y, Akira S. Identification and functions of pattern-recognition receptors. *J Allergy Clin Immunol.* 2010;125(5):985-992.

11. Salzman NH. Microbiota-immune system interaction: an uneasy alliance. *Curr Opin Microbiol.* 2011;14(1):99-105.

Chapter 6

Human Microflora and Chronic Diseases

KEY POINT

○ The composite human superorganism, including the trillions of intestinal bacteria, mimics a micro-universe that needs to be considered as a whole in the pathogenesis of any disease.

Any perturbation of the normal homeostatic mechanisms between the gut and bacteria can shift the balance from controlled to uncontrolled and self-perpetuated inflammation across the body.

The host immune system is a sort of sensory system that takes and assimilates the vital information. It is capable of learning and remembering the stimulus as well as the challenges it might pose. Modern lifestyles, including eating canned and processed foods, can reduce biodiversity within the gut microbiota. This leads to altered microbial input for immunosensory education. Such alterations in early life can pose a risk for developing allergic and inflammatory disorders in later years of life. Intestinal bacteria are critical for both the initiation and perpetuation of chronic intestinal inflammation.[1]

A dysregulation of homeostatic balance between bacteria- and host-derived signals leads to a disruption of the intestinal barrier and initiates the cascade, leading to mucosal immune disorders in genetically susceptible hosts. The effect of antibiotics on the immune system depends not just on the number, but rather the kind of microbial flora involved.[2]

SMALL BOWEL BACTERIAL OVERGROWTH

Abnormal expansion of gut microbial flora, leading to small intestinal bacterial overgrowth, has been implicated in numerous and diverse pathogenic disorders, such as acute pancreatitis, irritable bowel syndrome (IBS),[3] inflammatory bowel disease (IBD), hepatic encephalopathy, fibromyalgia, etc.

Small bowel bacterial overgrowth (SIBO) is amenable to antibiotic treatment. Gut-selective antibiotics are preferred over broad-spectrum antibiotics. In addition to measures to strengthen the intestinal barrier (see Chapters 10 and 11), SIBO may be treated with the following:

○ Probiotics

- ○ Prokinetic agents
- ○ Herbal microbials (eg, Dysbiocide [Biotics Research Corporation, Rosenberg, TX], FC-Cidal [Biotics Research Corporation], and ADP [Biotics Research Corporation])
- ○ Dietary modifications like trial of avoidance of FODMAPs (fermentable oligo-, di-, and monosaccharides, and polyols; see Chapter 10)

INFLAMMATORY BOWEL DISEASE

- ○ Numerous bacteria-related TLR/nod-like receptor-related genes have been described in IBD.
- ○ IBD and functional bowel disease have distinct dyshomeostasis of intestinal bacteria.[4]
- ○ There is reduced bacterial diversity in patients with IBD.
- ○ Colonization of germ-free IL-10-/- mice with *Escherichia coli* and *Enterococcus faecalis* results in proinflammatory responses; however, the same response does not occur when colonized by *Bacteroides vulgatus*.
- ○ Certain host features, like deletion of transcription factor T-beta involved in host immunity, results in development of a "colito-genic" flora capable of transferring colitis.

ALLERGIC DISORDERS[5]

Disturbance or irregularity in the development of these recognition patterns during the early years of life can result in ill health during later years. Skin barrier dysfunction and increased intestinal permeability appear to play a key role by allowing antigen migration through the gut mucosal barrier.

Atopic sensitization appears to be preceded by alterations in the unique fingerprint of gut bacteria or bacterial clusters.

HEPATIC ENCEPHALOPATHY[6]

- ○ Treatment for hepatic encephalopathy includes the use of laxatives, such as lactulose and/or antibiotics. These management strategies stand the test of time, suggesting a communication between the intestinal microbiota and the brain—albeit under pathological conditions.
- ○ Probiotics are beneficial in treating minimal hepatic encephalopathy.

PSYCHONEUROLOGICAL DISORDERS

○ There is bidirectional communication between the brain and commensal bacteria of the gut. This potentially modulates brain function and behavior.[7]

○ Changes in established behavioral patterns alter GI physiology, including the bacteria.

○ Intestinal bacteria produce neuroactive chemicals, such as serotonin, melatonin, catecholamines, histamine, and acetylcholine.

○ Bacteria are also involved in the synthesis of several gases (carbon monoxide, hydrogen sulphide, and nitric oxide) that are involved in neurotransmission in the enteric and central nervous systems.

The intestinal flora not only affect the development of the hypothalamic-pituitary response to stress, but also the development of normal cognitive function in animal models. Introduction of pathogenic organisms into the gut have been linked to the development of anxiety-like behavior.

Some experts have invoked the concept of infection and the hygiene hypothesis in the pathogenesis of disorders, such as autism and depression.[8-10]

○ Reserpine-induced depression-like behavior in mice increases susceptibility to acute colitis.

○ Restriction of certain carbohydrates, such as sucrose or fructose, improves behavior in some patients with depression. These effects are attributed to altered bacterial fermentation patterns.

○ There is a higher prevalence of GI disorders in autism compared to healthy controls.

○ Oral vancomycin provides short-term benefit of neuropsychological symptoms in autism.

○ Probiotics help in reducing anxiety in patients with chronic fatigue syndrome.

CHRONIC PAIN DISORDERS[8]

○ Healthy integrity of the mucosal immune system is vital for normal pain perception in the gut.

○ Absence of CD4 lymphocytes results in increased sensitivity to pain in animals. This can be reversed by restoring CD4 cells.

Table 6-1. Diseases Associated With Alterations in Gut Flora

- Inflammatory bowel disease, including ulcerative colitis[4] and Crohn's disease
- Atherosclerosis[11]
- Irritable bowel syndrome[9]
- Diabetes mellitus[11]
- Small bowel bacterial overgrowth
- Autism[12]
- Depression[10]
- Nonalcoholic fatty liver disease[11]
- Asthma, allergies[13]
- Antibiotic-associated diarrhea
- Cancer[14]
- Hepatic encephalopathy
- Autoimmune disorders[14]
- Necrotizing enterocolitis
- Chronic pain disorders (eg, fibromyalgia,[15] chronic fatigue syndrome[12,16])
- Obesity[17]
- Restless leg syndrome[18]

○ Use of oral antibiotics causing disturbances in the normal bacterial imprint in animals results in increased levels of the sensory neurotransmitter substance P, which is associated with enhanced pain perception.

Germ-free animals have a higher threshold of somatic pain perception compared to conventional mice. Restoration of bacteria reverses the pattern.

INFECTO-OBESITY[17]

○ Metabolic signals from the microbiota influence fat storage and composition.

○ There are differences in the gut bacteria in the obese versus the lean.

○ Obese microbiota harvest more energy from diet, and this is a transmissible trait.

○ The diet-microbe-host interactions influence the proinflammatory cytokine production and may also be involved in the adiposity-associated inflammatory disorders, including metabolic syndrome.

Table 6-1 shows the diseases associated with alterations in gut flora.

References

1. Sekirov I, Russell SL, Antunes LCM, Finlay BB. Gut microbiota in health and disease. *Physiol Rev.* 2010;90(3):859-904.

2. Sekirov I, Tam NM, Jogova M, et al. Antibiotic-induced perturbations of the intestinal microbiota alter host susceptibility to enteric infection. *Infect Immun.* 2008;76(10):4726-4736.

3. Spiller R, Garsed K. Infection, inflammation, and the irritable bowel syndrome. *Dig Liver Dis.* 2009;41(12):844-849.

4. Noor SO, Ridgway K, Scovell L, et al. Ulcerative colitis and irritable bowel patients exhibit distinct abnormalities of the gut microbiota. *BMC Gastroenterol.* 2010;10:134.

5. Kloepfer KM, Gern JE. Virus/allergen interactions and exacerbations of asthma. *Immunol Allergy Clin North Am.* 2010;30(4):553-563.

6. Riggio O, Mannaioni G, Ridola L, et al. Peripheral and splanchnic indole and oxindole levels in cirrhotic patients: a study on the pathophysiology of hepatic encephalopathy. *Am J Gastroenterol.* 2010;105(6):1374-1381.

7. Forsythe P, Sudo N, Dinan T, et al. Mood and gut feelings. *Brain Behav Immun.* 2010;24(1):9-16.

8. Rhee SH, Pothoulakis C, Mayer EA. Principles and clinical implications of the brain-gut-enteric microbiota axis. *Nat Rev Gastroenterol Hepatol.* 2009;6(5):306-314.

9. O'Mahony SM, Marchesi JR, Scully P, et al. Early life stress alters behavior, immunity, and microbiota in rats: implications for irritable bowel syndrome and psychiatric illnesses. *Biol Psychiatry.* 2009;65(3):263-267.

10. Raison CL, Lowry CA, Rook GA. Inflammation, sanitation, and consternation: loss of contact with coevolved, tolerogenic microorganisms and the pathophysiology and treatment of major depression. *Arch Gen Psychiatry.* 2010;67(12):1211-1224.

11. Erridge C. Diet, commensals and the intestine as sources of pathogen-associated molecular patterns in atherosclerosis, type 2 diabetes and non-alcoholic fatty liver disease. *Atherosclerosis.* 2011;216(1):1-6.

12. Bienenstock J, Collins S. 99th Dahlem conference on infection, inflammation and chronic inflammatory disorders: psycho-neuroimmunology and the intestinal microbiota: clinical observations and basic mechanisms. *Clin Exp Immunol.* 2010;160(1):85-91.

13. McLoughlin RM, Mills KH. Influence of gastrointestinal commensal bacteria on the immune responses that mediate allergy and asthma. *J Allergy Clin Immunol.* 2011;127(5):1097-1107; quiz 1108-1109.

14. Tlaskalová-Hogenová H, St Pánková R, Kozáková H, et al. The role of gut microbiota (commensal bacteria) and the mucosal barrier in the pathogenesis of inflammatory and autoimmune diseases and cancer: contribution of germ-free and gnotobiotic animal models of human diseases. *Cell Mol Immunol.* 2011;8(2):110-120.

15. Wallace DJ, Hallegua DS. Fibromyalgia: the gastrointestinal link. *Curr Pain Headache Rep.* 2004;8(5):364-368.

16. Rao AV, Bested AC, Beaulne TM, et al. A randomized, double-blind, placebo-controlled pilot study of a probiotic in emotional symptoms of chronic fatigue syndrome. *Gut Pathog.* 2009;1(1):6.

17. Pasarica M, Dhurandhar NV. Infectobesity: obesity of infectious origin. *Adv Food Nutr Res.* 2007;52:61-102.

18. Weinstock LB, Walters AS. Restless legs syndrome is associated with irritable bowel syndrome and small intestinal bacterial overgrowth. *Sleep Med.* 2011;12(6):610-613.

Chapter

Role of Probiotics in Health Maintenance

KEY POINTS

❍ All probiotics are not the same, and the beneficial effects are strain specific.

❍ Probiotic administration can play an important role in health maintenance and the prevention of disease.[1]

❍ Use of multistrain probiotic formulations is likely to be superior to single-strain formulations.

❍ Despite widespread use, reports of side effects related to probiotics have been exceedingly rare.[2]

Roman historian Plinio promoted the use of fermented milk for GI infections. In recent decades, increasing attention has focused on the role of probiotics in boosting immunity to prevent or treat infections, chronic inflammatory diseases, and allergic disorders.[3]

MECHANISM OF ACTION OF PROBIOTICS

❍ Inhibit growth and invasion by pathogenic organisms.

❍ Strengthen the leaky intestinal barrier.

❍ Modulate the immune system directly at the gut level and indirectly at the level of systemic immune system.

❍ Attenuate the pain perception via actions on opioid and cannabinoid receptors.

Not all strains are similar. The effects of any probiotic depends upon the particular strain used. Most benefits are derived from live probiotic bacteria. Killed bacteria may offer limited benefits via its DNA as well as proteins/cytokines.

Irritable Bowel Syndrome

Please refer to Chapter 44 for details.

Lactose Intolerance

A systematic review in 2010 on treatments of lactose intolerance concluded that there was insufficient evidence for the beneficial role of probiotics.[4,5]

Boosting Immunity Against Infections

Numerous animal studies have documented the immune-boosting properties of probiotics. McVay et al demonstrated that formula acidified with live *Lactococcus lactis* provides superior protection against pulmonary and GI bacterial colonization in rabbits.[6] Use of certain probiotics may elicit a faster immune response to vaccinations.

Effect on Immune System and Infections During Infancy

Some,[7] but not all,[8] studies have shown benefit. A double-blind trial demonstrated that probiotic treatment (*Lactobacillus casei*) given to women who had recently delivered babies and were breastfeeding reduces the risk of GI disturbances in the breastfed child.[7]

Infections in Children at Risk for Allergies

A randomized, placebo-controlled, double-blind trial examined the effect of feeding a synbiotic mixture of 4 probiotic species (*Lactobacillus rhamnosus GG* and *LC705, Bifidobacterium breve Bb99,* and *Propionibacterium freudenreichii ssp shermanii*) plus 0.8 g of galactooligosaccharides in pregnant women for allergy prevention in high-risk infants.[9] The women were given the synbiotic during the last 4 weeks of pregnancy and the infants were continued on the same for a period of 6 months. Over the 2 years of infancy, respiratory infections occurred less frequently in the synbiotic group.

Infections in Day Care Facilities

Use of probiotics in children attending day care reduces the number of infections, suggesting their impact on the spread of infections.[10,11] The *Lactobacillus reuteri* group displayed superior results compared with *Bifidobacterium lactis* or controls.

Infections in the Elderly[12,13]

Aging is generally associated with impaired immunity and a greater predisposition to infections. A controlled study (n = 360) reported that supplementation with milk fermented with yogurt cultures and *L casei DN-114001* resulted in a 20% reduction of the duration of winter infections in the elderly.[12]

Infections in Healthy Adults

Ingestion of probiotic bacteria *Lactobacillus gasseri PA 16/8, Bifidobacterium longum SP 07/3,* and *Bifidobacterium bifidum MF 20/5* significantly shortens common cold episodes by almost 2 days.[14] Another study using *L reuteri* or placebo for 80 days[15] showed that the probiotic group used significantly less sick leave. Limited data suggest a benefit of probiotics for protection against exercise-induced infections in athletes.[16,17]

Infections After Vaccinations

Oral consumption of *Lactobacillus fermentum* reduces the incidence of influenza-like illness after vaccination, suggesting that probiotic potentiates the immunologic response of the vaccine.[18]

Recurrent Otitis Media in Children

Studies examining the effect of probiotics on recurrent otitis media have shown mixed results.[19-21] Children with serous otitis media may get more benefits from probiotic use.[21]

Urinary Tract Infections

Data suggest a promising role for probiotics for preventing infections in patients with neurogenic bladder. Probiotics like *E coli 83972* and *E coli HU2117* reduce urinary tract infections in patients with indwelling catheters.[22,23]

Vulvovaginal Infections

Daily ingestion of yogurt containing *Lactobacillus acidophilus* results in a 3-fold reduction in vulvovaginal *Candida* infections.[24]

Infections Associated With Abdominal Surgeries

Several randomized, controlled trials (RCTs) have demonstrated the positive effect of probiotics plus prebiotics in preventing postoperative infections after major abdominal surgeries and even liver transplantation surgery.[25,26]

Pancreatitis

See Chapter 64 for details.

Nosocomial Infections

Currently, there are insufficient data to conclusively determine whether probiotics are beneficial in the prevention of nosocomial pneumonia.[27]

A Cochrane database meta-analysis concluded that enteral supplementation of probiotics reduces the risk of severe necrotizing enterocolitis and mortality in preterm infants.[28]

Small Bowel Bacterial Overgrowth[29,30]

Treatment of SIBO with *Bacillus clausii* normalizes the hydrogen breath test in 47% of the patients.[30] This success rate is comparable to that achieved with many antibiotics used in clinical practice.

Use of *L casei* or *L reuteri* for fighting infections appears to be promising.

Allergic Disorders

ATOPIC DERMATITIS

Results of the clinical studies in atopic dermatitis have been mixed.[31-37] A meta-analysis by Lee et al concluded that current evidence is more convincing for probiotic efficacy in prevention than treatment of pediatric atopic dermatitis.[38] In contrast, Betsi et al[39] concluded that more RCTs are needed to elucidate whether probiotics are useful for the treatment or prevention of atopic dermatitis.

RESPIRATORY ALLERGIES

Studies examining the role of prebiotics and probiotics in allergic rhinitis have been promising.[40-43] Early dietary intervention with a mixture of prebiotic oligosaccharides reduces the incidence of allergic manifestations and infections.[40] Administration of milk fermented with *Lactobacillus paracasei-33* results in improvement of rhinoconjunctivitis. On the other hand, the effect of *L rhamnosus* supplementation in children with birch pollen allergy is similar to placebo.[43]

L casei, L reuteri, and *L rhamnosus* strain *GG* (ATCC 53103) show promise for primary prevention of allergic disorders.

Enhancing Growth and Development

RATIONALE

Probiotics enhance the potential for growth by enhancing immunity and preventing allergies, infections, and a chronic inflammatory state.

Results of the clinical studies, although mixed, show promise.[44-49] Saran et al conducted a controlled trial to investigate the effect of probiotic supplementation on the growth of poor children with growth retardation.[44] The experimental group received yogurt containing *L acidophilus*, whereas the control group received an isocaloric supplement daily for a period of 6 months. There was a significant increase in weight and height in the probiotic group, and this was associated with fewer cases of diarrhea and fever.

Inflammatory Bowel Disease

See Chapters 45 and 46 for more details.

Collagenous Colitis

Wildt et al investigated the clinical effect of treatment with *L acidophilus LA-5* and *Bifidobacterium animalis subsp lactis BB-12* (AB-Cap-10) in patients in a randomized, double-blind, placebo-controlled study (n = 29) for 12 weeks.[50] Probiotics decreased the bowel frequency.

Diverticulitis and Diverticular Colitis

Diverticulitis reflects inflammation/infection of a diverticulum and usually involves a microperforation. Diverticular colitis, on the other hand, involves segmental colitis. Data indicate that probiotics may be of benefit.[51,52]

Diarrhea

Issues related to diarrhea are discussed in Chapters 47, 48, and 49.

Liver Cirrhosis and Encephalopathy

Please see Section XII for details.

Other Potential Uses

Tables 7-1 through 7-4 show the positive preventative impact of probiotics in various clinical states.

SAFETY OF PROBIOTICS

Whelan et al performed a systematic review of literature and found 20 case reports of adverse events in 32 patients.[2] Of the 53 trials, most showed either no effect or a positive effect on outcomes related to safety, such as mortality and infections.

Table 7-1. Preventing Orodental Disorders

Disorder	Probiotic	Study Design	Results
Dental caries[53]	L reuteri lozenge (1.1 x 10(8) CFU) once daily	Randomized, double-blind, placebo-controlled study	Significant reduction in salivary Streptococcus mutans levels
Dental caries[54]	B lactis Bb-12 in ice cream; 100 mL once daily	Double-blind, randomized, crossover trial	Significant reduction in salivary S mutans levels (P < 0.05)
Dental caries[55]	L reuteri ATCC 55730 once daily for 3 weeks	Placebo-controlled study design with parallel arms, n = 120	Significant reduction of S mutans levels
Dental caries[56]	B animalis DN-173 010 in yogurt	Double-blind, randomized crossover study, n = 21	Significant reduction of salivary S mutans after probiotic
Gingivitis and plaque[57]	L reuteri formulations (LR-1 or LR-2) per day	Randomized, placebo-controlled, double-blind study	Significant reduction in gingival and plaque index
Halitosis[58]	Streptococcus salivarius K12 or placebo lozenges	Placebo-controlled study, n = 23	Substantial (>100 ppb) reductions of volatile sulphur compounds

Table 7-2. Potential Future Uses for Disease Prevention

Disorder/Dysfunction	Impact of Probiotics
Cardiovascular disease	Mixed data on effect on lowering cholesterol[59-63]
Affect motility and relieve colic[64,65]	Improves GI motility and restores bacterial homeostasis
Bone and joint health[66,67]	Beneficial effects on mineral absorption, metabolism, and bone composition and architecture
Athletic performance[68]	Better recovery from fatigue and immune enhancement
Protecting against liver injury[69,70]	Alteration of intestinal microflora
Malnutrition[71]	Improves nutrient absorption
Aging processes[72-74]	Inhibits immunosenescence and lowers chronic inflammation
Restless leg syndrome[75]	Inhibits SIBO, which may be a common denominator in chronic pain syndromes
Obesity[76]	Intestinal flora vary in ability for nutrient extraction and probiotics alter the "obese" microbiota to "lean"
Manic depressive disorder[77]	Alters intestinal microflora to affect proinflammatory cytokines, oxidative stress, and improved nutrition
Chronic fatigue syndrome[78]	Effects via brain-gut axis
Attention deficit hyperactivity disorder (ADHD)[79]	ADHD may be an "allergic disorder" and probiotics may prevent allergy
HIV and sexually transmitted diseases[80]	Prevents HIV and sexually transmitted infections in women by treating and preventing recurrent bacterial vaginosis or directly by secreting substances that block infections

Table 7-3. Primary and Secondary Prevention of Cancer

Cancer Type	Study Design	Variable Studied	Control	Outcome
Colon cancer[81]	Double-blind RCT in colon cancer and poly-pectomized patients	Oligofructose-enriched inulin + L rhamnosus GG and B lactis Bb12	Placebo	Favorable impact on several colorectal cancer bio-markers
Colon cancer[82]	Double-blind RCT in colon cancer (n = 34) and polypectomized (n = 40) patients	L rhamnosus GG and B lactis Bb12, plus inulin enriched with oligofructose	Controls received encapsulated malto-dextrin and 10 g of maltodextrin	Minor stimulatory effects on the systemic immune system
Colon cancer[83]	RCT in subjects after removal of at least 2 colorectal tumors	Dietary fiber and L casei	No treatment	Reduced occurrence of tumors with a grade of moderate atypia or higher
Bladder cancer[84]	RCT following transure-thral resection of the bladder tumor	Oral L casei preparation or biolactis powder	Cases = 23; controls = 25	Prolonged 50% recurrence-free interval (350 versus 195 days)
Bladder cancer[85]	RCT of superficial tran-sitional cell carcinoma of the bladder following transurethral resection	Oral L casei preparation or biolactis powder	Placebo	Biolactis powder showed a better prophylactic effect in patients with primary multiple tumors, recurrent single tumors

(continued)

Table 7-3 (continued). Primary and Secondary Prevention of Cancer

Cancer Type	Study Design	Variable Studied	Control	Outcome
Bladder cancer[86]	Case control study (cases = 180)	*L casei*, taken as fermented milk	Controls = 445	Reduction in risk of bladder cancer with intake of fermented milk products
Breast cancer[87]	*Saccharomyces cerevisiae*-induced apoptosis of breast cancer MCF-7 cell line	Arabinoxylan rice bran (MGN-3/Biobran)		Yeast-induced apoptosis of MCF-7 cells is enhanced in the presence of MGN-3
Breast cancer[88]	Mice injected with breast tumor cells	*Lactobacillus helveticus* R389	Mice not injected with tumor cells	Increased IgA and CD4 positive cells in mammary glands

Table 7-4. Improving Immunity in Immunocompromised Subjects

Subjects	Design#	Variable Studied	Outcome
Children with HIV[89]	Double-blind RCT for 2 months; children aged 2 to 12 years	Formula containing *B bifidum* with *Streptococcus thermophilus*	Probiotics resulted in significant increase in CD4 counts (+118 cells mm^3 versus -42 cells mm^3, $p<0.05$)
Women with HIV[90]	Controlled, prospective study	Yogurt supplemented with probiotic *L rhamnosus GR-1* and *L reuteri RC-14*	Mean CD4 cell count remained the same or increased along with resolution of diarrhea
Children with cystic fibrosis[91]	Controlled, prospective study; (cystic fibrosis = 30; controls = 30; and IBD = 15)	*L rhamnosus GG*	Reduction in calprotectin and nitric oxide concentrations
Children with cystic fibrosis[92]	A prospective, randomized, placebo-controlled study	*L rhamnosus GG* or oral hydration solution	Reduction of pulmonary exacerbations and hospital admissions
Alcoholic cirrhosis[93]	Open-labeled trial; patients = 12; healthy subjects = 13	*L casei Shirota*	Normalization of neutrophil phagocytic capacity

Floch, in 2011, chaired a working group that gave an "A" recommendation for use of probiotics in acute childhood diarrhea, prevention of antibiotic-associated diarrhea, prevention and maintenance of remission in pouchitis, and treatment and prevention of atopic eczema associated with cow's milk allergy. These experts offered "B" grade recommendations in several other areas of treating IBD and IBS.[94]

The probiotics with the greatest number of proven benefits are *L rhamnosus* strain GG and *Saccharomyces boulardii*. We should not expect reproducible results from studies that employ different species or strains, variable formulations, and diverse dosing schedules. Use of multistrain formulations is more likely to be beneficial.

REFERENCES

1. Minocha A. Probiotics for preventive health. *Nutr Clin Pract.* 2009;24(2):227-241.

2. Whelan K, Myers CE. Safety of probiotics in patients receiving nutritional support: a systematic review of case reports, randomized controlled trials, and nonrandomized trials. *Am J Clin Nutr.* 2010;91(3):687-703.

3. Gupta V, Garg R. Probiotics. *Indian J Med Microbiol.* 2009;27:202-209.

4. Ojetti V, Gigante G, Gabrielli M, et al. The effect of oral supplementation with *Lactobacillus reuteri* or *tilactase* in lactose intolerant patients: randomized trial. *Eur Rev Med Pharmacol Sci.* 2010;14(3):163-170.

5. Shaukat A, Levitt MD, Taylor BC, et al. Systematic review: effective management strategies for lactose intolerance. *Ann Intern Med.* 2010;152(12):797-803.

6. McVay MR, Boneti C, Habib CM, et al. Formula fortified with live probiotic culture reduces pulmonary and gastrointestinal bacterial colonization and translocation in a newborn animal model. *J Pediatr Surg.* 2008;43(1):25-29.

7. Ortiz-Andrellucchi A, Sánchez-Villegas A, Rodríguez-Gallego C, et al. Immunomodulatory effects of the intake of fermented milk with *Lactobacillus casei* DN114001 in lactating mothers and their children. *Br J Nutr.* 2008;100(4):834-845.

8. Shadid R, Haarman M, Knol J, et al. Effects of galactooligosaccharide and long-chain fructooligosaccharide supplementation during pregnancy on maternal and neonatal microbiota and immunity—a randomized, double-blind, placebo-controlled study. *Am J Clin Nutr.* 2007;86(5):1426-1437.

9. Kukkonen K, Savilahti E, Haahtela T, et al. Long-term safety and impact on infection rates of postnatal probiotic and prebiotic (synbiotic) treatment: randomized, double-blind, placebo-controlled trial. *Pediatrics.* 2008;122(1):8-12.

10. Weizman Z, Asli G, Alsheikh A. Effect of a probiotic infant formula on infections in child care centers: comparison of two probiotic agents. *Pediatrics*. 2005;115(1):5-9.

11. Hojsak I, Snovak N, Abdovi S, et al. *Lactobacillus GG* in the prevention of gastrointestinal and respiratory tract infections in children who attend day care centers: a randomized, double-blind, placebo-controlled trial. *Clin Nutr*. 2010;29(3):312-316.

12. Turchet P, Laurenzano M, Auboiron S, Antoine JM. Effect of fermented milk containing the probiotic *Lactobacillus casei* DN-114001 on winter infections in free-living elderly subjects: a randomized, controlled pilot study. *J Nutr Health Aging*. 2003;7(2):75-77.

13. Fukushima Y, Miyaguchi S, Yamano T, et al. Improvement of nutritional status and incidence of infection in hospitalized, enterally fed elderly by feeding. *Br J Nutr*. 2007;98(5):969-977.

14. de Vrese M, Winkler P, Rautenberg P, et al. Effect of *Lactobacillus gasseri* PA 16/8, *Bifidobacterium longum* SP 07/3, *B. bifidum* MF 20/5 on common cold episodes: a double blind, randomized, controlled trial. *Clin Nutr*. 2005;24(4):481-491.

15. Tubelius P, Stan V, Zachrisson A. Increasing work-place healthiness with the probiotic *Lactobacillus reuteri*: a randomized, double-blind placebo-controlled study. *Environ Health*. 2005;4:25.

16. Tiollier E, Chennaoui M, Gomez-Merino D, Drogou C, Filaire E, Guezennec CY. Effect of a probiotics supplementation on respiratory infections and immune and hormonal parameters during intense military training. *Mil Med*. 2007;172(9):1006-1011.

17. Kekkonen RA, Vasankari TJ, Vuorimaa T, Haahtela T, Julkunen I, Korpela R. The effect of probiotics on respiratory infections and gastrointestinal symptoms during training in marathon runners. *Int J Sport Nutr Exerc Metab*. 2007;17(4):352-363.

18. Olivares M, Díaz-Ropero MP, Sierra S, et al. Oral intake of *Lactobacillus fermentum* CECT5716 enhances the effects of influenza vaccination. *Nutrition*. 2007;23(3):254-260.

19. Tano K, Grahn Håkansson E, Holm SE, Hellström S. A nasal spray with alpha-haemolytic streptococci as long term prophylaxis against recurrent otitis media. *Int J Pediatr Otorhinolaryngol*. 2002;62(1):17-23.

20. Hatakka K, Blomgren K, Pohjavuori S, et al. Treatment of acute otitis media with probiotics in otitis-prone children-a double-blind, placebo-controlled randomized study. *Clin Nutr*. 2007;26(3):314-321.

21. Skovbjerg S, Roos K, Holm SE, et al. Spray bacteriotherapy decreases middle ear fluid in children with secretory otitis media. *Arch Dis Child*. 2009;94(2):92-98.

22. Darouiche RO, Thornby JI, Cerra-Stewart C, Donovan WH, Hull RA. Bacterial interference for prevention of urinary tract infection: a prospective, randomized, placebo-controlled, double-blind pilot trial. *Clin Infect Dis*. 2005;41(10):1531-1534.

23. Trautner BW, Hull RA, Thornby JI, Darouiche RO. Coating urinary catheters with an avirulent strain of *Escherichia coli* as a means to establish asymptomatic colonization. *Infect Control Hosp Epidemiol.* 2007;28(1):92-94.

24. Hilton E, Isenberg HD, Alperstein P, France K, Borenstein MT. Ingestion of yogurt containing *Lactobacillus acidophilus* as prophylaxis for candidal vaginitis. *Ann Intern Med.* 1992;116(5):353-357.

25. Rayes N, Seehofer D, Theruvath T, et al. Effect of enteral nutrition and synbiotics on bacterial infection rates after pylorus-preserving pancreatoduodenectomy: a randomized, double-blind trial. *Ann Surg.* 2007;246(1):36-41.

26. Rayes N, Seehofer D, Theruvath T, et al. Supply of pre- and probiotics reduces bacterial infection rates after liver transplantation—a randomized, double-blind trial. *Am J Transplant.* 2005;5(1):125-130.

27. McNabb B, Isakow W. Probiotics for the prevention of nosocomial pneumonia: current evidence and opinions. *Curr Opin Pulm Med.* 2008;14(3):168-175.

28. Alfaleh K, Anabrees J, Bassler D, Al-Kharfi T. Probiotics for prevention of necrotizing enterocolitis in preterm infants. *Cochrane Database Syst Rev.* 2011;3:CD005496.

29. Schiffrin EJ, Parlesak A, Bode C, et al. Probiotic yogurt in the elderly with intestinal bacterial overgrowth: endotoxaemia and innate immune functions. *Br J Nutr.* 2009;101(7):961-966.

30. Gabrielli M, Lauritano EC, Scarpellini E, et al. *Bacillus clausii* as a treatment of small intestinal bacterial overgrowth. *Am J Gastroenterol.* 2009;104(5):1327-1328.

31. Huurre A, Laitinen K, Rautava S, Korkeamäki M, Isolauri E. Impact of maternal atopy and probiotic supplementation during pregnancy on infant sensitization: a double-blind placebo-controlled study. *Clin Exp Allergy.* 2008;38(8):1342-1348.

32. Kuitunen M, Kukkonen K, Juntunen-Backman K, et al. Probiotics prevent IgE-associated allergy until age 5 years in cesarean-delivered children but not in the total cohort. *J Allergy Clin Immunol.* 2009;123(2):335-341.

33. Kalliomäki M, Salminen S, Poussa T, Arvilommi H, Isolauri E. Probiotics and prevention of atopic disease: 4-year follow-up of a randomized placebo-controlled trial. *Lancet.* 2003;361(9372):1869-1871.

34. Kalliomäki M, Salminen S, Arvilommi H, Kero P, Koskinen P, Isolauri E. Probiotics in primary prevention of atopic disease: a randomized placebo-controlled trial. *Lancet.* 2001;357(9262):1076-1079.

35. Kirjavainen PV, Salminen SJ, Isolauri E. Probiotic bacteria in the management of atopic disease: underscoring the importance of viability. *J Pediatr Gastroenterol Nutr.* 2003;36(2):223-227.

36. Abrahamsson TR, Jakobsson T, Böttcher MF, et al. Probiotics in prevention of IgE-associated eczema: a double-blind, randomized, placebo-controlled trial. *J Allergy Clin Immunol.* 2007;119(5):1174-1180.

37. Kopp MV, Hennemuth I, Heinzmann A, Urbanek R. Randomized, double-blind, placebo-controlled trial of probiotics for primary prevention: no clinical effects of *Lactobacillus GG* supplementation. *Pediatrics.* 2008;121(4):e850-856.

38. Lee J, Seto D, Bielory L. Meta-analysis of clinical trials of probiotics for prevention and treatment of pediatric atopic dermatitis. *J Allergy Clin Immunol.* 2008;121(1):116-121.

39. Betsi GI, Papadavid E, Falagas ME. Probiotics for the treatment or prevention of atopic dermatitis: a review of the evidence from randomized controlled trials. *Am J Clin Dermatol.* 2008;9(2):93-103.

40. Arslanoglu S, Moro GE, Schmitt J, et al. Early dietary intervention with a mixture of prebiotic oligosaccharides reduces the incidence of allergic manifestations and infections during the first two years of life. *Nutrition.* 2007;137(11):2420-2424.

41. Tamura M, Shikina T, Morihana T, et al. Effects of probiotics on allergic rhinitis induced by Japanese cedar pollen: randomized double-blind, placebo-controlled clinical trial. *Int Arch Allergy Immunol.* 2007;143(1):75-82.

42. Giovannini M, Agostoni C, Riva E, et al; Felicita Study Group. A randomized prospective double blind controlled trial on effects of long-term consumption of fermented milk containing *Lactobacillus casei* in pre-school children with allergic asthma and/or rhinitis. *Pediatr Res.* 2007;62(2):215-220.

43. Helin T, Haahtela S, Haahtela T. No effect of oral treatment with an intestinal bacterial strain, *Lactobacillus rhamnosus* (ATCC 53103), on birch-pollen allergy: a placebo-controlled double-blind study. *Allergy.* 2002;57(3):243-246.

44. Saran S, Gopalan S, Krishna TP. Use of fermented foods to combat stunting and failure to thrive. *Nutrition.* 2002;18(5):393-396.

45. He M, Yang YX, Han H, Men JH, Bian LH. Effects of yogurt supplementation on the growth of preschool children in Beijing suburbs. *Biomed Environ Sci.* 2005;18(3):192-197.

46. Vendt N, Grünberg H, Tuure T, et al. Growth during the first 6 months of life in infants using formula enriched with *Lactobacillus rhamnosus GG*: double-blind, randomized trial. *J Hum Nutr Diet.* 2006;19(1):51-58.

47. Chouraqui JP, Grathwohl D, Labaune JM, et al. Assessment of the safety, tolerance, and protective effect against diarrhea of infant formulas containing mixtures of probiotics. *Am J Clin Nutr.* 2008;87(5):1365-1373.

48. Indrio F, Riezzo G, Raimondi F, Bisceglia M, Cavallo L, Francavilla R. The effects of probiotics on feeding tolerance, bowel habits, and gastrointestinal motility in preterm newborns. *J Pediatr.* 2008;152(6):801-806.

49. Velaphi SC, Cooper PA, Bolton KD, et al. Growth and metabolism of infants born to women infected with human immunodeficiency virus and fed acidified whey-adapted starter formulas. *Nutrition.* 2008;24(3):203-211.

50. Wildt S, Munck LK, Vinter-Jensen L, et al. Probiotic treatment of collagenous colitis: a randomized, double-blind, placebo-controlled trial with *Lactobacillus acidophilus* and *Bifidobacterium animalis subsp lactis*. *Inflamm Bowel Dis.* 2006;12(5):395-401.

51. Tursi A, Brandimarte G, Giorgetti GM, Elisei W, Aiello F. Balsalazide and/or high-potency probiotic mixture (VSL#3) in maintaining remission after attack of acute, uncomplicated diverticulitis of the colon. *Int J Colorectal Dis.* 2007;22(9):1103-1108.

52. Tursi A, Brandimarte G, Giorgetti GM, Elisei W. Beclomethasone dipropionate plus VSL#3 for the treatment of mild to moderate diverticular colitis: an open, pilot study. *J Clin Gastroenterol.* 2005;39(7):644-645.

53. Caglar E, Kuscu OO, Cildir SK, Kuvvetli SS, Sandalli N. A probiotic lozenge administered medical device and its effect on salivary *mutans streptococci* and *lactobacilli*. *Int J Paediatr Dent.* 2008;18(1):35-39.

54. Caglar E, Kuscu OO, Selvi Kuvvetli S, Kavaloglu Cildir S, Sandalli N, Twetman S. Short-term effect of ice-cream containing *Bifidobacterium lactis* Bb-12 on the number of salivary *mutans streptococci* and *lactobacilli*. *Acta Odontol Scand.* 2008;66(3):154-158.

55. Caglar E, Cildir SK, Ergeneli S, Sandalli N, Twetman S. Salivary *mutans streptococci* and *lactobacilli* levels after ingestion of the probiotic bacterium *Lactobacillus reuteri* ATCC 55730 by straws or tablets. *Acta Odontol Scand.* 2006;64(5):314-318.

56. Caglar E, Sandalli N, Twetman S, Kavaloglu S, Ergeneli S, Selvi S. Effect of yogurt with *Bifidobacterium* DN-173 010 on salivary *mutans streptococci* and *lactobacilli* in young adults. *Acta Odontol Scand.* 2005;63(6):317-320.

57. Krasse P, Carlsson B, Dahl C, Paulsson A, Nilsson A, Sinkiewicz G. Decreased gum bleeding and reduced gingivitis by the probiotic *Lactobacillus reuteri*. *Swed Dent J.* 2006;30(2):55-60.

58. Burton JP, Chilcott CN, Moore CJ, Speiser G, Tagg JR. A preliminary study of the effect of probiotic *Streptococcus salivarius* K12 on oral malodour parameters. *J Appl Microbiol.* 2006;100(4):754-764.

59. Bouhnik Y, Achour L, Paineau D, Riottot M, Attar A, Bornet F. Four-week short chain fructo-oligosaccharides ingestion leads to increasing fecal bifidobacteria and cholesterol excretion in healthy elderly volunteers. *J Nutr.* 2007;6:42.

60. Greany KA, Bonorden MJ, Hamilton-Reeves JM, et al. Probiotic capsules do not lower plasma lipids in young women and men. *Eur J Clin Nutr.* 2008;62(2):232-237.

61. Greany KA, Nettleton JA, Wangen KE, Thomas W, Kurzer MS. Probiotic consumption does not enhance the cholesterol-lowering effect of soy in postmenopausal women. *J Nutr.* 2004;134(12):3277-3283.

62. Kekkonen RA, Sysi-Aho M, Seppanen-Laakso T, et al. Effect of probiotic *Lactobacillus rhamnosus GG* intervention on global serum lipidomic profiles in healthy adults. *World J Gastroenterol.* 2008;14(20):3188-3194.

63. Xiao JZ, Kondo S, Takahashi N, et al. Effects of milk products fermented by *Bifidobacterium longum* on blood lipids in rats and healthy adult male volunteers. *J Dairy Sci.* 2003;86(7):2452-2461.

64. Indrio F, Riezzo G, Raimondi F, Bisceglia M, Cavallo L, Francavilla R. Effects of probiotic and prebiotic on gastrointestinal motility in newborn. *J Physiol Pharmacol*. 2009;60(Suppl 6):27-31.

65. Savino F, Cordisco L, Tarasco V, et al. *Lactobacillus reuteri* DSM 17938 in infantile colic: a randomized, double-blind, placebo-controlled trial. *Pediatrics*. 2010;126(3):e526-533.

66. Scholz-Ahrens KE, Ade P, Marten B, et al. Prebiotics, probiotics, and synbiotics affect mineral absorption, bone mineral content, and bone structure. *J Nutr*. 2007;137(3 Suppl 2):838S-846S.

67. Hatakka K, Martio J, Korpela M, et al. Effects of probiotic therapy on the activity and activation of mild rheumatoid arthritis—a pilot study. *Scand J Rheumatol*. 2003;32(4):211-215.

68. Nichols AW. Probiotics and athletic performance: a systematic review. *Curr Sports Med Rep*. 2007;6(4):269-273.

69. Ewaschuk J, Endersby R, Thiel D, et al. Probiotic bacteria prevent hepatic damage and maintain colonic barrier function in a mouse model of sepsis. *Hepatology*. 2007;46(3):841-850.

70. Gerbitz A, Schultz M, Wilke A, et al. Probiotic effects on experimental graft-versus-host disease: let them eat yogurt. *Blood*. 2004;103(11):4365-4367.

71. Parra D, Martínez JA. Amino acid uptake from a probiotic milk in lactose intolerant subjects. *Br J Nutr*. 2007;98(Suppl 1):S101-104.

72. Guigoz Y, Doré J, Schiffrin EJ. The inflammatory status of old age can be nurtured from the intestinal environment. *Curr Opin Clin Nutr Metab Care*. 2008;11(1):13-20.

73. Candore G, Balistreri CR, Colonna-Romano G, et al. Immunosenescence and anti-immunosenescence therapies: the case of probiotics. *Rejuvenation Res*. 2008;11(2):425-432.

74. Schiffrin EJ, Parlesak A, Bode C, et al. Probiotic yogurt in the elderly with intestinal bacterial overgrowth: endotoxaemia and innate immune functions. *Br J Nutr*. 2009;101(7):961-966.

75. Weinstock LB, Fern SE, Duntley SP. Restless legs syndrome in patients with irritable bowel syndrome: response to small intestinal bacterial overgrowth therapy. *Dig Dis Sci*. 2008;53(5):1252-1256.

76. Zhang H, DiBaise JK, Zuccolo A, et al. Human gut microbiota in obesity and after gastric bypass. *Proc Natl Acad Sci*. 2009;106(7):2365-2370.

77. Logan AC, Katzman M. Major depressive disorder: probiotics may be an adjuvant therapy. *Med Hypotheses*. 2005;64(3):533-538.

78. Rao AV, Bested AC, Beaulne TM, et al. A randomized, double-blind, placebo-controlled pilot study of a probiotic in emotional symptoms of chronic fatigue syndrome. *Gut Pathog*. 2009;1(1):6.

79. Pelsser LM, Buitelaar JK, Savelkoul HF. ADHD as a (non) allergic hypersensitivity disorder: a hypothesis. *Pediatr Allergy Immunol*. 2009;20(2):107-112.

80. Bolton M, van der Straten A, Cohen CR. Probiotics: potential to prevent HIV and sexually transmitted infections in women. *Sex Transm Dis*. 2008;35(3):214-225.

81. Rafter J, Bennett M, Caderni G, et al. Dietary synbiotics reduce cancer risk factors in polypectomized and colon cancer patients. *Am J Clin Nutr.* 2007;85(2):488-496.

82. Roller M, Clune Y, Collins K, Rechkemmer G, Watzl B. Consumption of prebiotic inulin enriched with oligofructose in combination with the probiotics *Lactobacillus rhamnosus* and *Bifidobacterium lactis* has minor effects on selected immune parameters in polypectomised and colon cancer patients. *Br J Nutr.* 2007;97(4):676-684.

83. Ishikawa H, Akedo I, Otani T, et al. Randomized trial of dietary fiber and *Lactobacillus casei* administration for prevention of colorectal tumors. Int J Cancer. 2005;116(5):762-767.

84. Aso Y, Akazan H. Prophylactic effect of a *Lactobacillus casei* preparation on the recurrence of superficial bladder cancer. BLP Study Group. *Urol Int.* 1992;49(3):125-129.

85. Aso Y, Akaza H, Kotake T, Tsukamoto T, Imai K, Naito S. Preventive effect of a *Lactobacillus casei* preparation on the recurrence of superficial bladder cancer in a double-blind trial. BLP Study Group. *Eur Urol.* 1995;27(2):104-109.

86. Ohashi Y, Nakai S, Tsukamoto T, et al. Habitual intake of lactic acid bacteria and risk reduction of bladder cancer. *Urol Int.* 2002;68(4):273-280.

87. Ghoneum M, Gollapudi S. Synergistic role of arabinoxylan rice bran (MGN-3/Biobran) in *S. cerevisiae*-induced apoptosis of monolayer breast cancer MCF-7 cells. *Anticancer Res.* 2005;25(6B):4187-4196.

88. de Moreno de LeBlanc A, Matar C, LeBlanc N, Perdigón G. Effects of milk fermented by *Lactobacillus helveticus* R389 on a murine breast cancer model. *Breast Cancer Res.* 2005;7(4):R477-486.

89. Trois L, Cardoso EM, Miura E. Use of probiotics in HIV-infected children: a randomized double-blind controlled study. *J Trop Pediatr.* 2008;54(1):19-24.

90. Anukam KC, Osazuwa EO, Osadolor HB, Bruce AW, Reid G. Yogurt containing probiotic *Lactobacillus rhamnosus* GR-1 and *L. reuteri* RC-14 helps resolve moderate diarrhea and increases CD4 count in HIV/AIDS patients. *J Clin Gastroenterol.* 2008;42(3):239-243.

91. Bruzzese E, Raia V, Gaudiello G, et al. Intestinal inflammation is a frequent feature of cystic fibrosis and is reduced by probiotic administration. *Aliment Pharmacol Ther.* 2004;20(7):813-819.

92. Bruzzese E, Raia V, Spagnuolo MI, et al. Effect of *Lactobacillus GG* supplementation on pulmonary exacerbations in patients with cystic fibrosis: a pilot study. *Clin Nutr.* 2007;26(3):322-328.

93. Stadlbauer V, Mookerjee RP, Hodges S, Wright GA, Davies NA, Jalan R. Effect of probiotic treatment on deranged neutrophil function and cytokine responses in patients with compensated alcoholic cirrhosis. *J Hepatol.* 2008;48(6):945-951

94. Floch MH, Walker WA, Madsen K, et al. Recommendations for probiotic use-2011 update. *J Clin Gastroenterol.* 2011;45 Suppl:S168-171.

Chapter 8
Select Probiotics Available on the Market

KEY POINTS

○ Avoid taking probiotics with food so the probiotic bacteria are not subjected to peak digestive acid and juices.

○ Since the administered probiotic bacteria are transient inhabitants in the gut, I recommend taking probiotics twice a day in order to maintain a steady state and avoid sharp fluctuations.

○ Data suggest that even killed probiotic bacteria may provide some health benefits.

○ Multistrain formulations may be superior to single-strain products.

○ The contents of the various formulations are based on information provided by the manufacturer of the product or on the Internet and is NOT guaranteed.

○ Studies have shown that the information provided by manufacturers may not be entirely accurate, so do your own due diligence.

My opinion on benefits of selected probiotic species (*Note*: This list is not exhaustive):

○ *Bifidobacterium infantis:* IBS

○ *L casei:* Boosts immunity, relieves digestive distress

○ *L reuteri:* Boosts immunity to fight infections, prevents infant colic

○ *L rhamnosus:* Skin eczema

○ *S boulardii:* Antibiotic-induced diarrhea

○ VSL#3: Ulcerative colitis

A wide variety of probiotics are currently available on the market.[1] Development of tailor-made probiotics designed for specific aberrations that are associated with microbial dysbiosis continues worldwide.[2] The young science of proteonomics is being increasingly used in research for the future.[3]

LISTING OF SELECT PROBIOTICS ON THE MARKET

Activia Yogurt (4-oz Single-Serving Cups, Also Available as 24-oz Tubs)

○ Manufactured by Dannon Inc (White Plains, NY)

○ Multiple related products: Activia Light, Activia Fiber, Activia drinks, Activia Dessert, etc

○ Contains *B animalis DN-173010,* aka *Bifidus regularis,* in addition to *S thermophilus* and *Lactobacillus bulgaricus*

○ Contains 2.5 g saturated fat per 4 oz

○ Each serving contains 10 billion CFUs of live bacteria

Adult Formula CP-1

○ Manufactured by Custom Probiotics Inc (Glendale, CA)

○ Five probiotic strains: *L acidophilus, L rhamnosus, Lactobacillus plantarum, B lactis,* and *B bifidum*

○ Each capsule has 50 billion CFUs

Align Capsules

○ Manufactured by Procter & Gamble (Cincinnati, OH)

○ Contains *B infantis 35624* in a vegetarian capsule shell

○ Each capsule contains 1 billion CFUs of bacteria

○ Manufacturer recommends 1 capsule per day

Attune Nutrition Bars

○ Manufactured by Attune Foods (San Francisco, CA) (This is different from the granola munch that is also made by this company, which contains 1 billion CFUs of *L acidophilus*)

○ Contains Kosher *L acidophilus NCFM, L casei Lc-11,* and *B lactis HN019*

○ Comes in several flavors

○ Contains 3 g fiber

○ Each serving contains 6.1 billion CFUs

BifoViden ID

○ Manufactured by Metagenics (San Clemente, CA)

○ A proprietary blend of *B lactis Bi-07, B lactis Bi-04* (formerly known as BI-01), and *S thermophilus St-21*

○ 15 billion live organisms per capsule

Bio-K+ Probiotic Capsules (Regular and Extra Strength)

○ Manufactured by Bio-K+ International Inc (Laval, Canada)
○ Contains *L acidophilus CL1285* and *L casei LBC804*
○ Contains 30 billion CFUs per capsule (extra strength has 50 billion CFUs)

Colon Health Capsules

○ Manufactured by Procter & Gamble
○ Probiotic bacteria include a proprietary blend of *L gasseri KS-13, B bifidum G9-1,* and *B longum MM-2*
○ Each capsule contains 1.5 billion cells
○ Capsules also available as a synbiotic formulation called Colon Health Probiotic + fiber that contains 3 g of inulin in addition to the probiotic blend

Culturelle Capsules

○ Manufactured by Amerifit Nutrition, Inc (Windsor, CT)
○ Contains *L rhamnosus GG*
○ Each capsule contains 10 billion CFUs

DanActive Cultured Milk (100-mL Bottles)

○ Manufactured by Dannon Inc
○ Marketed in Europe as Actimel
○ Contains *S thermophilus* and *L bulgaricus,* in addition to *L casei DN-114 001.* The latter is also marketed as *L casei* Defensis or Immunitas.
○ Different flavors are available
○ Each serving contains 10 billion CFUs

Florastor Capsules (250 mg)

○ Manufactured by Biocodex, Inc (San Bruno, CA)
○ Contains *S boulardii*
○ Each 250-mg capsule contains 5 billion CFUs
○ Dose is 500 mg bid

Gerber Good Start Protect Plus Powdered Infant Milk Formula

○ Manufactured by Nestlé (Vevey, Switzerland)
○ Contains *B lactis Bb-12*
○ Contains 1×10^6 CFUs per gram of powder

Good Belly Fruit Drink

- ○ Manufactured by NextFoods (Boulder, CO)
- ○ Contains *L plantarum 299v*
- ○ Each serving contains 20 billion CFUs

Kefir Drinks

- ○ One brand is Lifeway Foods Inc (Morton Grove, IL)
- ○ Contains 10 to 12 different probiotics
- ○ Has 7 to 10 billion CFUs per cup

LactoViden ID

- ○ Manufactured by Metagenics
- ○ A multistrain proprietary blend of *L acidophilus NCFM* strain, *Lactobacillus salivarius Ls-33*, *L paracasei Lpc-37*, *L plantarum Lp-115*, and *S thermophilus St-21*
- ○ 15 billion live organisms per capsule

OWP Probiotics

- ○ Manufactured by One Wellness Place (Macon, GA)
- ○ Multistrain blend of *B longum*, *B breve*, *B infantis*, *L plantarum*, *L rhamnosus*, and *L acidophilus*
- ○ Each capsule has 15 billion CFUs

Proboulardi (275 mg)

- ○ Manufactured by Metagenics
- ○ Contains *S boulardii* plus *B lactis HN019* and *L rhamnosus HN001*
- ○ A 3:1 blend of: *B lactis HN019*, *L rhamnosus HN001* with 4 billion live organisms
- ○ *S boulardii* (providing 5.5 billion live organisms)

Stonyfield Farm Yogurt

- ○ Manufactured by Stonyfield Farms (Londonderry, NH), a subsidiary of Dannon Inc
- ○ Also makes other probiotic products like Oikos and Soy yogurt
- ○ Contains multiple strains of bacteria, such as *L rhamnosus HN001*, *B lactis*, *L acidophilus*, and *L casei* in addition to *S thermophilus* and *L bulgaricus*

Ultimate Probiotic Formula

○ Manufactured by Swanson Health Products (Fargo, ND)

○ Probiotic strains: *B lactis, B longum, L plantarum, L acidophilus, L casei,* Kyo-Dophilus blend (Wakunaga of America Co Ltd, Mission Viejo, CA), *L salivarius, L rhamnosus, L bulgaricus,* and *Lactobacillus sporogenes*

○ Contains 60 billion CFUs per capsule, plus 100 mg of prebiotic NutraFlora short chain fructooligosaccharides (FOS)

VSL#3 Packets

○ Manufactured by Sigma-Tau Pharmaceuticals (Gaithersburg, MD)

○ Contains 8 different strains of bacteria: *B breve, B infantis, B longum, L acidophilus, L bulgaricus, L casei, L plantarum,* and *S thermophilus*

○ Each packet contains 450 billion CFUs

○ Manufacturer recommends different doses for different disorders. These include: IBS 0.5 to 1 packet/d; ulcerative colitis 1 to 2 packets/d; and pouchitis 2 to 4 packets per day. In difficult-to-maintain remission of ulcerative colitis, 4 to 8 packets per day are recommended

Yakult Cultured Milk

○ A Japanese probiotic milk product manufactured by Yakult Honsha Co (Minato-ku, Tokyo, Japan)

○ Probiotic *L casei Shirota*

○ Each serving contains 8 billion CFUs

Yo-Plus Yogurt

○ Manufactured by Yoplait Inc (Minneapolis, MN)

○ Contains *B animalis subsp lactis Bb-12,* in addition to *S thermophilus* and *L bulgaricus* plus prebiotic inulin 3 g per serving

○ Each serving contains greater than 5 billion CFUs

References

1.   Aureli P, Capurso L, Castellazzi AM, et al. Probiotics and health: an evidence-based review. *Pharmacol Res.* 2011;63(5):366-376.

2. Gerritsen J, Smidt H, Rijkers GT, de Vos WM. Intestinal microbiota in human health and disease: the impact of probiotics. *Genes Nutr.* 2011;6(3):209-240.

3. Aires J, Butel MJ. Proteomics, human gut microbiota and probiotics. *Expert Rev Proteomics.* 2011;8(2):279-288.

Chapter

Prebiotics and Synbiotics

KEY POINTS
❍ Prebiotics are colonic foods.
❍ Prebiotics maintain mucosal growth and stimulate growth of intestinal flora.

PROBIOTIC VERSUS SYNBIOTIC

Prebiotics are also known as colonic food.[1] Synbiotic, in contrast, is a combination of prebiotic and probiotic.[2,3] The combination has the potential to provide at least additive, and possibly synergistic, beneficial effects.

PREBIOTIC FUNCTIONS IN THE INTESTINES

❍ Maintain gut wall integrity
❍ Water electrolyte homeostasis
❍ Provide energy/nutrients for host/bacteria
❍ Stimulate growth of flora

TYPES OF PREBIOTICS

❍ Dietary fiber is a common prebiotic.
❍ Fructo-oligosaccharides (FOS) are promising prebiotics because of their selective fermentation toward more healthy gut bacteria.[4]
❍ Both FOS and galactooligosaccharides fulfill the criteria of successful prebiotics.
❍ Inulin-type fructans have positive prebiotic effects
❍ Isomaltooligosaccharides may be regarded as a quasi-prebiotic since they are partially metabolized in human gut.

POSSIBLE HEALTH BENEFITS OF PREBIOTICS[5]

○ Improved resistance to pathogens, resulting in a decrease in GI infections and respiratory infections
○ Decrease in cholesterol
○ Weight control and obesity-related disorders
○ Increased bacterial synthesis of vitamins
○ Protection against allergies by reducing gut inflammation
○ Improved absorption of calcium and magnesium
○ Improved glycemic control

TYPES OF PREBIOTIC PRODUCTS ON THE MARKET

Products on the market that may be fortified with prebiotics include dairy products, health drinks, infant formula, cereal, dried instant (as well as canned) foods, pet foods, etc.

Always consider health benefits of prebiotics in the context of FODMAP hypothesis. Optimizing the mix of different types of indigestible carbohydrates may yield the best results. See Chapter 10 for more details.

REFERENCES

1. Roberfroid M, Gibson GR, Hoyles L, et al. Prebiotic effects: metabolic and health benefits. *Br J Nutr*. 2010;104(Suppl 2):S1-63.

2. Gourbeyre P, Denery S, Bodinier M. Probiotics, prebiotics, and synbiotics: impact on the gut immune system and allergic reactions. *J Leukoc Biol*. 2011;89(5):685-695.

3. Vitali B, Ndagijimana M, Cruciani F, et al. Impact of a synbiotic food on the gut microbial ecology and metabolic profiles. *BMC Microbiol*. 2010;7:10:4.

4. Sabater-Molina M, Larqué E, Torrella F, Zamora S. Dietary fructo-oligosaccharides and potential benefits on health. *J Physiol Biochem*. 2009;65(3):315-328.

5. Bosscher D, Breynaert A, Pieters L, Hermans N. Food-based strategies to modulate the composition of the intestinal microbiota and their associated health effects. *J Physiol Pharmacol*. 2009;60(Suppl 6):5-11.

LEAKY GUT SYNDROME

Chapter

10 *Leaky Gut: Fact or Fiction?*

KEY POINTS

○ The human body is constantly being subjected to a barrage of chemical, physical, and biological insults from the gastrointestinal (GI) lumen. The body is protected by the so-called intestinal barrier.[1]

○ The epithelial barrier is highly selective and semipermeable. It is a complex, dense mucous layer composed of IgA, antimicrobial peptides, and junctional complexes, including tight junctions (TJs).

○ Intestinal epithelium safeguards the mucosal barrier immunity.[2]

○ A disruption of the intestinal barrier exposes the gut and, indirectly, the rest of the body to the trillions of microbes, toxins, and other metabolic/toxic products.

Access to the gut immune system via the disrupted barrier creates the potential for pathologic immune stimulation, uncontrolled inflammation, and even acute sepsis.

POTENTIAL CHRONIC CONSEQUENCES OF LEAKY GUT

Perturbations of gut bacteria in early life during a critical maturation period can lead to a disruption in the gut's ability to recognize commensal from enteropathogens.[3] This can trigger uncontrolled

Minocha A. *A Guide to Alternative Medicine
and the Digestive System* (pp 47-76).
© 2013 Taylor & Francis Group.

pathologic inflammation in an otherwise predisposed subject, setting the stage for increased intestinal permeability in a vicious cycle. This creates a perfect environment for the individual to suffer from a diverse variety of chronic allergic and immune-mediated disorders in later life.

> The epithelial barrier is a complex dense mucous layer composed of IgA antibodies, antimicrobial peptides, and junctional complexes. Junctional complexes bind the epithelial cells and maintain the barrier. This arrangement permits signaling mechanisms and facilitates selective permeability.

STRUCTURE OF JUNCTIONAL COMPLEX

This complex is composed of the following:
- TJs[4] are dynamic, multiprotein complexes that maintain a selective, semipermeable barrier.
- Adherens junctions,[5] also known as *zonula adherens*, are protein complexes occurring at points of intercellular contact. They provide mechanical linkage.
- Desmosomes[6] provide intercellular mechanical linkage.

Inflammation disrupts the intestinal TJ, increasing intestinal permeability and creating "leaky gut." This allows luminal toxins/antigens access to the body across the gut wall. Inhibition of cytokine-induced increase in intestinal permeability protects against intestinal mucosal damage and intestinal inflammation.

ROLE OF INTESTINAL EPITHELIAL CELLS[7]

Intestinal epithelial cells (IECs) are involved in a dynamic crosstalk with the gut bacteria. IECs must adapt to constant changes in their environment by processing both bacterial and host-derived immune signals.

ROLE OF MAST CELLS

Activated mast cells release numerous inflammatory mediators. *Trichinella spiralis* infection in animal models results in intestinal mastocytosis, accompanied by increased intestinal permeability.

ROLE OF EOSINOPHILS

Eosinophils have been implicated in the pathogenesis of inflammatory bowel disease (IBD) and decreased barrier function. An in vitro culture of IECs with eosinophils increases permeability.

ROLE OF BACTERIA NORMALLY PRESENT IN THE GUT

A delicate equilibrium between the bacterial flora and intestinal immune system must exist. Interactions with commensals are essential to maintaining the architectural integrity of the intestinal surface. The gut barrier and immune system does not simply tolerate commensal bacteria but is dependent on them. The pathogenic bacteria and/or viruses, in contrast to commensals, can disrupt the TJs and the gut barrier via a variety of virulence factors.[8]

Some degree of bacterial translocation across the gut wall may be a normal phenomenon meant to allow the body to sample luminal antigens, so the gut may mount a controlled immune response.[9]

EFFECT OF PATHOGENS ON BARRIER INTEGRITY

Pathogenic microflora affect barriers directly by binding to cell-surface molecules and inducing changes in TJ proteins, or indirectly by generating toxins leading to cell damage. *Cholera toxin* induces TJ barrier dysfunction via its toxins, causing an increased permeability along with changes in intestinal ion and fluid transport. *Clostridium perfringens* toxin directly interacts with TJs, causing an increase in intestinal permeability. Zonulin[10] regulates functioning of TJs, and its abnormalities are involved in the pathogenesis of several inflammatory diseases, including IBD, type I diabetes, and celiac disease.

PHYSIOLOGICAL AND ENVIRONMENTAL FACTORS

Table 10-1 shows some factors affecting intestinal permeability, whereas Table 10-2 enlists measures to protect and strengthen the intestinal barrier.

Age

Intestinal permeability is higher at both extremes of life: infancy and old age. The permeability is especially high in premature babies and has been implicated in the pathogenesis of necrotizing enterocolitis.

Table 10-1. Factors Increasing Intestinal Permeability

- ❖ Formula feeding during infancy[11]
- ❖ Food allergies
- ❖ Dysbiosis
- ❖ Allergenic versus low allergenic diet[12]
- ❖ Infection/inflammation[1,2,8,13]
- ❖ Unhealthy cooking practices such as frying[14,15]
- ❖ Small intestine bacterial overgrowth
- ❖ Unhealthy diet, food additives/preservatives[15]
- ❖ Ischemia
- ❖ Alcoholism[16]
- ❖ Sustained strenuous exercise[17,18]
- ❖ Chemotherapy and radiation therapy
- ❖ Fasting and total parenteral nutrition[19]
- ❖ Emotional stress[17,20]
- ❖ Nonsteroidal anti-inflammatory drugs[16,21,22]
- ❖ Smoking[21,22]
- ❖ Surgery
- ❖ Medications like iron, acid blockers, broad spectrum antibiotics
- ❖ Types of diet and malnutrition[23,24]
- ❖ Dehydration

Pregnancy

The stress-induced increase in intestinal permeability provides opportunity for the passage of bacteria and their components and is believed to be a risk factor for spontaneous abortion by impeding fetomaternal tolerance.

Evidence from experimental animal models implicates products of abnormal bacteria that modulate the stress-signaling cascade, causing abnormal immune activation and pregnancy loss.

Table 10-2. Measures to Prevent Leakiness and Strengthen Intestinal Barrier

❖ Avoid the worsening factors in Table 10-1 as much as possible, in consultation with a physician

❖ Probiotics[3,25]

❖ Good orodental hygiene, including regular dental visits for prevention and treatment

❖ *High fiber diet/prebiotics[13,26]

❖ Breastfeed[11] in early infancy if possible, or use milk banks

❖ Gut-selective antibiotics and herbal antimicrobials in case of small intestine bacterial overgrowth

❖ Avoid and treat constipation

❖ Regular exposure to farm animals as children

❖ Adequate fluid intake

❖ Avoid frequent snacking between meals

❖ Avoid and treat infection

❖ Vitamins A and D (check levels)

❖ *Butyrate[27]

❖ Calcium[28] and magnesium

❖ Aged garlic extract

❖ Zinc[29]

❖ Elimination/exclusion diet as appropriate (see Tables 10-3 and 10-4)

❖ Glutamine[15,30,31]

❖ N-acetylcysteine

❖ Turmeric

❖ Bovine colostrum

❖ Optimize stress coping mechanisms

❖ Omega-3 fatty acids[25]

❖ Low sodium

❖ Avoid extremes of temperature, especially cold

❖ Minimize exposure to environmental toxins: grass, ragweed, pollens, dust mites, cats, roaches

Note: Any changes in medications or significant changes in lifestyle and diet need to be undertaken under appropriate physician supervision.

*Too much may worsen symptoms in some individuals.

Exercise Stress[17]

Exercise-heat stress causes intestinal barrier dysfunction, leading to GI symptoms accompanied by an increased production of proinflammatory cytokines. Prolonged exercise alone in marathon runners can produce GI symptoms.[18]

Farming Versus Urban Environment

Regular exposure to farm animals reduces the prevalence of allergic disorders. Even maternal exposure to barns during pregnancy offers protective benefit.

Farm effect, especially among animal farmers, provides a more pronounced protective benefit. The most benefit is seen among pig and cattle farmers.[32]

DIET AND NUTRITION

Dietary components can affect TJ permeability, metabolic enzymes, as well as immune functions. Intestinal barrier is impaired in uremic patients and returns toward normal on low protein diets.[23] Potato glycoalkaloids, especially the potato skins, worsen intestinal permeability and aggravate IBD in animals.[14] Avoid french fries.

An elemental diet ameliorates drug-induced small bowel inflammation, suggesting an important role for eliminating certain dietary proteins. An elemental diet also ameliorates Crohn's disease (CD) activity in humans. Low-mineral water ameliorates the intestinal permeability of patients with atopic dermatitis.[12]

A Six Food Elimination Diet may be an easy option to eliminate many likely allergenic food components (cow's milk protein, eggs, soy, wheat, peanut/tree nuts, and seafood). It has been successfully used to ameliorate eosinophilic esophagitis.

FODMAP Diet Concept

FODMAP is an acronym applied to a group of short-chain carbohydrates and sugar alcohols composed of fermentable oligo-, di- and monosaccharides, and polyols. These are osmotically active small molecules. The smaller the length of carbohydrate, the faster the fermentation. Table 10-3 displays some foods involved in the high and low FODMAP categories. The threshold for low versus high FODMAP content has not been scientifically standardized and validated.

Table 10-3. Food Classes Based on FODMAP Concepts

FODMAP Food Class[33-35]	Comment
Fructose: May be consumed in diet, free fructose, part of sucrose, or one component of fructans. Examples: honey, a variety of fruits, and high fructose corn syrup.	Thirty percent of the population has fructose malabsorption due to limited capacity of transport mechanisms across epithelium. Fructose restriction is needed only in those with fructose intolerance; this can be tested with hydrogen breath tests.
Lactose: Present in milk and other dairy products like margarine, yogurt, and soft unripe cheeses (ricotta, cottage).	Prevalence of lactase deficiency due to reduced activity of brush border hydrolases may vary from 5% to 90% depending upon ethnicity. Low FODMAP options include use of lactose-free dairy products, rice milk, sorbet, etc.
Fructans: Shorter molecules are called fructooligosaccharides (FOS) or oligofructose, longer ones are inulins. FODMAP-rich sources include wheat, rye, and many vegetables, like artichokes, asparagus, beets, and onions.	Lack of hydrolases limits intestinal absorptive capacity to less than 5%. Dietary fructans are mostly FOS. FOS and inulin are frequently added for putative health benefits.
Galactans or galactooligosaccharides present in a variety of lentils, beans, and vegetables.	Limited absorptive capacity due to lack of hydrolases. Galactans are present in diet in the form of raffinose and stachyose.
Polyols: Naturally present in a variety of fruit (apples, pears, peaches, cherries, plums, and stone fruits).	Polyols do not have active absorptive mechanisms and are absorbed by simple diffusion. Absorption depends upon molecule size. Smaller erythritol is absorbed well, others (like sorbitol) are too large for simple diffusion. Examples include sorbitol, xylitol, mannitol, maltitol, erythritol, and arabitol. May be present as additives, such as humectants and artificial sweeteners.

Note: Cut-off levels of high versus low FODMAP content have not been standardized or validated.

Excess intake, rapid delivery, and bacterial fermentation of undigested carbohydrates produces increased organic acids (short-chain fatty acids or SCFAs), increased surfactant activity, increased gases (hydrogen, carbon dioxide, methane, and hydrogen sulfide), and gut distension that injures the intestinal barrier. While butyrate is mostly beneficial, other SCFAs can cause more damage. The gas content of the gut plays an important role in GI symptoms. The process, if rapid, can be especially "explosive." The speed of bacterial fermentation and generation of metabolic products varies according to substrate (lactulose > inulin > resistant starch).

FODMAPS POTENTIAL DRAWBACKS

- ○ FODMAPs have been implicated in the rising tide of a variety of disorders, such as CD, celiac disease, irritable bowel syndrome (IBS), chronic fatigue syndrome (CFS), and autism.
- ○ A low FODMAP diet diminishes access to the benefits of prebiotics.
- ○ Legumes and milk products are a major source of nutrition for vegetarians. Since the goal of FODMAP strategy is overall reduction, greater cuts need to be made in other categories in order to accomplish the desired goals.

HARM VERSUS BENEFITS OF FODMAP MAY BE INDIVIDUAL SPECIFIC

Consumption of a lower proportion of rapidly fermentable carbohydrates, along with a greater amount of slowly fermentable carbohydrates, shifts the balance toward benefits. Ingestion of raw potato starch, guar gum, and arabinoxylan causes intestinal injury. The deleterious effects of these foods do not occur if they are consumed along with slowly fermentable wheat bran.

Breast Milk Versus Formula[11]

Preterm infants receiving greater than 75% of feedings from human milk have significantly lower intestinal permeability (3.8-fold lower) compared to those consuming less than 25% of feedings from human milk. Prolonged feeding with a hydrolyzed formula, compared to a cow's milk formula, reduces childhood allergies and infant cow milk allergy.

Unprocessed Cow Milk

Consumption of unprocessed cow's milk in early life has been documented to have a protective effect. This protection is also seen in nonfarm children ingesting unpasteurized cow's milk. *Note*: This is not meant to be a recommendation for consuming unpasteurized milk.

Hot Spices

Spicy food improves nutrient absorption by causing alterations in the intestinal barrier, along with increases in microvilli length and perimeter. This, in turn, increases the absorptive capacity. Hot spices also have anti-inflammatory effects. However, the effects in the damaged epithelium may be quite the opposite due to components like capsaicin and piperine having opposing effects on permeability.[36]

Dehydration

Dehydration increases intestinal permeability, and this is attenuated in subjects receiving fluids during exercise.

Fasting and Enteral and Parenteral Nutrition[19]

Fasting, combined with stress, leads to intestinal damage as well as translocation of microorganisms and toxins. Surgery has similar effects. Endotoxemia worsens the inflammatory response in postoperative patients on parenteral nutrition. Carbohydrate administration prior to surgery maintains the integrity of the intestinal barrier and protects against postoperative dysfunction.

> While total parenteral nutrition increases the potential for translocation across the gut wall, enteral nutrition may not reduce it.

Dietary Fructooligosaccharide Worsen Barrier Function

Results of studies of harm versus benefits from FOS have been mixed. FOS is a source of prebiotic benefits. On the other hand, ingestion of short-chain FOS may increase intestinal permeability.[28]

Gliadin

Celiac sprue represents a classical prototype, demonstrating a breakdown of TJs with increased permeability because of the food protein gliadin. Gliadin, because of its actions in disrupting intercellular junctions, has also been implicated in the pathogenesis of a variety of other autoimmune disorders.

Food Surfactants

Food-grade surfactants cause separation of the TJs and increase absorption of food antigens.

Lipids

Excessive dietary fat causes an increase in small intestinal permeability by suppressing TJ proteins. While certain lipids dilate the TJs, omega-3 fatty acids actually strengthen the barrier. SCFAs enhance the barrier function, although too much nonbutyrate SCFAs may worsen it.

LIFESTYLE FACTORS

Alcohol

Alcohol intake, both acute and chronic, causes barrier dysfunction due to the influx of inflammatory cells and the release of cytokines and reactive oxygen molecules.[16]

Smoking

Studies on the role of smoking in intestinal permeability have yielded mixed results.[21,22]

THERAPEUTIC INTERVENTIONS

The more complex the surgery, the more impaired the intestinal barrier. Medications like nonsteroidal anti-inflammatory drugs (NSAIDs), and even supplements like iron, worsen barrier function.

STRESS, ANXIETY, AND INTESTINAL BARRIER FUNCTION[20]

Stress, whether physiological, pathological, or psychological, affects fluid, electrolyte secretion and absorption, GI motility, as well as visceral sensitivity. Stress also causes structural and functional changes of intestinal barrier.

Stress-induced changes occur via temporary redistribution of TJ proteins and they worsen colitis in animals. Rats separated from their mothers have increased stress-induced defecation and mucosal damage. Stressed patients are more likely to suffer relapses of functional and inflammatory disorders. Stress-induced increase in permeability has been implicated in a variety of chronic disorders and offers an attractive target for intervention.

ROLE OF COMPLEMENTARY AND ALTERNATIVE THERAPIES IN LEAKY GUT SYNDROME

Probiotics

The beneficial effects of probiotics during health and sickness occur, in part, due to their effects on barrier function augmentation. This also allows them to modulate the inflammatory reactions in response to luminal antigens and toxins. Mechanism of action includes competitive adherence to the mucus and epithelium.

Prebiotics[13,26,37]

Effects of inulin-type fructans on the microbial balance of the intestinal microflora, along with effect on intestinal permeability, result in a favorable impact on immune responses. Such changes have been associated with several health benefits, including the prevention of infections and inflammatory disorders in animal models and human studies.[37] Green banana and pectin reduce intestinal permeability and improve diarrhea in children in developing countries.

Traditional Chinese Medicine

Da Cheng Qi decoction, used in traditional Chinese medicine, decreases intestinal permeability and multiorgan dysfunction in patients with acute severe pancreatitis when compared to controls.[38]

Bovine Colostrum

Bovine colostrum strengthens the intestinal barrier and reduces bacterial translocation in multiple animal models of inflammation, including NSAID or ischemia.

Glutamine[30,31]

Glutamine maintains and restores the intestinal barrier in critically ill patients. It also improves the prognosis of critically ill patients by reducing the frequency of infections. Of note, glutamine supplementation is widely used in sick patients in Europe.

Arginine

Arginine serves as a precursor for nitric oxide. Some data suggest that it may actually be harmful in severe sepsis.

Taurine

Relative taurine deficiency during the neonatal period has been implicated in adverse neurodevelopmental outcomes in preterm infants. While evidence from randomized, controlled trials showing the benefit of taurine is lacking, it is used as a supplement because of positive observational data.

Diets Supplemented With Spray-Dried Plasma or Plasma Protein Fractions

Plasma protein supplements reduce proinflammatory cytokines and modulate the mucosal immune response in gut-associated lymphoid tissue. These diets improve the growth performance of farm animals.

Alanyl-Glutamine Supplemented Formula

Children taking alanyl-glutamine supplemented enteral formula have a greater weight and height for their age, along with improved intestinal permeability when compared to controls.

Enzyme-Modified Cheese

Enzyme-modified cheese inhibits the translocation of allergens (eg, ovalbumin) via its effects on the intestinal barrier.

A Cochrane database review studied the impact of feeding multinutrient-fortified human breast milk and concluded that feeding preterm or low birth weight infants following hospital discharge with multinutrient-fortified breast milk compared with unfortified breast milk increases growth rates during infancy.[39] However, fortifying breast milk for infants fed directly from the breast is logistically difficult and would impede breast feeding, which, in addition to nutritional implications, plays a vital role in maternal bonding.

Immunonutrition

A large meta-analysis on the role of immune-nutrient feeds concluded that they decrease the risk of infectious complications, suggesting that beneficial function involves an improvement in intestinal permeability.

Butyrate[27]

Colonocytes derive their nutrition in part from SCFAs (mainly propionate, butyrate, and acetate) produced by bacterial fermentation in the colon. Bacterial fermentation of ingested germinated barley foodstuff results in increased butyrate production, strengthens intestinal barrier, and ameliorates colitis in rats.

N-Acetylcysteine

Administration of N-acetylcysteine protects animals against drug-induced intestinal damage and ameliorates intestinal barrier dysfunction.

Aged Garlic Extract

This prevents intestinal barrier disruption and protects against drug-induced damage to the crypt cells.

Vitamin A

Supplementation to children in developing countries helps reduce the frequency of infections and promotes growth.

Zinc

Zinc supplements improve markers of intestinal permeability in patients with diarrhea. Zinc supplementation in quiescent CD attenuates intestinal permeability in subjects with documented increased permeability.[29] This is associated with a decrease in relapses.

Calcium

Dietary calcium strengthens the intestinal epithelial mucosal barrier and ameliorates experimental colitis in animals.

Herbs and Herbal Extracts

A variety of phytobotanicals, like crude rhubarb[40] and berberine, reduce intestinal barrier permeability.

Nutritional Approach to Strengthen Barrier

A nutritional approach to restore impaired intestinal barrier function and growth after neonatal stress in rats can be accomplished by a diet containing specific long-chain polyunsaturated fatty acids, prebiotics and probiotics, glutamine, and curcumin.[15,25]

CONCLUSION

The intestinal barrier is a highly complex structure that allows for selective permeability.[24,41] Luminal contents (including diet, drugs, and intestinal bacteria) interacting with this barrier on one side and the host immune and nervous system on the other play a critical role in health and sickness.[42] Table 10-4 provides a general guide of foods with a higher likelihood of individual sensitivities as well as alternate options. *Note*: The sensitivities are individual-specific; it is possible for an individual to be sensitive to an alternate option while being able to tolerate a product from the "high likelihood" category. A hit and trial strategy based on individual experiences needs to be adopted to discern one's optimal pattern. Simple things, such as being fed breast milk versus formula milk during infancy, may have long-term consequences.[11,43]

REFERENCES

1. Catalioto RM, Maggi CA, Giuliani S. Intestinal epithelial barrier dysfunction in disease and possible therapeutical interventions. *Curr Med Chem*. 2011;18(3):398-426.

Table 10-4. Guide to Exclusion Diet Based on
Likelihood of Food Sensitivities

Foods to Exclude	Alternate Options
Milk[43,44]	Rice milk; kefir and plain yogurt brands with live cultures that include more than 2 standard bacterial strains
Eggs[43]	Alternate sources of proteins
Fruits: Apples, strawberries, oranges, mangoes, nectarines, lychee, plums, pears; avoid frozen, canned, or sweetened products because of potential reaction to additives/preservatives[45]	Bananas, blueberries, raspberries, grapes, honeydew melon, cantaloupe, cranberries, grapes, resins, figs, papaya
Fish: Shark, tuna, sword fish, orange roughy. *Note*: Also keep in mind the potential mercury content of the fish you are consuming (see Chapter 69)[44]	Sardines, salmon, shrimp. *Note*: farmed fish may provide less benefits than wild
Pork, beef[46]	Skinless chicken, turkey; preferably organic
Canned meats	Fresh meats, especially organic
Corn; gluten-containing foods (wheat,[43,46] barley, rye, spelt, bulgur, farina, kamut, semolina, triticale). Role of oats is controversial and best avoided. Beware of breaded foods; read labels carefully—gluten may be in anything from beer to imitation meats	Amaranth, arrowroot, buckwheat, maize, rice, soy, beans, quinoa (see Chapter 67), tapioca, potatoes[47]
Vegetables/condiments: Potatoes, tomatoes, peas, peppers, paprika, chili pepper, cayenne, soy sauce, barbecue sauce, teriyaki, vinegar, mayonnaise, cinnamon[45,48]	Most vegetables (ie, cauliflower, broccoli, green onions, lettuce), low sodium salt, basil, cumin, garlic, ginger, mint, parsley, cumin, rosemary, thyme, dill (Baltic spice), mustard, tarragon
For vegetarians only: soy[43] and its products, tofu, tempeh[44]	Split peas, lentils/legumes (many people are actually sensitive to legumes as well), quinoa
Raw vegetables	Steam/boil, lightly sauté

(continued)

Table 10-4 (continued). Guide to Exclusion Diet Based on Likelihood of Food Sensitivities

Foods to Exclude	Alternate Options
Deep fried cooking	Steamed/boiling; grilled/roasted also acceptable
Oils: Butter, margarine, shortening, olive oil[49]	Clarified butter, ghee; since extra virgin olive oil is devoid of additives, some who are sensitive to olive oil may be able to handle extra virgin olive oil
Nuts and seeds: peanuts,[46] walnuts, sesame, sunflower, pecans, hazelnuts. *Note*: cross-reactivity among nuts is common	Coconut, pine nuts, flax seeds, cashews
Alcohol: Alcohol itself and the nonalcoholic components can be harmful. Wine is the worst culprit due to biogenic amines and sulphite additives. Avoid dark beers/alcohols	Distilled alcohols (ie, sherry or whiskey) may have fewer reactions than wine. Light beer is better than dark beer
Chocolate, caffeine	Carob, decaf products
Sweeteners: Minimize refined sugar intake; avoid high FODMAP sweeteners	Low FODMAP artificial sweeteners; use in patients with chronic diseases is controversial
Drinks: Minimize alcohol, carbonated and caffeinated beverages, mineral water	Filtered/distilled water, decaffeinated herbal teas
Food additives like monosodium glutamate,[50] benzoic acid[48]	Benzoate-free diet; use fresh products as much as possible
Six Food Elimination Diet: cow's milk protein, eggs, soy, wheat, peanut/tree nuts, seafood[51]	Reintroduce one at a time after a trial of at least 8 weeks. Cow's milk is worst and should be reintroduced last
High glycemic food load: refined sugar, white wheat products, white rice, potatoes, high fructose corn syrup, etc	Low glycemic foods like nuts, meats, yogurt, bananas, legumes, whole grains, most (but not all) vegetables, etc

Note: A product may appear on both sides, based on category. Also, responses may vary based on genetic predisposition and exposure to foods during childhood. Subjects may outgrow their sensitivity with age.[46] Unbalanced exclusion diet increases potential for nutrient deficiencies.

2.   Cario E. Heads up! How the intestinal epithelium safeguards mucosal barrier immunity through the inflammasome and beyond. *Curr Opin Gastroenterol.* 2010;26(6):583-590.

3.   Ohland CL, Macnaughton WK. Probiotic bacteria and intestinal epithelial barrier function. *Am J Physiol Gastrointest Liver Physiol.* 2010;298(6):G807-819.

4.   Furuse M. Molecular basis of the core structure of tight junctions. *Cold Spring Harb Perspect Biol.* 2010;2(1):a002907.

5.   Harris TJ, Tepass U. Adherens junctions: from molecules to morphogenesis. *Nat Rev Mol Cell Biol.* 2010;11(7):502-514.

6.   Thomason HA, Scothern A, McHarg S, Garrod DR. Desmosomes: adhesive strength and signalling in health and disease. *Biochem J.* 2010;429(3):419-433.

7.   Maldonado-Contreras AL, McCormick BA. Intestinal epithelial cells and their role in innate mucosal immunity. *Cell Tissue Res.* 2011;343(1):5-12.

8.   Guttman JA, Samji FN, Li Y, Vogl AW, Finlay BB. Evidence that tight junctions are disrupted due to intimate bacterial contact and not inflammation during attaching and effacing pathogen infection in vivo. *Infect Immun.* 2006;74(11):6075-6084.

9.   García de Lorenzo y Mateos A, Acosta Escribano J, Rodríguez Montes JA. Clinical importance of bacterial translocation. *Nutr Hosp.* 2007;22(Suppl 2):50-55.

10. Fasano A. Zonulin and its regulation of intestinal barrier function: the biological door to inflammation, autoimmunity, and cancer. *Physiol Rev.* 2011;91(1):151-175.

11. Le Huërou-Luron I, Blat S, Boudry G. Breast- v. formula-feeding: impacts on the digestive tract and immediate and long-term health effects. *Nutr Res Rev.* 2010;23(1):23-36.

12. Dupuy P, Cassé M, André F, Dhivert-Donnadieu H, Pinton J, Hernandez-Pion C. Low-salt water reduces intestinal permeability in atopic patients. *Dermatology.* 1999;198(2):153-155.

13. Guarner F. Studies with inulin-type fructans on intestinal infections, permeability, and inflammation. *J Nutr.* 2007;137(11 Suppl):2568S-2571S.

14. Patel B, Schutte R, Sporns P, Doyle J, Jewel L, Fedorak RN. Potato glycoalkaloids adversely affect intestinal permeability and aggravate IBD. *Inflamm Bowel Dis.* 2002;8(5):340-346.

15. Rapin JR, Wiernsperger N. Possible links between intestinal permeability and food processing: a potential therapeutic niche for glutamine. *Clinics (Sao Paulo).* 2010;65(6):635-643.

16. Farhadi A, Keshavarzian A, Kwasny MJ, et al. Effects of aspirin on gastroduodenal permeability in alcoholics and controls. *Alcohol.* 2010;44(5):447-456.

17. Lambert GP. Stress-induced gastrointestinal barrier dysfunction and its inflammatory effects. *J Anim Sci.* 2009;87(Suppl 14):E101-108.

18. Smetanka RD, Lambert GP, Murray R, Eddy D, Horn M, Gisolfi CV. Intestinal permeability in runners in the 1996 Chicago marathon. *Int J Sport Nutr.* 1999;9(4):426-433.

19. MacFie J. Enteral versus parenteral nutrition: the significance of bacterial translocation and gut-barrier function. *Nutrition*. 2000;16(7-8):606-611.

20. Gareau MG, Silva MA, Perdue MH. Pathophysiological mechanisms of stress-induced intestinal damage. *Curr Mol Med*. 2008;8(4):274-281.

21. Suenaert P, Bulteel V, Den Hond E, Hiele M. The effects of smoking and indomethacin on small intestinal permeability. *Aliment Pharmacol Ther*. 2000;14(6):819-822.

22. Suenaert P, Bulteel V, Den Hond E, et al. In vivo influence of nicotine on human basal and NSAID-induced gut barrier function. *Scand J Gastroenterol*. 2003;38(4):399-408.

23. Magnusson M, Magnusson KE, Sundqvist T, Denneberg T. Increased intestinal permeability to differently sized polyethylene glycols in uremic rats: effects of low- and high-protein diets. *Nephron*. 1990;56(3):306-311.

24. Ménard S, Cerf-Bensussan N, Heyman M. Multiple facets of intestinal permeability and epithelial handling of dietary antigens. *Mucosal Immunol*. 2010;3(3):247-259.

25. García-Ródenas CL, Bergonzelli GE, Nutten S, et al. Nutritional approach to restore impaired intestinal barrier function and growth after neonatal stress in rats. *J Pediatr Gastroenterol Nutr*. 2006;43(1):16-24.

26. Shiau SY, Chang GW. Effects of certain dietary fibers on apparent permeability of the rat intestine. *J Nutr*. 1986;116(2):223-32.

27. Hamer HM, Jonkers D, Venema K, Vanhoutvin S, Troost FJ, Brummer RJ. Review article: the role of butyrate on colonic function. *Aliment Pharmacol Ther*. 2008;27(2):104-119.

28. Schepens MA, Rijnierse A, Schonewille AJ, et al. Dietary calcium decreases but short-chain fructo-oligosaccharides increase colonic permeability in rats. *Br J Nutr*. 2010;104(12):1780-1786.

29. Sturniolo GC, Di Leo V, Ferronato A, D'Odorico A, D'Incà R. Zinc supplementation tightens "leaky gut" in Crohn's disease. *Inflamm Bowel Dis*. 2001;7(2):94-98.

30. Tubman TR, Thompson SW, McGuire W. Glutamine supplementation to prevent morbidity and mortality in preterm infants. *Cochrane Database Syst Rev*. 2008;(1):CD001457.

31. Weitzel LR, Wischmeyer PE. Glutamine in critical illness: the time has come, the time is now. *Crit Care Clin*. 2010;26(3):515-525.

32. Braun-Fahrländer C. Environmental exposure to endotoxin and other microbial products and the decreased risk of childhood atopy: evaluating developments since April 2002. *Curr Opin Allergy Clin Immunol*. 2003;3(5):325-329.

33. Barrett JS, Gibson PR. Development and validation of a comprehensive semi-quantitative food frequency questionnaire that includes FODMAP intake and glycemic index. *J Am Diet Assoc*. 2010;110(10):1469-1476.

34. Gibson PR, Shepherd SJ. Evidence-based dietary management of functional gastrointestinal symptoms: the FODMAP approach. *J Gastroenterol Hepatol*. 2010;25(2):252-258.

35. Gibson PR, Shepherd SJ. Personal view: food for thought--Western lifestyle and susceptibility to Crohn's disease. The FODMAP hypothesis. *Aliment Pharmacol Ther.* 2005;21(12):1399-1409.

36. Jensen-Jarolim E, Gajdzik L, Haberl I, Kraft D, Scheiner O, Graf J. Hot spices influence permeability of human intestinal epithelial monolayers. *J Nutr.* 1998;128(3):577-581.

37. Veereman G. Pediatric applications of inulin and oligofructose. *Nutrition.* 2007;137(11 Suppl):2585S-2589S.

38. Chen H, Li F, Jia JG, Diao YP, Li ZX, Sun JB. Effects of traditional Chinese medicine on intestinal mucosal permeability in early phase of severe acute pancreatitis. *Chin Med J (Engl).* 2010;123(12):1537-1542.

39. McCormick FM, Henderson G, Fahey T, McGuire W. Multinutrient fortification of human breast milk for preterm infants following hospital discharge. *Cochrane Database Syst Rev.* 2010;(7):CD004866.

40. Chen DC, Wang L. Mechanisms of therapeutic effects of rhubarb on gut origin sepsis. *Chin J Traumatol.* 2009;12(6):365-369.

41. Rhee SH, Pothoulakis C, Mayer EA. Principles and clinical implications of the brain-gut-enteric microbiota axis. *Nat Rev Gastroenterol Hepatol.* 2009;6(5):306-314.

42. Visser J, Rozing J, Sapone A, Lammers K, Fasano A. Tight junctions, intestinal permeability, and autoimmunity: celiac disease and type 1 diabetes paradigms. *Ann NY Acad Sci.* 2009;1165:195-205.

43. Gonsalves N. Food allergies and eosinophilic gastrointestinal illness. *Gastroenterol Clin North Am.* 2007;36(1):75-91.

44. Guandalini S, Newland C. Differentiating food allergies from food intolerances. *Curr Gastroenterol Rep.* 2011;13(5):426-434.

45. Ballmer-Weber BK, Hoffmann-Sommergruber K. Molecular diagnosis of fruit and vegetable allergy. *Curr Opin Allergy Clin Immunol.* 2011;11(3):229-235.

46. Kagalwalla AF, Shah A, Li BU, et al. Identification of specific foods responsible for inflammation in children with eosinophilic esophagitis successfully treated with empiric elimination diet. *J Pediatr Gastroenterol Nutr.* 2011;53(2):145-149.

47. Vega-Gálvez A, Miranda M, Vergara J, et al. Nutrition facts and functional potential of quinoa (*Chenopodium quinoa willd.*), an ancient Andean grain: a review. *J Sci Food Agric.* 2010;90(15):2541-2547.

48. Campbell HE, Escudier MP, Patel P, et al. Review article: cinnamon- and benzoate-free diet as a primary treatment for orofacial granulomatosis. *Aliment Pharmacol Ther.* 2011;34(7):687-701.

49. Unsel M, Ardeniz O, Mete N, et al. Food allergy due to olive. *J Investig Allergol Clin Immunol.* 2009;19(6):497-499.

50. Genuis SJ. Sensitivity-related illness: the escalating pandemic of allergy, food intolerance and chemical sensitivity. *Sci Total Environ.* 2010;408(24):6047-6061.

51. Gonsalves N, Yang GY, Doerfler B, et al. Elimination diet effectively treats eosinophilic esophagitis in adults; food reintroduction identifies causative factors. *Gastroenterology.* 2012;142(7):1451-1459.

Chapter 11   *Disorders Associated With Leaky Gut*

KEY POINTS

○ Clinical and experimental evidence is consistent with the involvement of the intestinal epithelial barrier in the pathogenesis of many GI and non-GI disorders.[1]

○ Seemingly diverse disorders result when the interaction of the dysfunctional intestinal barrier, altered intestinal flora, and deranged intestinal immune responsiveness in genetically predisposed patients creates a "perfect storm" critical to the disease.

○ Leaky gut may be just one part of the overall pathogenic pathway of various diseases, and other exogenous factors, including bacterial pathogens, are involved.

Table 11-1 lists some of the GI and extragastrointestinal disorders associated with intestinal hyperpermeability or leaky gut.

CELIAC DISEASE[2]

Celiac disease is a classic example of manifestation of leaky gut syndrome. It is an immune-mediated GI disorder with extragastrointestinal manifestations. The offending component in gluten is gliadin. Most patients have a genetic component.

Abnormal tight junctions (TJs) in genetically predisposed subjects permits the gliadin contained in gluten to be absorbed and accessible to the intestinal immune system. This, in turn, triggers an inappropriate immune response to the ingested gluten. Abnormalities of the intestinal barrier are seen even in asymptomatic patients. Increased intestinal permeability precedes exposure to gluten and the development of celiac disease, and persists in asymptomatic patients with celiac disease treated with a gluten-free diet. Healthy first-degree relatives of the patients have altered increased permeability.

Celiac disease has multiple extragastrointestinal manifestations, including liver injury. Such distant manifestations may be due to shared genetic factors, as well as the systemic effects of abnormal intestinal permeability, cytokines, and autoantibodies.

Table 11-1. Some of the Disorders Potentially Involved With Leaky Gut Syndrome

Digestive Disorders	Nondigestive Disorders
Celiac disease[2]	Type 1 diabetes mellitus[16]
Inflammatory bowel disease[3]	Atopic dermatitis[17]
Necrotizing enterocolitis	Asthma[18-20]
Severe pancreatitis[4]	Autism[21-25]
Irritable bowel syndrome[5,6]	Cognitive decline in dementia[26]
NSAID-induced enteropathy[7,8]	Infections
Food allergies[9,10]	Congestive heart failure[27]
Alcoholic liver disease	Sepsis syndrome, multiorgan failure[28]
Nonalcoholic fatty liver disease[11]	Schizophrenia
Infections in liver cirrhosis	Chronic fatigue syndrome[29,30]
Obstructive jaundice[12]	Fibromyalgia[31]
Hepatic encephalopathy	HIV[32,33]
Liver cirrhosis[13,14]	Psoriasis[34-38]
Intrahepatic cholestasis of pregnancy[15]	Uremia
Chemotherapy-induced mucositis	Cancer[39]
Collagenous colitis	Depression[40,41]
Graft versus host disease	Multiple sclerosis
Primary biliary cirrhosis	Chronic inflammatory demyelinating polyneuropathy
Intestinal infections	Ankylosing spondylitis
Nonerosive gastroesophageal reflux disease	Restless leg syndrome

TYPE 1 DIABETES MELLITUS[16]

A combination of dysregulated intestinal barrier function causing leaky gut, aberrations of intestinal microflora, and altered intestinal immune responsiveness in genetically predisposed patients appears to play a central role in pathogenesis of type 1 diabetes mellitus. The leaky gut allows increased passage of luminal antigens across the intestinal barrier, which in turn triggers an autoimmune response causing damage to the pancreas.

Altered intestinal barrier is seen in biobreeding diabetes-prone rats, which develop diabetes with exposure to normal diet.

Prediabetic, normoglycemic subjects show subclinical enhanced permeability. The increase in permeability is at the highest just prior to the development of clinical manifestations.

AGING-ASSOCIATED DEMENTIA[26]

While controlled data of aging in humans show no differences in usual intestinal parameters, data from animals suggest otherwise. Puppies (12 weeks old) and large dogs have higher intestinal permeability than adults (60 weeks old) and small dogs.

Inflammatory Bowel Disease[3]

The disrupted barrier in a predisposed individual results in exposure of luminal factors to lamina propria and an exaggerated immune response. Patients show abnormal TJ proteins and increased intestinal inflammation.

Experimental models of IBD using knockout mice first have increased intestinal permeability, which is then followed by the development of colitis. Patients at an increased risk for IBD show an exaggerated intestinal permeability in response to stimulation. Hyperpermeability precedes the development of the disease. Increasing permeability predicts a clinical relapse in patients in remission.

The CARD15 gene is involved in the pathogenesis of Crohn's disease (CD). The increase in intestinal permeability in relatives of patients with CD correlates with the number of mutations in the CARD15 gene.

Mechanisms common to multiple organ involvement in IBD include genetic susceptibility to abnormal antigen presentation, the presence of autoantibodies against shared antigens, and enhanced intestinal permeability.

Disrupted intestinal barrier function is, by itself, not sufficient to cause IBD. While spontaneous colitis does not develop in some transgenic animal models exhibiting increased permeability, the onset and severity of colitis is accelerated in such transgenic mice when exposed to experimental insults.

Nonsteroidal Anti-Inflammatory Drug-Induced Enteropathy[7,8]

Increased intestinal permeability can be seen within 24 hours of nonsteroidal anti-inflammatory drug (NSAID) ingestion and is key to biochemical changes and tissue damage in NSAID-induced enteropathy.

Liver Diseases

Liver Cirrhosis

Altered intestinal function precedes the appearance of bacterial DNA in serum and ascites in patients with cirrhosis.[13,14] The increased intestinal permeability correlates with progression of the liver disease. Antibiotic prophylaxis is associated with reduced incidence of spontaneous bacterial peritonitis. Antibiotics are effective for the treatment and prevention of hepatic encephalopathy.

Nonalcoholic Fatty Liver Disease[11]

Intestinal permeability is increased in obese mice. Even genetically obese mice have enhanced intestinal permeability. Patients with nonalcoholic fatty liver disease and metabolic syndrome display increased intestinal permeability, along with an increased bacterial lipopolysaccharide (LPS) level leading to increased liver damage.

Primary Biliary Cirrhosis

There is increased intestinal permeability in primary biliary cirrhosis. Antimitochondrial antibodies seen in primary biliary cirrhosis cross-react with bacterial antigens. This molecular mimicry indicates that increased intestinal permeability plays an important role.

Obstructive Jaundice[12]

Complications of obstructive jaundice include increased bacterial toxin due to disruption of the immunologic, biological, and mechanical intestinal barrier. Ringer's ethyl pyruvate solution maintains intestinal barrier function and decreases intestinal oxidative injury and inflammatory reaction in rats with obstructive jaundice.

Intrahepatic Cholestasis of Pregnancy[15]

GI permeability, plasma levels of anti-lipopolysacharide (LPS), and proinflammatory cytokines in intrahepatic cholestasis of pregnancy were compared between 22 normal pregnant women and 29 nonpregnant women. Intestinal permeability was increased in intrahepatic cholestasis of pregnancy (ICP), and the abnormalities persisted long past pregnancy.

IRRITABLE BOWEL SYNDROME

IBS is being increasingly recognized as an activated adaptive immune response characterized by low-grade inflammation. Increased epithelial barrier permeability and an abnormal gut flora have been implicated.[5,6] Patients with self-reported food hypersensitivity have a high prevalence of IBS and allergic disorders. There may be a subgroup of patients with IBS (atopic IBS) who have typical IBS symptoms in association with atopic manifestations and may be characterized as atopic IBS.

CONGESTIVE HEART FAILURE

Congestive heart failure is being increasingly recognized as a multisystem disorder that includes hormonal derangements, as well as alterations in intestinal morphology, permeability, and absorptive function.[27] The disruption of the intestinal barrier, associated with translocation of bacterial endotoxin, contributes to an inflammatory state seen in congestive heart failure that further exacerbates cardiac dysfunction.

> The disturbed intestinal barrier may be caused by a chronic low-grade systemic inflammatory state and resultant cardiac cachexia, which is a marker for poor prognosis.

FOOD ALLERGIES

Most cases of childhood food allergy[9,10] do not persist into adulthood. However, once food allergy is established in an adult, it is rarely cured. Dietary antigens disrupt the intestinal barrier. Once sensitized, increased intestinal permeability persists in subjects even in the absence of continued food antigen stimulation.

Infants with a food allergy demonstrate increased intestinal permeability. Severity of clinical symptoms is directly proportional to the degree of disruption of the intestinal barrier. Food protein-induced enterocolitis syndrome occurs in children up to the age of 3 years. Usually cow's milk and soy are the offending factors, although grains (rice, oat, and barley), vegetables, and chicken and fish may be involved.

Patients who have undergone liver transplantation have increased levels of food antigen-specific IgE, and some of these subjects even develop food allergies for the first time. This occurs even when the donor had no prior history of food allergies.

ATOPIC DERMATITIS[17]

An impaired intestinal barrier allows luminal antigens to get into the subepithelial space and stimulate inflammatory cascade.

Distinct foods may trigger isolated skin manifestations in some patients. Symptoms occur within minutes of ingestion without any correlation with atopic dermatitis. Food challenge in atopic subjects shows increased levels of immune complexes that contain food proteins as antigens. Probiotics can reverse an increase in intestinal permeability and help in the prevention of atopic dermatitis in genetically predisposed high-risk infants.

MAJOR DEPRESSION

Major depression[40,41] is associated with an activation of the inflammatory response system. Proinflammatory cytokines and translocated bacterial LPS may induce depressive symptoms. Leaky gut thus offers a potential new target for the treatment of depression.

An interplay of discreet factors, like intestinal permeability, inflammation, and stress, creates a "perfect storm" leading to multiple multisystem manifestations of major depression in some animal models.

Increased intestinal permeability is seen in animal models of depression due to maternal separation, along with increased susceptibility to the development of colitis. Use of antidepressants improves the markers of depression and reduces susceptibility to the development of colitis. Serum antibodies against LPS of gut bacteria are significantly greater in patients with major depression than in normal volunteers. This suggests that disrupted intestinal barrier function plays a role in the inflammatory pathophysiology of depression.

SEPSIS SYNDROME AND MULTIORGAN FAILURE[28]

Intra-abdominal sepsis is associated with severe immunological imbalance, accompanied by intestinal barrier dysfunction and endotoxemia. Fasting, combined with the stress of sickness, worsens barrier function and causes a translocation of microorganisms and toxins. However, some degree of bacterial translocation may also be a normal phenomenon meant to allow the body to sample luminal antigens so that the gut may mount a controlled immune response. Selective gut decontamination reduces both the intestinal bacterial load and respiratory infections in critically ill patients.

There is often an absence of a discreet focus of infection in many patients of sepsis with systemic inflammatory response syndrome, indicating an abnormal intestinal barrier.

SEVERE ACUTE PANCREATITIS

Intestinal permeability is seen early in the course of severe acute pancreatitis. Gram-negative bacteremia is seen in infected pancreatic necrosis and sepsis syndrome associated with severe pancreatitis. Multiorgan failure and mortality are linked to altered intestinal barrier function in early acute pancreatitis.[4] Some but not all data suggest that immune-enhanced enteral nutrition ameliorates the severity of acute pancreatitis associated with reduction in the intestinal permeability. Da Cheng Qi decoction decreases intestinal permeability as well as bacterial infections in patients with pancreatitis when compared to controls.

CHRONIC FATIGUE SYNDROME

CFS[29] is associated with immune dysfunction and increased oxidative stress, along with increased intestinal permeability. Serum antibodies against the LPS of gram-negative bacteria are significantly increased in patients with CFS. The increase is directly proportional to the severity of illness. This suggests that the gut bacteria are involved in the pathogenesis of CFS.

Anecdotal reports indicate that treating such patients with antioxidants and a "leaky gut diet" results in normalizing the increased translocation of the LPS of gram-negative bacteria accompanied by a complete remission of the CFS symptoms.[30]

FIBROMYALGIA

The pain intensity of patients with fibromyalgia correlates with the degree of small intestinal bacterial overgrowth. This, in turn, is associated with an increased intestinal permeability. Goebel et al[31] studied patients with fibromyalgia, complex regional pain syndrome, and healthy controls. The intestinal permeability was increased both in fibromyalgia and complex regional pain syndrome patients when compared to healthy controls.

AUTISM

Children with autism[21,22] demonstrate intestinal hyperpermeability. Increased intestinal permeability allows the breakdown products of food to enter the circulation, and these then interact with the brain directly or via antigenic response. Nonallergic activation of GI and brain mast cells could contribute to the pathologic findings and provide targets for autism therapy.[23]

Patients with autism display an increased cellular immune reactivity to common dietary proteins. Seventy percent of children with autistic spectrum disorder have a history of GI problems, compared to 28% of neurotypical controls and 42% with other developmental abnormalities. One-third of patients with autism give a history of cow's milk and/or soy protein intolerance during infancy.[24] A Cochrane database review found that dietary intervention has significant effects on overall autistic traits, social isolation, and the overall ability to communicate and interact.[25]

PSORIASIS

There are common chromosomal risk loci for GI diseases characterized by leaky gut (eg, IBD, celiac disease) that are also related to type 1 diabetes as well as psoriasis.[34] The claudins of tight junctions are not only altered in IBD but also in psoriasis.[35,36]

There is an increased permeability in psoriatic patients when compared to controls, suggesting that leaky gut is involved. Microscopic colonic abnormalities are seen in patients with psoriasis even when the colonic mucosa appears grossly normal.[37] There is a high incidence of celiac disease in patients with psoriasis. Malabsorption is present more often in psoriatic patients than in controls.[38]

ASTHMA

Intestinal permeability is increased in patients with bronchial asthma.[18] High intestinal IgA in early life predicts a lower risk for

IgE-associated allergic diseases, such as asthma and food allergies.[19] Boosting airway T-regulatory cells by GI stimulation has been advocated as a strategy for better control of asthma.[20]

HIV

Leaky gut has been implicated in mucosal transmission, as well as in the immune activation seen in HIV-1–infected individuals.[32] Increased gut permeability is seen in HIV infection as indicated by increased circulating bacterial LPS levels. The levels decline in patients on antiretroviral therapy. Glutamine administration may help restore the AIDS-associated increased intestinal permeability to its baseline.[33]

REFERENCES

1. Turner JR. Intestinal mucosal barrier function in health and disease. *Nat Rev Immunol.* 2009;9(11):799-809.

2. Schuppan D, Junker Y, Barisani D. Celiac disease: from pathogenesis to novel therapies. *Gastroenterology.* 2009;137(6):1912-33.

3. Salim SY, Söderholm JD. Importance of disrupted intestinal barrier in inflammatory bowel diseases. *Inflamm Bowel Dis.* 2011;17(1):362-381.

4. Besselink MG, van Santvoort HC, Renooij W, et al; Dutch Acute Pancreatitis Study Group. Intestinal barrier dysfunction in a randomized trial of a specific probiotic composition in acute pancreatitis. *Ann Surg.* 2009;250(5):712-719.

5. Barbara G, Cremon C, De Giorgio R, et al. Mechanisms underlying visceral hypersensitivity in irritable bowel syndrome. *Curr Gastroenterol Rep.* 2011;13(4):308-315.

6. Park JH, Park DI, Kim HJ, et al. The relationship between small-intestinal bacterial overgrowth and intestinal permeability in patients with irritable bowel syndrome. *Gut Liver.* 2009;3(3):174-179.

7. Bjarnason I, Takeuchi K. Intestinal permeability in the pathogenesis of NSAID-induced enteropathy. *J Gastroenterol.* 2009;44(Suppl 19):23-29.

8. Troost FJ, Saris WH, Brummer RJ. Recombinant human lactoferrin ingestion attenuates indomethacin-induced enteropathy in vivo in healthy volunteers. *Eur J Clin Nutr.* 2003;57(12):1579-1585.

9. Ménard S, Cerf-Bensussan N, Heyman M. Multiple facets of intestinal permeability and epithelial handling of dietary antigens. *Mucosal Immunol.* 2010;3(3):247-259.

10. Perrier C, Corthésy B. Gut permeability and food allergies. *Clin Exp Allergy.* 2011;41(1):20-28.

11. Miele L, Valenza V, La Torre G, et al. Increased intestinal permeability and tight junction alterations in nonalcoholic fatty liver disease. *Hepatology.* 2009;49(6):1877-1887.

12. Assimakopoulos SF, Tsamandas AC, Louvros E, et al. Intestinal epithelial cell proliferation, apoptosis and expression of tight junction proteins in patients with obstructive jaundice. *Eur J Clin Invest.* 2011;41(2):117-125.

13. Ancel D, Barraud H, Peyrin-Biroulet L, Bronowicki JP. Intestinal permeability and cirrhosis. *Gastroenterol Clin Biol.* 2006;30(3):460-468.

14. Cesaro C, Tiso A, Del Prete A, et al. Gut microbiota and probiotics in chronic liver diseases. *Dig Liver Dis.* 2011;43(6):431-438.

15. Reyes H, Zapata R, Hernández I, et al. Is a leaky gut involved in the pathogenesis of intrahepatic cholestasis of pregnancy? *Hepatology.* 2006;43(4):715-722.

16. Vaarala O. Leaking gut in type 1 diabetes. *Curr Opin Gastroenterol.* 2008;24(6):701-706.

17. Proksch E, Fölster-Holst R, Jensen JM. Skin barrier function, epidermal proliferation and differentiation in eczema. *J Dermatol Sci.* 2006;43(3):159-169.

18. Hijazi Z, Molla AM, Al-Habashi H, Muawad WM, Molla AM, Sharma PN. Intestinal permeability is increased in bronchial asthma. *Arch Dis Child.* 2004;89(3):227-229.

19. Kukkonen K, Kuitunen M, Haahtela T, Korpela R, Poussa T, Savilahti E. High intestinal IgA associates with reduced risk of IgE-associated allergic diseases. *Pediatr Allergy Immunol.* 2010;21(1 Pt 1):67-73.

20. Strickland DH, Judd S, Thomas JA, Larcombe AN, Sly PD, Holt PG. Boosting airway T-regulatory cells by gastrointestinal stimulation as a strategy for asthma control. *Mucosal Immunol.* 2011;4(1):43-52.

21. de Magistris L, Familiari V, Pascotto A, et al. Alterations of the intestinal barrier in patients with autism spectrum disorders and in their first-degree relatives. *J Pediatr Gastroenterol Nutr.* 2010;51(4):418-424.

22. Galiatsatos P, Gologan A, Lamoureux E. Autistic enterocolitis: fact or fiction? *Can J Gastroenterol.* 2009;23(2):95-98.

23. Theoharides TC, Doyle R, Francis K, Conti P, Kalogeromitros D. Novel therapeutic targets for autism. *Trends Pharmacol Sci.* 2008;29(8):375-382.

24. Horvath K, Perman JA. Autistic disorder and gastrointestinal disease. *Curr Opin Pediatr.* 2002;14(5):583-587.

25. Millward C, Ferriter M, Calver S, Connell-Jones G. Gluten- and casein-free diets for autistic spectrum disorder. *Cochrane Database Syst Rev.* 2008;(2):CD003498

26. Brenner SR. Hypothesis: intestinal barrier permeability may contribute to cognitive dysfunction and dementia. *Age Ageing.* 2010;39(2):278-279.

27. Sandek A, Bauditz J, Swidsinski A, et al. Altered intestinal function in patients with chronic heart failure. *J Am Coll Cardiol.* 2007;50(16):1561-1569.

28. Soeters PB, Luyer MD, Greve JW, Buurman WA. The significance of bowel permeability. *Curr Opin Clin Nutr Metab Care.* 2007;10(5):632-638.

29. Maes M, Mihaylova I, Kubera M, Leunis JC. An IgM-mediated immune response directed against nitro-bovine serum albumin (nitro-BSA) in chronic fatigue syndrome (CFS) and major depression: evidence that nitrosative stress is another factor underpinning the comorbidity between major depression and CFS. *Neuro Endocrinol Lett.* 2008;29(3):313-319.

30. Maes M, Coucke F, Leunis JC. Normalization of the increased translocation of endotoxin from gram negative enterobacteria (leaky gut) is accompanied by a remission of chronic fatigue syndrome. *Neuro Endocrinol Lett.* 2007;28(6):739-744.

31. Goebel A, Buhner S, Schedel R, Lochs H, Sprotte G. Altered intestinal permeability in patients with primary fibromyalgia and in patients with complex regional pain syndrome. *Rheumatology (Oxford).* 2008;47(8):1223-1227.

32. Maingat F, Halloran B, Acharjee S, et al. Inflammation and epithelial cell injury in AIDS enteropathy: involvement of endoplasmic reticulum stress. *FASEB J.* 2011;25(7):2211-2220.

33. Noyer CM, Simon D, Borczuk A, Brandt LJ, Lee MJ, Nehra V. A double-blind placebo-controlled pilot study of glutamine therapy for abnormal intestinal permeability in patients with AIDS. *Am J Gastroenterol.* 1998;93(6):972-975.

34. Festen EA, Goyette P, Scott R, et al. Genetic variants in the region harboring IL2/IL21 associated with ulcerative colitis. *Gut.* 2009;58(6):799-804.

35. Watson RE, Poddar R, Walker JM, et al. Altered claudin expression is a feature of chronic plaque psoriasis. *J Pathol.* 2007;212(4):450-458.

36. Kirschner N, Poetzl C, von den Driesch P, et al. Alteration of tight junction proteins is an early event in psoriasis: putative involvement of proinflammatory cytokines. *Am J Pathol.* 2009;175(3):1095-1106.

37. Scarpa R, Manguso F, D'Arienzo A, et al. Microscopic inflammatory changes in colon of patients with both active psoriasis and psoriatic arthritis without bowel symptoms. *J Rheumatol.* 2000;27(5):1241-1246.

38. Ojetti V, De Simone C, Aguilar Sanchez J, et al. Malabsorption in psoriatic patients: cause or consequence? *Scand J Gastroenterol.* 2006;41(11):1267-1271.

39. Ullman TA, Itzkowitz SH. Intestinal inflammation and cancer. *Gastroenterology.* 2011;140(6):1807-1816.

40. Maes M. The cytokine hypothesis of depression: inflammation, oxidative & nitrosative stress (IO&NS) and leaky gut as new targets for adjunctive treatments in depression. *Neuro Endocrinol Lett.* 2008;29(3):287-291.

41. Maes M, Kubera M, Leunis JC. The gut-brain barrier in major depression: intestinal mucosal dysfunction with an increased translocation of LPS from gram negative enterobacteria (leaky gut) plays a role in the inflammatory pathophysiology of depression. *Neuro Endocrinol Lett.* 2008;29(1):117-124.

TYPES OF COMPLEMENTARY AND ALTERNATIVE THERAPIES USED

Chapter

12

Overview of Complementary and Alternative Medicine Therapies

KEY POINTS

- ○ The demarcation between complementary and alternative medicine (CAM) and conventional medicine is not absolute.
- ○ Alternative medicine and complimentary medicine are not the same, although they are frequently grouped together.
- ○ Many CAM therapies, despite defying biological plausibility, have withstood the test of time as well as more recent scientific scrutiny.

Complementary medicine implies treatment strategies or regimens used in addition to the conventional therapies (ie, relaxation exercise in addition to antianxiety medicine).

Alternative medicine is the label for therapies used instead of conventional medicine. These do not include treatments seen in conventional medicine (ie, this might mean getting Ayurvedic or acupuncture treatment instead of seeing your physician).

Conventional medicine refers to the typical modern Western medicine practiced by holders of MD (medical doctor) or DO (doctor of osteopathy) degrees. Specific CAM practices may, over time, become widely accepted (eg, cognitive behavioral therapy [CBT]).

Minocha A. *A Guide to Alternative Medicine and the Digestive System* (pp 77-116).
© 2013 Taylor & Francis Group.

INTEGRATIVE MEDICINE

Integrative medicine is defined as the use of a combination and permutation of conventional and evidence-based complementary and alternative therapies (in addition to or in lieu of conventional medicine) that are backed by some scientific evidence for their efficacy. Cost savings could be realized by incorporating it into general practice.[1]

Examples of integrative medicine include the following:

○ Use of fiber and CBT plus Amitiza (lubiprostone) for some patients with irritable bowel syndrome (IBS)
○ Use of yoga exercises, omega-3 fatty acids, and statins for cardiovascular disease

A strict application of this principle denies the fact that while some CAM strategies have been tested in humans or animals, many of the mainstream practices lack solid evidence for their use.

COMPLEMENTARY AND ALTERNATIVE MEDICINE

These 2 terms, *complementary medicine* and *alternative medicine*, are frequently grouped together and called CAM.

The National Center for Complementary and Alternative Medicine defines CAM as "a group of diverse medical and health care systems, practices, and products, that are not currently part of conventional medicine."[2]

A practice that may be complementary or alternative in one culture may be part of conventional medical practice in another.

Mainstream Versus Complementary and Alternative Medicine Therapies

CAM therapies are based largely on time-tested observations and cultural practices. At the same time, almost half of mainstream medical treatments are used despite lack of solid evidence provided by rigorous randomized, controlled trials (RCTs) and/or approval by the Food and Drug Administration.

TYPES OF COMPLEMENTARY AND ALTERNATIVE MEDICINE

Different organizations and societies have divided CAM therapies in different manners. The National Center for Complementary and Alternative Medicine divides CAM into 5 loosely divided and

Table 12-1. Mind-Body Treatment Strategies

❖ Biofeedback
❖ Relaxation and art strategies
❖ Mental/guided imagery
❖ Hypnosis

overlapping categories: whole medical systems, mind-body medicine, biologically based practices, manipulative and body-based practices, and energy medicine. Others have added additional categories to bring about more clarity, therefore an overlap may be seen.

Whole Body Systems

These are systems involving multiple strategies including lifestyle, herbals, etc, and are based on cultural background. They include traditional Chinese medicine (eg, acupuncture), homeopathy, Ayurveda, and naturopathy.

Mind-Body Medicine

Mind-body treatment strategies are based on the concept of integration of the mind, body, and spirit. This concept is consistent with the biopsychosocial model invoked in the pathogenesis of many chronic ailments (Table 12-1).[3-9]

Lifestyle Strategies

This category overlaps a lot with some of the other ones including whole body systems and mind-body medicine.
○ Diet
○ Exercise and physical therapy

Biologically Based Therapies

Most of the ancient pharmacotherapy of whole body systems falls in the herbal category. The new knowledge gained from dietary patterns has led to an explosion of dietary supplements and the relatively young science of functional medicine.[10]
○ Herbals/phytobotanicals
○ Dietary supplements, including vitamins and minerals
○ Probiotics
○ Functional foods

Manipulative and Body-Based Practices

○ Massage
○ Chiropractic and spinal manipulation
○ Osteopathic manipulation
○ Craniosacral therapy
○ Acupressure

Energy Medicine[11]

This is based on the concept of "invisible energy" and is known by different names like *qi, prana, life force,* etc in different ancient health systems. Energy therapy may involve presumed energy (biofields) on one extreme, to well-demonstrable and measurable bioelectromagnetic energy fields on the other. The therapeutic relief is accomplished by "unclogging" the flow of this critical energy or vital intrinsic power and restoring it to a dynamic equilibrium for attaining or maintaining optimal health. Two types of energy therapies are in vogue:

○ Biofield therapies are meant to affect, manipulate, and modulate the various energy fields that purportedly encircle and diffuse into the body. There is a paucity of scientific evidence supporting the existence of such energy fields. Examples of such therapies include reflexology, therapeutic touch, healing touch, Reiki, qi gong, and crystal healing.

○ Bioelectromagnetic-based treatments, also known as *veritable energy medicine,* are based on demonstrable and reproducible electromagnetic fields. Energy fields may be affected by a variety of electrical magnetic currents. Modalities include electrical nerve stimulation, magnet therapy, light therapy, or bioelectromagnetic field therapies (eg, pulsed, alternating-current, or direct-current fields).

REFERENCES

1. Guarneri E, Horrigan BJ, Pechura CM. The efficacy and cost effectiveness of integrative medicine: a review of the medical and corporate literature. *Explore (NY).* 2010;6(5):308-312.

2. National Center for Complementary and Alternative Medicine. What Is Complementary and Alternative Medicine? Available at: http://nccam.nih.gov/health/whatiscam. Accessed June 25, 2012.

3. Lackner JM, Mesmer C, Morley S, Dowzer C, Hamilton S. Psychological treatments for irritable bowel syndrome: a systematic review and meta-analysis. *J Consult Clin Psychol.* 2004;72(6):1100-1113.

4. Zijdenbos IL, de Wit NJ, van der Heijden GJ, Rubin G, Quartero AO. Psychological treatments for the management of irritable bowel syndrome. *Cochrane Database Syst Rev.* 2009;(1):CD006442.

5.   Chang FY, Lu CL. Treatment of irritable bowel syndrome using comple-
     mentary and alternative medicine. *J Chin Med Assoc.* 2009;72(6):294-300.

6.   Huertas-Ceballos A, Logan S, Bennett C, Macarthur C. Psychosocial
     interventions for recurrent abdominal pain (RAP) and irritable bowel
     syndrome (IBS) in childhood. *Cochrane Database Syst Rev.*
     2008;(1):CD003014.

7.   Hutton J. Cognitive behaviour therapy for irritable bowel syndrome.
     Eur J Gastroenterol Hepatol. 2005;17(1):11-14.

8.   Gonsalkorale WM, Whorwell PJ. Hypnotherapy in the treatment of
     irritable bowel syndrome. *Eur J Gastroenterol Hepatol.* 2005;17(1):15-20.

9.   Kearney DJ, Brown-Chang J. Complementary and alternative medicine
     for IBS in adults: mind-body interventions. *Nat Clin Pract Gastroenterol
     Hepatol.* 2008;5(11):624-636.

10. Hyman M. Systems biology, toxins, obesity, and functional medicine.
     Altern Ther Health Med. 2007;13(2):S134-139.

11. Rosch PJ. Bioelectromagnetic and subtle energy medicine: the interface
     between mind and matter. *Ann N Y Acad Sci.* 2009;1172:297-311.

Chapter

13 *Acupuncture*

KEY POINTS

O Acupuncture is based on the premise of imbalance of yin and
   yang and the problems/imbalance associated with the flow of
   vital energy through the body.

O There are no anatomical or histological correlates of acupoints,
   and this system of medicine defies plausibility because of difficulty reconciling with current medical knowledge.

O Multiple studies have documented the benefit of acupuncture
   in a variety of disorders.

Acupuncture[1,2] refers to the stimulation of focal points on the body
using a variety of techniques. It is an ancient practice that originated
when soldiers injured by arrows found relief of pain in other parts of
the body. Stone-based acupuncture needles were used in 3000 BC.

Acupuncture for strengthening health requires a quick in-and-out
insertion of needles. Healing complex diseases may require as long as
1 hour or more. A meta-analysis and systematic review in 2010 reported that an effective response rate of acupuncture in asthma is better

than the control.[3] A Cochrane database review concluded that acupuncture is effective in relieving pain.[4]

Acupuncture has been shown to be beneficial in the treatment of nausea and vomiting, gastroparesis, functional dyspepsia, and constipation.[5] It has the potential for benefit in IBS and motion sickness.

ACUPUNCTURE POINTS

○ Lie along pathways of flow of qi, the vital energy
○ Defy plausibility because of difficulty reconciling with current medical knowledge

Multiple variations of acupuncture are in vogue, including classical Chinese, Japanese, Tibetan, Vietnamese, Korean, and French acupuncture. While the Japanese use extremely thin needles, the French use acupuncture based on the modern neuroendocrine concepts.

ACUPUNCTURE TREATMENT

○ Recreates balance by application of needles, pressure, heat, etc in acupuncture points
○ An average of a dozen needles are inserted in each session
○ May take place over weeks to months
○ Some insurance companies cover the cost of acupuncture treatment while others do not

MODIFICATIONS OF ACUPUNCTURE

Moxibustion
○ Uses needles warmed by burning a combination of herbs

Acupressure
○ Manual technique

○ Utilizes physical pressure by hands/elbows instead of a needle puncture at acupoints

Electroacupuncture

○ Modern version of acupuncture utilizing the same acupoints
○ May enhance positive effects of acupuncture
○ Utilizes needles with continuous electric pulses
○ Has been referred to as *percutaneous electrical nerve stimulation*

Auriculotherapy

○ Needle punctures of ears
○ Different body systems are represented in the ear

BIOCHEMICAL BASIS OF ACUPUNCTURE AS ANALGESIC

Actions at multiple levels, depending upon the clinical state:[6]
○ Low-frequency electroacupuncture activates the mu- and delta-opioid receptors by stimulating increased endorphins and cytokines
○ High-frequency electroacupuncture acts on the kappa-opioid receptor via dynorphin
○ Endogenous opiates act in conjunction with the serotoninergic descending inhibitory pathway for the analgesic effects

Complications of acupuncture are rare but can be serious.[7] These include bleeding, transmission of infections (hepatitis, HIV, and bacterial), pneumothorax, cardiac tamponade, and spinal cord injuries. It may affect the functioning of demand pacemakers.

REFERENCES

1. Diehl DL. Acupuncture for gastrointestinal and hepatobiliary disorders. *J Altern Complement Med.* 1999;5:27-45.
2. Li HY, Cui L, Cui M, Tong YY. Active research fields of acupuncture research: a document co-citation clustering analysis of acupuncture literature. *Altern Ther Health Med.* 2010;16(6):38-45.
3. Yu L, Zhang Y, Chen C, Cui HF, Yan XK. Meta-analysis on randomized controlled clinical trials of acupuncture for asthma. *Zhongguo Zhen Jiu.* 2010;30(9):787-792.

4.   Lee MS, Ernst E. Acupuncture for pain: an overview of Cochrane reviews. *Chin J Integr Med*. 2011;17(3):187-189. Epub Feb 27, 2011.

5.   Larson JD, Gutowski KA, Marcus BC, et al. The effect of electroacu-stimulation on postoperative nausea, vomiting, and pain in outpatient plastic surgery patients: a prospective, randomized, blinded, clinical trial. *Plast Reconstr Surg*. 2010; 125(3):989-994.

6.   Lin JG, Chen WL. Review: acupuncture analgesia in clinical trials. *Am J Chin Med*. 2009;37(1):1-18.

7.   Ernst E, Lee MS, Choi TY. Acupuncture: does it alleviate pain and are there serious risks? A review of reviews. *Pain*. 2011;152(4):755-764.

Chapter

14 *Aquatic Therapy*

KEY POINTS

○   Aquatic therapy provides low impact exercises and is especially targeted at subjects with disabilities or chronic pain disorders.

○   It involves synchronization of breathing with physical movements and, in addition to physical benefits, provides a better sense of well being.

○   It has the potential for benefit in patients with irritable bowel syndrome and cancer rehabilitation.

Aquatic therapy, also known as *water aerobic therapy* or *pool therapy*, refers to the physical therapy and rehabilitation performed in water without the need for weights.[1]

PRINCIPLES OF AQUATIC THERAPY

Its popularity is based on the belief that it is healthier than the use of weights.[2] Water buoyancy helps support the weight of the patient. The combination of water resistance and buoyancy reduces weight-bearing and stress placed on the joints, allowing low-impact exercises with reduced joint stress compared to exercises on land. Not just a remedy for adults, it is being increasingly used in children as well.[3]

TYPES OF AQUATIC THERAPY

Water enthusiasts have many options regarding not only depth of water (ie, shallow versus deep water therapy), but also the format of exercises that they may enjoy and find easy to perform consistent with their health. Various types of aquatic therapy are available including Ai Chi, Ai Chi Ne, BackHab, Bad Raga and the Burdenko method, and Feldenkrais.[4]

Halliwick is a 10-point program of motor learning and mental adjustments that specializes in teaching patients with a variety of physical or mental disabilities to get involved with water activity exercises.

Wassertanzen means "water dance" and involves the patient surrendering control of his or her breath to go underwater.

Watsu is a combination of water and shiatsu, where the subject is held in warm water by the therapist and moved around using water resistance as the source of massage. It has been successfully used for the rehabilitation of patients with stroke.

Yogalates uses a combination of yoga, Pilates, and Ai Chi.

CONTRAINDICATIONS

- ❍ Significant cardiac or respiratory disease
- ❍ Fevers and active infections
- ❍ Urinary or stool incontinence
- ❍ Consult your physician prior to any exercise program

SIGNIFICANCE IN GASTROINTESTINAL DISEASES

While there are lack of data on the role of aquatic therapy in digestive health, data on its beneficial effect in chronic pain disorders, like fibromyalgia, indicate that it may have the potential for therapeutic benefit in chronic functional bowel disorders.

REFERENCES

1. Moerles KM. Water works. Baby boomers drive trend toward state-of-the-art aquatic therapy. *Rehab Manag.* 2010;23(7):14-17.

2. Cowan SM, Blackburn MS, McMahon K, Bennell KL. Current Australian physiotherapy management of hip osteoarthritis. *Physiotherapy.* 2010;96(4):289-295.

3. Hillier S, McIntyre A, Plummer L. Aquatic physical therapy for children with developmental coordination disorder: a pilot randomized controlled trial. *Phys Occup Ther Pediatr.* 2010;30(2):111-124.

4. Connors KA, Galea MP, Said CM, Remedios LJ. Feldenkrais method balance classes are based on principles of motor learning and postural control retraining: a qualitative research study. *Physiotherapy.* 2010;96(4):324-336.

Chapter

15 *Aromatherapy*

KEY POINTS

○ Aromatherapy massage is effective in several medical disorders.

○ Evidence for its benefit in cancer palliative care is encouraging.

Aromatherapy[1] employs a variety of scents as a means of attaining therapeutic goals on the body system. Common sources of aromatherapy include botanical oils such as rose, lemon, lavender, and peppermint.

Aromatherapy is most widely used at home for stress and pain relief, although an increasing number of clinics and emergency rooms are starting to employ this strategy.[2] It has been used in the management of anxiety,[3] especially cancer palliation states[4] and is widely accepted among women.[5] Some businesses pump in these scents to customer areas to calm the waiting customers.

> The aroma of these oils is believed to produce distinctive therapeutic, psychological, and physiological actions on the mind-body and restore harmony, relieving sickness or fatigue.

EVIDENCE

Aromatherapy helps reduce blood pressure in patients with hypertension.[6] Aromatherapy massage is an effective treatment of menopausal symptoms, such as hot flashes, depression, and pain in climacteric women.[7] Aromatherapy using topically applied lavender, clary sage, and rose is effective in decreasing the severity of menstrual cramps.[8]

Aromatherapy helps relieve constipation in the elderly.[9] Aromatherapy massage reduces abdominal subcutaneous fat, waist circumference, and improves body image in postmenopausal women.

A Cochrane database review concluded that massage and aromatherapy massage confer short-term benefits on psychological well being, with possible benefits on anxiety in patients with cancer. There may also be positive effects on physical symptoms.

REFERENCES

1. Stringer J, Donald G. Aromasticks in cancer care: an innovation not to be sniffed at. *Complement Ther Clin Pract.* 2011;17(2):116-121.

2. Holm L, Fitzmaurice L. Emergency department waiting room stress: can music or aromatherapy improve anxiety scores? *Pediatr Emerg Care.* 2008;24(12):836-838.

3. Lee YL, Wu Y, Tsang HW, Leung AY, Cheung WM. A systematic review on the anxiolytic effects of aromatherapy in people with anxiety symptoms. *J Altern Complement Med.* 2011;17(2):101-108. Epub Feb 10, 2011.

4. Ernst E. Massage therapy for cancer palliation and supportive care: a systematic review of randomised clinical trials. *Support Care Cancer.* 2009;17(4):333-227.

5. Tillett J, Ames D. The uses of aromatherapy in women's health. *J Perinat Neonatal Nurs.* 2010;24(3):238-245.

6. Hur MH, Lee MS, Kim C, Ernst E. Aromatherapy for treatment of hypertension: a systematic review. *J Eval Clin Pract.* 2012;18(1):37-41.

7. Hur MH, Yang YS, Lee MS. Aromatherapy massage affects menopausal symptoms in Korean climacteric women: a pilot-controlled clinical trial. *Evid Based Complement Alternat Med.* 2008;5(3):325-328.

8. Han SH, Hur MH, Buckle J, Choi J, Lee MS. Effect of aromatherapy on symptoms of dysmenorrhea in college students: a randomized placebo-controlled clinical trial. *J Altern Complement Med.* 2006;12(6):535-541.

9. Kim MA, Sakong JK, Kim EJ, et al. Effect of aromatherapy massage for the relief of constipation in the elderly. *Taehan Kanho Hakhoe Chi.* 2005;35(1):56-64.

Chapter

16 *Ayurveda*

KEY POINTS

○ Ill-health is not natural and represents a disrupted homeostatic balance and disharmony.

○ Therapeutic strategy involving multidimensional options, including nutrition and digestion, is directed at restoring the healthy balance needed for a healthy state.

CAM is widely popular in India.[1] Of those, Ayurveda (which is an ancient Indian system of medicine) is the most widely practiced, and there are medical schools offering degree courses in this system of medicine.[2,3]

The word *Ayurveda* is derived from 2 Sanskrit words: *ayus*, meaning life, and *veda*, meaning science.

MULTIDIMENSIONAL NUTRITION AND DIGESTION IS THE KEY

Healthy digestion is fundamental to a healthy body. Nourishment is derived not just from ingested food, but also through the mind-body system (ie, what we hear, feel, smell, etc).

GREAT ELEMENTS OF THE UNIVERSE

The human body is a microcosm of the universe and is a grouping of the 5 great elements plus the "immaterial self"; each body has a unique constitution. These elements are as follows:

○ *Earth* represents the solid state of matter in our universe. In our body, it is represented by bones, teeth, etc.

○ *Water* represents the fluid state of universe and the body. Within the body, it manifests as water, blood, lymph, and other bodily fluids. It is essential for carrying nutritive and immune substances and expelling wastes.

○ *Fire* represents the metabolic processes, whether they are releasing energy or storing food. It is also involved in the neurochemical reactions of thoughts, impulses, reactions, etc.

○ *Air* is the gaseous form of matter. Air, primarily oxygen, is needed for numerous metabolic reactions involving energy.

○ *Ether/space* is where everything happens and in which everything exists.

VITAL FORCES KNOWN AS DOSHAS

There are 3 vital forces or interactions, called *doshas*.[4] They represent the unique body constitution derived from the combination of 5 elements, in pairs.

Tridosha Balance and Health

○ Each person contains all 3 doshas
○ Proportion of doshas varies in each individual
○ A balanced Tridosha maintains a healthy mind-body equilibrium, resulting in positive health

The Three Doshas

The 3 active doshas and their elements are as follows:
1. Vata (air and ether)
2. Pitta (fire and water)
3. Kapha (water and earth)

VATA

Vata is primarily concerned with movement. The body function correlates of Vata include drying, cooling, agitating, breathing, GI motility, etc.

PITTA

Pitta represents the transformation involved with modulating and regulating the mind-body unit. Pitta is involved with most metabolic processes, including digestion, absorption, assimilation, temperature, intelligence, etc.

KAPHA

Kapha epitomizes the stirring forces involved in body structure and lubrication. It is the glue that helps build the physical structure of the body and maintains its resistance. Kapha organs include the chest, throat, head, sinuses, nose, mouth, joints, as well as fluid secretions. Kapha emotions include attachment, greed, love, calmness, and jealousy.

The body is the same, but each person is unique. Within each person, there is constant and, at the same time, ever-changing interactions among the vital forces, or the doshas, depending upon the circumstances. This explains why people can have so much in common, but also have an endless variety of individual differences in the way they behave and respond to their environment.

Role of Food and Taste in Health, Sickness, and the Doshas

Different foods, tastes, etc affect the doshas in different ways. One food or herb may aggravate one dosha while harmonizing another.

THE CONCEPT OF PRAKRUTI AND VIKRUTI

○ Prakruti[5] represents the basic constitution and is determined at the time of conception. The proportion of the doshas is maintained throughout one's lifetime.

○ Vikruti represents the current condition.

○ Interactions with external environment attempt to alter the dynamic equilibrium of the basic constitution all the time, while innate regulatory influences resist the change.

○ A substantial deviation from the Prakruti results in an imbalance and, thus, sickness.[6]

○ Appropriate therapies including herbs, diet (type of foods), and lifestyle changes can bring the Vikruti closer to the Prakruti by correcting the imbalance. This brings the body back to a healthy state.

AYURVEDIC TREATMENTS[7]

○ Medications are usually of plant origin, although rarely animal sources are used and include milk, bones, and gallstones.

○ Minerals like sulfur, lead, and gold are also used as part of therapeutic strategies.

○ Alcohol has been used as a sedative for surgery.

REFERENCES

1. Kiefer D, Pitluk J, Klunk K. An overview of CAM: components and clinical uses. *Nutr Clin Pract.* 2009;24(5):549-559.

2. Patwardhan B. Ayurveda, evidence-base and scientific rigor. *J Ayurveda Integr Med.* 2010;1(3):169-170.

3. Mishra L, Singh BB, Dagenais S. Ayurveda: a historical perspective and principles of the traditional healthcare system in India. *Altern Ther Health Med.* 2001;7(2):36-42.

4. Hankey A. Ayurvedic physiology and etiology: Ayurvedo Amritanaam. The doshas and their functioning in terms of contemporary biology and physical chemistry. *J Altern Complement Med.* 2001;7(5):567-574.

5. Patwardhan B, Bodeker G. Ayurvedic genomics: establishing a genetic basis for mind-body typologies. *J Altern Complement Med.* 2008;14(5):571-576.

6. Sharma H, Chandola HM, Singh G, Basisht G. Utilization of Ayurveda in health care: an approach for prevention, health promotion, and treatment of disease. Part 1—Ayurveda, the science of life. *J Altern Complement Med.* 2007;13(9):1011-1019.

7. Khalsa KP. The practitioner's perspective: introduction to Ayurvedic herbalism. *J Herb Pharmacother.* 2007;7(3-4):129-142.

Chapter

17 *Biofeedback*

KEY POINTS

- ○ Conscious mind needs to see/hear what is abnormal and normal physiological function.
- ○ Subjects practice normalizing the body function with the aid of a machine.
- ○ Biofeedback has been widely used for gastrointestinal (GI) as well as non-GI disorders.[1-4]

USE OF BIOFEEDBACK IN DIGESTIVE DISORDERS

- ○ Pelvic dyssynergia[5,6]
- ○ Constipation[7,8]
- ○ Fecal incontinence[9]
- ○ Solitary rectal ulcer syndrome
- ○ Recurrent abdominal pain in children

PRINCIPLES OF BIOFEEDBACK

- ○ Conscious mind has the ability to and needs to see/hear what is abnormal and normal physiological function.
- ○ Accomplished through the use of biofeedback machines that display the abnormal rhythm of the dysfunctional/distressed organ.
- ○ Patients, with instructions from therapist, then correct the abnormality to restore the normal functioning.
- ○ Biofeedback instruments for home use are available.

BIOFEEDBACK DEVICES

These include electromyogram, anorectal manometry, electrogastrogram, electroencephalogram, and galvanic skin response.

REFERENCES

1. Nagai Y. Biofeedback and epilepsy. *Curr Neurol Neurosci Rep.* 2011;11(4):443-50.

2. McGrady A. The effects of biofeedback in diabetes and essential hypertension. *Cleve Clin J Med.* 2010;77(Suppl 3):S68-71.

3. Cutshall SM, Wentworth LJ, Wahner-Roedler DL, et al. Evaluation of a biofeedback-assisted meditation program as a stress management tool for hospital nurses: a pilot study. *Explore (NY).* 2011;7(2):110-112.

4. Chiarioni G, Whitehead WE. The role of biofeedback in the treatment of gastrointestinal disorders. *Nat Clin Pract Gastroenterol Hepatol.* 2008;5(7):371-382.

5. Adams MA, Chey WD. Biofeedback training for dyssynergic defecation: an approach whose time has come? *Gastroenterology.* 2011;140(5):1682-1685.

6. Desantis DJ, Leonard MP, Preston MA, Barrowman NJ, Guerra LA. Effectiveness of biofeedback for dysfunctional elimination syndrome in pediatrics: a systematic review. *J Pediatr Urol.* 2011;7(3):342-348.

7. Shim LS, Jones M, Prott GM, Morris LI, Kellow JE, Malcolm A. Predictors of outcome of anorectal biofeedback therapy in patients with constipation. *Aliment Pharmacol Ther.* 2011;33(11):1245-1251.

8. Camilleri M, Bharucha AE. Behavioural and new pharmacological treatments for constipation: getting the balance right. *Gut.* 2010;59(9):1288-1296.

9. Norton C, Cody JD, Hosker G. Biofeedback and/or sphincter exercises for the treatment of faecal incontinence in adults. *Cochrane Database Syst Rev.* 2006;3:CD002111.

Chapter

18 *Cognitive Behavioral Therapy*

KEY POINTS

- ○ CBT is based on the principle that thoughts mediate between external stimuli and emotional reactions.
- ○ Subjects can modify their thoughts and, consequently, the reaction.
- ○ CBT has been shown to be effective in many chronic pain disorders, including functional bowel diseases.

CBT promotes healing by helping the patient discover and accordingly modify anomalies of thought, conceptions, perceptions, actions, and reactions that cause distress, and thus promote healing.

CBT techniques can be learned and self-applied. Internet-delivered CBT is also effective.[1]

BENEFITS IN GASTROINTESTINAL DISORDERS

- ○ Bulimia nervosa[2]
- ○ Irritable bowel syndrome[3]
- ○ Inflammatory bowel disease[3,4]
- ○ Functional abdominal pain[5]

BENEFITS IN NONGASTROINTESTINAL DISORDERS[6-10]

These include tinnitus, chronic fatigue syndrome, generalized anxiety disorder, attention deficit hyperactivity disorder, post-traumatic stress disorder, sleep disorders, mood disorders, schizophrenia, substance abuse disorders, chronic orofacial pain (including temporomandibular disorders), fibromyalgia, and chronic pain disorders.

OVERVIEW OF COGNITIVE BEHAVIORAL THERAPY

- ○ Helps "unlearn" undesirable responses to adverse situations
- ○ Involves modification of thinking processes of how we feel and what we do

Compared to the other psychotherapies, CBT involves briefer and fewer sessions and does not require the therapist to be present all the time. The patient may do CBT exercises him- or herself at home alone with appropriate instructions.

WHAT IS INVOLVED IN A COGNITIVE BEHAVIORAL THERAPY SESSION

- ○ Involves thinking, behaving, and responding in ways to attain the objectives (eg, being pain-free)
- ○ Frequently encourages a stoic approach to difficult situations
- ○ Teaches how an adverse situation may be modified to an advantage

○ For example, it would teach that being upset about a problem creates another issue besides the "problem" (ie, that the subject is upset as well). However, a calmer or pleasant approach may help rationalize the problem and facilitate approaches/solutions to resolve them

○ Self-learning is the key

REFERENCES

1. Palermo TM, Wilson AC, Peters M, Lewandowski A, Somhegyi H. Randomized controlled trial of an internet-delivered family cognitive-behavioral therapy intervention for children and adolescents with chronic pain. *Pain*. 2009;146(1-2):205-213.

2. Hay PP, Bacaltchuk J, Stefano S, Kashyap P. Psychological treatments for bulimia nervosa and binging. *Cochrane Database Syst Rev*. 2009;(4):CD000562.

3. Ford AC, Talley NJ, Schoenfeld PS, Quigley EM, Moayyedi P. Efficacy of antidepressants and psychological therapies in irritable bowel syndrome: systematic review and meta-analysis. *Gut*. 2009;58(3):367-378.

4. Grover M, Drossman DA. Psychopharmacologic and behavioral treatments for functional gastrointestinal disorders. *Gastrointest Endosc Clin N Am*. 2009;19(1):151-170.

5. Levy RL, Langer SL, Walker LS, et al. Cognitive-behavioral therapy for children with functional abdominal pain and their parents decreases pain and other symptoms. *Am J Gastroenterol*. 2010;105(4):946-956.

6. Hesser H, Weise C, Westin VZ, Andersson G. A systematic review and meta-analysis of randomized controlled trials of cognitive-behavioral therapy for tinnitus distress. *Clin Psychol Rev*. 2011;31(4):545-553.

7. Price JR, Mitchell E, Tidy E, Hunot V. Cognitive behaviour therapy for chronic fatigue syndrome in adults. *Cochrane Database Syst Rev*. 2008;(3):CD001027.

8. Safren SA, Sprich S, Mimiaga MJ, et al. Cognitive behavioral therapy vs relaxation with educational support for medication-treated adults with ADHD and persistent symptoms: a randomized controlled trial. *JAMA*. 2010;304(8):875-880.

9. Babson KA, Feldner MT, Badour CL. Cognitive behavioral therapy for sleep disorders. *Psychiatr Clin North Am*. 2010;33(3):629-640.

10. Sarzi-Puttini P, Atzeni F, Cazzola M. Neuroendocrine therapy of fibromyalgia syndrome: an update. *Ann N Y Acad Sci*. 2010;1193:91-97.

Chapter

19 *Energy Medicine*

KEY POINTS

○ Energy medicine strategies aim to unclog the clogged up vital energy that is causing the diseased state.

○ Reorientation of the vital energy returns the body to a healthy state.

○ Reiki involves transfer of positive energy from the healer to the patients, which, in turn, promotes body defenses and restores the body and soul to its harmonious balance.

THE ENERGY

Invisible energy has been invoked in several systems of medicine in one form or the other as therapeutic modalities. It is known by different names like *qi* (Chinese), *prana* (Ayurveda), *ki* (Reiki), *life force*, etc.

THERAPEUTIC GOALS

The goal of these therapies is to unclog this "constipated" vital energy and redirect this critical power or force in the complex network of channels in optimal fashion and a dynamic equilibrium. This reorientation of the vital energy forces results in the sick attaining and maintaining optimal health.

A select few energy-based therapies are described next.

Static Magnets

A large amount of money is spent on magnets by patients with chronic pain, like arthritis and fibromyalgia. Application on different parts of the body is based on the illness and goal. A meta-analysis concluded that while there is no convincing evidence to support their use, a positive benefit could not be excluded in patients with osteoarthritis.[1]

A pooled analysis showed a correlation between magnetic fields and childhood leukemia. A recent Cochrane database review found that high frequency transcranial magnetic stimulation is effective in chronic pain.[2]

Electromagnetic Field

External electromagnetic field affects the body by modulating its endogenous electromagnetic activity.[3] Therapeutic microwave resonance may be an electromagnetic version of acupuncture.

Electromagnetic pelvic stimulation in women with urinary incontinence results in improvement in provocative pad testing, without associated symptomatic relief.[4]

A double-blind RCT showed that the application of a low-frequency magnetic field improves chronic musculoskeletal pain.[5]

Reiki

The word *Reiki*[6] is derived from 2 words: *rei*, implying some universal spirit or supreme power, and *ki*, being life energy (analogous to qi in Chinese medicine and prana in Ayurveda). Transfer of positive energy promotes body defenses and restores the body and soul to its harmonious balance.

The effectiveness of Reiki has been questioned in scientific circles. A systematic review of therapeutic use of Reiki found that 9 of the 12 trials meeting inclusion criteria showed benefit. However, the quality of studies was poor.[6]

REFERENCES

1. Pittler MH, Brown EM, Ernst E. Static magnets for reducing pain: systematic review and meta-analysis of randomized trials. *CMAJ.* 2007;177(7):736-742.

2. O'Connell NE, Wand BM, Marston L, Spencer S, Desouza LH. Noninvasive brain stimulation techniques for chronic pain. *Cochrane Database Syst Rev.* 2010;(9):CD008208.

3. Hyland GJ. Physical basis of adverse and therapeutic effects of low intensity microwave radiation. *Indian J Exp Biol.* 2008;46(5):403-419.

4. Gilling PJ, Wilson LC, Westenberg AM, et al. A double-blind randomized controlled trial of electromagnetic stimulation of the pelvic floor vs sham therapy in the treatment of women with stress urinary incontinence. *BJU Int.* 2009;103(10):1386-1390.

5. Thomas AW, Graham K, Prato FS, et al. A randomized, double-blind, placebo-controlled clinical trial using a low-frequency magnetic field in the treatment of musculoskeletal chronic pain. *Pain Res Manag.* 2007;12(4):249-258.

6. vanderVaart S, Gijsen VM, de Wildt SN, Koren G. A systematic review of the therapeutic effects of Reiki. *J Altern Complement Med.* 2009;15(11):1157-1169.

Chapter

20 *Fasting*

"Humans live on one-quarter of what they eat; on the other three-quarters lives their doctor."

Egyptian pyramid inscription, 3800 BC

KEY POINTS

○ Fasting has been promoted as a medical remedy against disease across cultures since ancient times.

○ The health benefits of calorie restriction include delayed onset of numerous chronic disorders (eg, cardiovascular disease, diabetes, and cancer).

Fasting involves a voluntary avoidance or restriction of food, with or without fluids. Thus a subject may undertake a partial or total abstention from all foods, or a select abstention of specific foods.

EFFECT ON HEALTH

Fasting has been promoted as a medical remedy against disease across cultures since ancient times. This includes the forefathers of medicine: Hippocrates, Galen, and Paracelsus. Practitioners of integrative medicine prescribe fasts for detoxification/cleansing the body for health maintenance, as well as a treatment for disease.

Much experimental data have been derived from animals. In addition to observation of religious diets,[1] human data about health effects have been derived from 3 types of diets:

○ Caloric restriction involves reduction of calories by 20% to 40%

○ Alternate-day fasting with consumption ad lib on eating days

○ Dietary restriction or reduction of a dietary component, usually a macronutrient

BENEFITS OF CALORIE RESTRICTION

In addition to enhanced longevity,[2,3] health benefits of calorie restriction include delayed onset of numerous chronic disorders,[4] including the following:

○ Autoimmune disorders
○ Coronary artery disease
○ Cardiomyopathies
○ Cancer
○ Diabetes[5]
○ Chronic kidney disease
○ Obesity

A calorie-restricted diet results in improved markers of health, especially cardiovascular and metabolic function.[6] It results in a decrease in heart rate, blood pressure, body fat, along with improved cardiac muscle function, glycemic control, lipid profile, and aging processes.[7] The mechanism may include resetting of the circadian clock, leading to synchronized metabolism.

Fasting on alternate days while consuming twice the amount of food on nonfasting days improves longevity, as well as glycemic control, and the effects are similar to calorie restriction every day. Even fasting for a day once a month may improve the markers for risk of cardiovascular disease.

Protein restriction in animals results in a 20% increase in life span, in contrast to fat or carbohydrate restriction that has no such effect. The beneficial effect of protein restriction is related primarily to the reduced intake of methionine.

Fasting to Lose Weight

Fasting on alternate days allows the subject to lose weight over short to medium term, although it is not sustained over the long term. On the other hand, an alternate day diet is superior to a daily restriction for retaining lean mass.

Punctuated fasting is superior to continued calorie restriction, and also increases life span.

Safety of Fasting

Healthy persons can fast for a few days without any adverse long-term adverse health effects, as long as adequate hydration is maintained. Diabetics and women who are pregnant or breastfeeding should not practice fasts. Excessive fasting, like anorexia nervosa, may cause severe systemic disturbances.

REFERENCES

1. Trepanowski JF, Bloomer RJ. The impact of religious fasting on human health. *Nutr J.* 2010;9:57.

2. Froy O, Miskin R. Effect of feeding regimens on circadian rhythms: implications for aging and longevity. *Aging.* 2010;2(1):7-27.

3. Froy O, Chapnik C, Miskin R. Relationship between calorie restriction and the biological clock: lessons from long-lived transgenic mice. *Rejuvenation Res.* 2008;1192:467-471.

4. Omodei D, Fontana L. Calorie restriction and prevention of age-associated chronic disease. *FEBS Lett.* 2011;585(11):1537-1542.

5. O'Keefe JH, Gheewala NM, O'Keefe JO. Dietary strategies for improving post-prandial glucose, lipids, inflammation, and cardiovascular health. *J Am Coll Cardiol.* 2008;51(3):249-255.

6. Fontana L. Calorie restriction and cardiometabolic health. *Eur J Cardiovasc Prev Rehabil.* 2008;15(1):3-9.

7. Minor RK, Allard JS, Younts CM, et al. Dietary interventions to extend life span and health span based on calorie restriction. *J Gerontol A Biol Sci Med Sci.* 2010;65(7):695-703.

Chapter

21 *Homeopathy*

KEY POINTS

○ Homeopathy is based on the principle of similars.
○ Since the formulations are so dilute, to the tune of molecules or even none, it continues to defy medical plausibility.

Homeopathy is widely practiced across the world, especially in Europe and India.

THEORY

In contrast to the principle of contraries used in allopathy, homeopathy is based on the principle of similars. This implies that a substance that can produce symptoms similar to a disease would also cure the disease. In order to reduce the toxic effects, the substance is highly diluted, some exceeding Avogadro's number (6×10^{23} molecules per mole).

Treating an infection with a highly diluted antibiotic medication may be considered malpractice in conventional medicine but not so in homeopathy.

The science of dilutions used in homeopathy defies biological plausibility and continues to baffle scientists. There has been and continues to be an ongoing, passionate debate on its effectiveness.

EVIDENCE

While there is a paucity of data examining the effect of homeopathy on digestive disorders, many of the independent systematic reviews and meta-analysis of placebo-controlled trials on homeopathy have concluded that its effects seem to be more than placebo.[1] There is also evidence from RCTs that homeopathy may be effective for the treatment of influenza, allergies, postoperative ileus, and childhood diarrhea.

A 6-year, university hospital outpatient observational study[2] of homeopathic treatment for chronic disease (n = 6544) including GI diseases found that 71% of the patients reported positive health changes, with 51% recording their improvement as better or much better.

A negative meta-analysis[3] and an accompanying editorial on the utility of homeopathy caused quite a furor, drawing numerous letters to the editor[4] critical of not only the study but also the journal for its editorial decrying homeopathy.

CONCLUSION

According to Sir William Osler, "Medicine is a science of uncertainty and an art of probability."[5(p125)] The usefulness of prescribing homeopathic medicine is no different than the use of allopathic prescriptions for unapproved indications, or prescribing nothing at all, and has not been studied. Perhaps it is difficult for many of us to understand since the homeopathic practitioners think and manage patients differently than modern medical practitioners do.

REFERENCES

1. Jonas WB, Kaptchuk TJ, Linde K. A critical overview of homeopathy. *Ann Intern Med.* 2003;138(5):393-399.

2. Spence DS, Thompson EA, Barron SJ. Homeopathic treatment for chronic disease: a 6-year, university-hospital outpatient observational study. *J Altern Complement Med.* 2005;11(5):793-798.

3. Shang A, Huwiler-Müntener K, Nartey L, et al. Are the clinical effects of homoeopathy placebo effects? Comparative study of placebo-controlled trials of homoeopathy and allopathy. *Lancet.* 2005;366(9487):726-732.

4. Linde K, Jonas W. Are the clinical effects of homoeopathy placebo effects? *Lancet.* 2005;366(9503):2081-2082.

5. Bean WB (Ed.). *Sir William Osler: Aphorisms from His Bedside Teachings and Writings.* NY: Henry Schuman, Inc.; 1950.

Chapter

22 *Hypnotherapy*

KEY POINTS

○ Hypnosis has been used for military intelligence in modern times.

○ Hypnosis represents an artificially induced trance, or an altered state of consciousness, which is distinct from normal sleep and wakefulness.

○ Optimal results in GI conditions can only be obtained if gut-oriented hypnotherapy is used; however, such training is not widely available.

POSSIBLE MECHANISM OF ACTIONS IN GASTROINTESTINAL DISORDERS

○ Can modify gastric acid secretion in healthy subjects

○ Hypnotic relaxation increases orocecal transit time[1]

○ Shortens gastric emptying time

○ Reduces visceral sensitivity; however, data are conflicting

○ Modulates autonomic imbalance with a generalized reduction of sympathetic activity and a wakeful hypometabolic state

○ Improves symptom-related cognition in functional bowel disorders[2]

Benefit in Gut

○ Reduces inflammatory response in active ulcerative colitis toward levels found previously in the inactive disease. These effects may in part be responsible for anecdotal evidence of benefits of hypnotherapy in ulcerative colitis[3]

○ Nausea and vomiting associated with chemotherapy

○ Hyperemesis gravidarum

○ Irritable bowel syndrome[4]

○ Prevents relapse in patients with duodenal ulcer (relapse rate of 53% compared to 100% in controls)

○ Improves symptoms and quality of life, and reduces need for medication in functional dyspepsia[5,6]

○ 80% of patients with noncardiac chest pain feel better with hypnosis treatment compared to 23% in controls

○ Helps patients cope with inflammatory bowel disease

○ Reduces need for sedation during endoscopy

References

1.   Beaugerie L, Burger AJ, Cadranel JF, Lamy P, Gendre JP, Le Quintrec Y. Modulation of orocaecal transit time by hypnosis. *Gut.* 1991;32(4):393-394.

2.   Gonsalkorale WM, Toner BB, Whorwell PJ. Cognitive change in patients undergoing hypnotherapy for irritable bowel syndrome. *J Psychosom Res.* 2004;56(3):271-278.

3.   Mawdsley JE, Jenkins DG, Macey MG, et al. The effect of hypnosis on systemic and rectal mucosal measures of inflammation in ulcerative colitis. *Am J Gastroenterol.* 2008;103(6):1460-1469.

4.   Miller V, Whorwell PJ. Hypnotherapy for functional gastrointestinal disorders: a review. *Int J Clin Exp Hypn.* 2009;57(3):279-292.

5.   Kandulski A, Venerito M, Malfertheiner P. Therapeutic strategies for the treatment of dyspepsia. *Expert Opin Pharmacother.* 2010;11(15):2517-25.

6.   Sharma RL. Functional dyspepsia: at least recommend hypnotherapy. *BMJ.* 2008;337:a1972.

Chapter

23 *Manipulative and Body-Based Therapies*

KEY POINTS

- ○ A diverse range of therapies form this group, including and not limited to acupressure, bone setting, craniosacral therapy, joint/spinal manipulation, massage, reflexology, shiatsu, etc.
- ○ Such therapies have been shown to be beneficial in a variety of ailments (eg, constipation and pain).

Manual or manipulative therapies utilize hands-on physical intervention for the treatment of a diverse group of diseases. It is the third common of all CAM therapies used by patients. Much of the evidence pertains to non-GI illnesses.

POSSIBLE BENEFITS OF MANUAL THERAPY IN GASTROINTESTINAL ILLNESS

These include constipation,[1] infantile colic,[2,3] chronic abdominal pain, and gastroesophageal reflux disease, based on anecdotal reports.[4]

REFERENCES

1. Harrington KL, Haskvitz EM. Managing a patient's constipation with physical therapy. *Phys Ther.* 2006;86(11):1511-1519.
2. Miller JE, Phillips HL. Long-term effects of infant colic: a survey comparison of chiropractic treatment and nontreatment groups. *J Manipulative Physiol Ther.* 2009;32(8):635-638.
3. Ernst E. Chiropractic spinal manipulation for infant colic: a systematic review of randomised clinical trials. *Int J Clin Pract.* 2009;63(9):1351-1353.
4. Alcantara J, Anderson R. Chiropractic care of a pediatric patient with symptoms associated with gastroesophageal reflux disease, fuss-cry-irritability with sleep disorder syndrome and irritable infant syndrome of musculoskeletal origin. *J Can Chiropr Assoc.* 2008;52(4):248-255.

Chapter

24 *Mindfulness and Meditation*

KEY POINTS

- ❍ Meditation has a profound effect on the body, especially in cardiopulmonary physiology.
- ❍ Mindfulness-based stress reduction (MBSR) is a secular clinical practice and results in overt alteration of grey matter.

DIFFERENCES BETWEEN MIND-BODY MEDICINE AND PSYCHOTHERAPY

Conventional psychotherapy tends to focus on a single therapy and a specific outcome. On the other hand, the mind-body medicine therapeutic approach tends to consider the role of human and environmental/social factors in the overall healing processes, and involves the patient-healer interactions (eg, empathy, compassion, etc) in order to address those factors.

MEDITATION

Meditation has a profound impact on physiological function, including reduction in heart rate, blood pressure, and respiratory rates, along with changes in blood flow.

Mindfulness practice is the technique that empties the mind without constraining thoughts or attention to any sensation, emotion, or perception in particular. It allows the person to become more aware of his or her inner self. The currently popular clinical equivalents of mindfulness meditation are MBSR and mindfulness-based cognitive therapy, which follow consistent and standardized techniques.

Mindfulness-Based Stress Reduction

MBSR was originally developed as a group program for pain management. It is a secular clinical practice and does not require any particular religious beliefs. The subject needs to be motivated and determined. It results in alterations in gray matter density in the brain regions involved in learning, memory, emotion, etc.[1] No negative side effects from MBSR have been documented.[2]

MBSR as an adjunct treatment results in coping better with symptoms, an improved sense of well-being and quality of life, as well as possibly better health outcomes.[3]

CLINICAL USE OF MINDFULNESS-BASED STRESS REDUCTION[4-6]

MBSR may be considered as a therapeutic option for insomnia, hot flashes, anxiety disorders, failed back surgery, depression, chronic fatigue syndrome, and fibromyalgia. A meta-analysis concluded that MBSR may improve cancer patients' psychosocial adjustment to their disease.

A meta-analysis concluded that MBSR results in decreased stress levels in healthy people. Another meta-analysis concluded that MBSR has small positive effects on depression, anxiety, and psychological distress in patients with chronic somatic diseases.[7]

REFERENCES

1. Hölzel BK, Carmody J, Vangel M, et al. Mindfulness practice leads to increases in regional brain gray matter density. *Psychiatry Res.* 2011;191(1):36-43.

2. Praissman S. Mindfulness-based stress reduction: a literature review and clinician's guide. *J Am Acad Nurse Pract.* 2008;20(4):212-216.

3. Merkes M. Mindfulness-based stress reduction for people with chronic diseases. *Aust J Prim Health.* 2010;16(3):200-210.

4. Schmidt S, Grossman P, Schwarzer B, Jena S, Naumann J, Walach H. Treating fibromyalgia with mindfulness-based stress reduction: results from a 3-armed randomized controlled trial. *Pain.* 2011;152(2):361-369.

5. Ledesma D, Kumano H. Mindfulness-based stress reduction and cancer: a meta-analysis. *Psychooncology.* 2009;18(6):571-579.

6. Sampalli T, Berlasso E, Fox R, Petter M. A controlled study of the effect of a mindfulness-based stress reduction technique in women with multiple chemical sensitivity, chronic fatigue syndrome, and fibromyalgia. *J Multidiscip Health.* 2009;2:53-59.

7. Bohlmeijer E, Prenger R, Taal E, Cuijpers P. The effects of mindfulness-based stress reduction therapy on mental health of adults with a chronic medical disease: a meta-analysis. *J Psychosom Res.* 2010;68(6):539-544.

Chapter

25 *Prayer and Spirituality*

KEY POINTS

- ○ Some studies have shown clinical benefit accruing from prayer.
- ○ Prayer is a matter of personal preference and should not be prescribed.

The National Center for Complementary and Alternative Medicine defines prayer as an active process of communicating with and appealing to a higher spiritual power.[1]

Potential mechanisms of prayer include relaxation response, a placebo effect, or expression of positive emotions. Supernatural intervention, although frequently invoked, is highly speculative and not scientifically verifiable.

Evidence from many studies, albeit somewhat conflicting, indicates benefit of distant, intercessory prayer in critically ill patients, defying biological plausibility.[2-5] A meta-analysis report in 2009 concluded that their findings were equivocal and that the evidence does not support a recommendation either in favor or against the use of intercessory prayer.[6]

EVIDENCE

There are very limited data examining the effect of prayer in healing disease. Studies have been criticized for serious design flaws.

- ○ Tsubono et al conducted a double-blind RCT on the effects of distant healing performed by a spiritual healer on chronic pain and found that treatment group had reduced pain intensity.[7]
- ○ A prospective double-blind RCT of patients admitted to a coronary care unit found that the intercessory prayer group had a significantly lower severity score and better outcomes based on the hospital course.[2] Results of studies have been mixed.[4,5]
- ○ O'Laoire showed that distant, intercessory prayer has a beneficial effect on self-esteem, anxiety, and depression.[3]

○ Intercessory prayer may affect outcomes of in vitro fertilization embryo transfer. The prayer group had a response rate of 50% compared to 26% in the controls.[8]

A systematic review concluded that, while studies for distant healing are flawed, there may be merit to their claims for benefit.[9]

REFERENCES

1. Jantos M, Kiat H. Prayer as medicine: how much have we learned? *Med J Aust.* 2007;186(10 Suppl):S51-35.

2. Byrd RC. Positive therapeutic effects of intercessory prayer in a coronary care unit population. *South Med J.* 1988;81:826-829.

3. O'Laoire S. An experimental study of the effects of distant, intercessory prayer on self-esteem, anxiety, and depression. *Altern Ther Health Med.* 1997;3:38-53.

4. Harris WS, Gowda M, Kolb JW, et al. A randomized, controlled trial of the effects of remote, intercessory prayer on outcomes in patients admitted to the coronary care unit. *Arch Intern Med.* 1999;159(19):2273-2278.

5. Benson H, Dusek JA, Sherwood JB, et al. Study of the therapeutic effects of intercessory prayer (STEP) in cardiac bypass patients: a multicenter randomized trial of uncertainty and certainty of receiving intercessory prayer. *Am Heart J.* 2006;151(4):934-942.

6. Roberts L, Ahmed I, Hall S, Davison A. Intercessory prayer for the alleviation of ill health. *Cochrane Database Syst Rev.* 2009;(2):CD000368.

7. Tsubono K, Thomlinson P, Shealy CN. The effects of distant healing performed by a spiritual healer on chronic pain: a randomized controlled trial. *Altern Ther Health Med.* 2009;15(3):30-34.

8. Cha KY, Wirth DP. Does prayer influence the success of in vitro fertilization-embryo transfer? Report of a masked, randomized trial. *J Reprod Med.* 2001;46:781-787.

9. Astin JA, Harkness E, Ernst E. The efficacy of "distant healing": a systematic review of randomized trials. *Ann Intern Med.* 2000;132(11):903-910.

Chapter

26 *Traditional Chinese Medicine*

KEY POINTS

○ Herbal therapies and acupuncture are the most widely known aspects of traditional Chinese medicine in the Western world.

○ Traditional Chinese medicine considers body functions based on the concept of a meridian system.

○ Traditional Chinese medicine is a highly individualized treatment program based on subjective, objective, and intuitive impressions.

The term *traditional Chinese medicine* is used for the many diverse medical practices all across the world, with or without modification.[1,2] Traditional Chinese medicine has the potential to play a vital role in the Western system of integrative medicine.[1,2] *Note*: Acupuncture is described in Chapter 13.

PRINCIPLES OF TRADITIONAL CHINESE MEDICINE

Traditional Chinese medicine considers body functions with its meridian system.

The body is composed of systems of function, rather than specific organs themselves. These systems are called *Zang-Fu*, where *Zang* involves solid organs and *Fu* represents the hollow viscus (ie, the gut).

Health is based on optimal balance of yin and yang and the free and balanced flow of qi, the vital energy essential for a healthy body.

In contrast to Ayurveda, not just dried plants but also animal parts may be used in traditional Chinese medicines.

Good quality evidence indicates the benefit of traditional Chinese medicine in IBS, functional dyspepsia, gastroparesis, and constipation.[3-5] Several therapies have shown benefit in liver disorders.[6]

REFERENCES

1. Dobos G, Tao I. The model of Western integrative medicine: the role of Chinese medicine. *Chin J Integr Med*. 2011;17(1):11-20.

2. Liu EH, Qi LW, Li K, Chu C, Li P. Recent advances in quality control of traditional Chinese medicines. *Comb Chem High Throughput Screen.* 2010;13(10):869-884.

3. Bensoussan A, Talley NJ, Hing M, Menzies R, Guo A, Ngu M. Treatment of irritable bowel syndrome with Chinese herbal medicine: a randomized controlled trial. *JAMA.* 1998;280(18):1585-1589.

4. Braden B, Caspary W, Börner N, Vinson B, Schneider AR. Clinical effects of STW 5 (Iberogast) are not based on acceleration of gastric emptying in patients with functional dyspepsia and gastroparesis. *Neurogastroenterol Motil.* 2009;21(6):632-638.

5. Cheng CW, Bian ZX, Wu TX. Systematic review of Chinese herbal medicine for functional constipation. *World J Gastroenterology.* 2009;15(39):4886-4895.

6. Luk JM, Wang X, Liu P, et al. Traditional Chinese herbal medicines for treatment of liver fibrosis and cancer: from laboratory discovery to clinical evaluation. *Liver Int.* 2007;27(7):879-890.

Chapter

27 *Vegetarianism*

KEY POINTS

○ Consumption of a variety of plant foods eaten in different meals during the day can adequately meet all essential protein needs in healthy adults. Any specific meal does not require all diverse plant proteins.[1]

○ The American Dietetic Association[2] has concluded that based on limited evidence,[3] macronutrient intake of pregnant vegetarian females is similar to that of nonvegetarians and there appears to be no significant health differences in babies born to nonvegan vegetarian mothers versus nonvegetarians.

○ Well-planned vegetarian diets, including a vegan diet, may be undertaken during any and all stages of the life cycle, including childhood,[4] pregnancy, and lactation.

HISTORICAL PERSPECTIVE

Pythagoras is considered to be the founder of vegetarianism. The proponents from modern history include Benjamin Franklin from the 18th century. Until then, vegetarianism was promoted based on moral and metaphysical grounds.[5]

WHAT IS VEGETARIANISM?

○ Lacto-vegetarian excludes eggs as well as meat, fish, and poultry.

○ Lacto-ovo-vegetarians do eat eggs.

○ Vegan, or a total vegetarian diet, is the most restrictive. Subjects do not ingest eggs, dairy, and other animal products. Some vegans also avoid honey and the use of animal products such as leather or wool.

○ Macrobiotic diet followers consume mostly grains, legumes, and vegetables, while fruits, nuts, and seeds are avoided. At the same time, some of these people do not exclude fish from the diet.

○ Raw foods diet, also known as a "living food diet," consists mainly of uncooked and unprocessed foods, including fruits, vegetables, nuts, seeds, grains and beans. Some followers may consume unpasteurized dairy products and even raw meat and fish.

○ Fruitarian diet involves use of fruits, nuts, and seeds. Subjects avoid vegetables, grains, beans, and animal products. Vegetables that are otherwise fruit, like avocado and tomatoes, are included in the diet.

○ Semi-vegetarians do consume some fish, chicken, or even meat. These self-described vegetarians may be identified in research studies as semi-vegetarians. Individual assessment is required to accurately evaluate the nutritional quality of the diet of a vegetarian or a self-described vegetarian.

In our overfed society, vegetarianism is a plus—unless it results in a nutritional deficiency (Table 27-1). Availability of numerous fortified food products in the market reflects an improvement of the vegetarian diet of the past.

POTENTIAL NUTRIENT DEFICIENCIES

These include vitamins (B_{12}, D), zinc,[6] long chain n-3 fatty acids, calcium (in vegans), iodine, and riboflavin.

Table 27-1. Advantages of Vegetarian Diet

- ❖ Reduced serum cholesterol[7]
- ❖ Reduced risk of obesity[8]
- ❖ Decreased risk and mortality of cardiovascular disease[9]
- ❖ Reduced risk of hypertension[10]
- ❖ Protection against cancers[11]
- ❖ Improved glucose control[12]
- ❖ Reduced risk of dementia[13]
- ❖ Reduced risk of diverticulitis[14]
- ❖ Reduced risk of gallstones[15]
- ❖ Improvement in rheumatoid arthritis[16]

Direct comparison of cholesterol-lowering foods with a statin in hypercholesterolemic participants found that a near-vegan diet rich in fiber, nuts, and soy protein reduces serum LDL-cholesterol levels as much as a low-saturated fat diet and a statin.[17]

SPECIAL DIETARY ADJUSTMENTS AND CIRCUMSTANCES

Proteins

Most nitrogen balance studies do not show significant difference in the protein based on a source of dietary protein.[18] Even vegetarian athletes can meet their protein needs well.[19]

Iron

The Institute of Medicine recommends almost twice the iron intake by vegetarians, compared to nonvegetarians.[20]

Older Adults

Dietary intake of vegetarian older adults is similar to nonvegetarians.[21] There may be reduced absorption due to atrophic gastritis, and fortified supplements may be used. Similarly, vitamin D production declines and supplements are helpful.

Athletes

A well-planned vegetarian diet provides adequate nutritional intake to athletes without requiring supplements.[22] Creatine supplementation may be of benefit in athletes that are involved in high-intensity exercise.

Renal Failure

The vegetarian diet is high in phosphorus, and increased use of phosphate binders may be needed. Plant proteins contain higher amounts of nonessential amino acids and thus generate more urea and pose a difficult challenge in severe renal failure. A carefully designed vegan diet can be effectively used in mild chronic renal failure and, in fact, may be the diet of choice when a patient is unable to tolerate a conventional low-protein diet. Ingestion of low potassium fruits, vegetables, and grains is needed to compensate for the relatively higher potassium content of plant foods like legumes and nuts.

REFERENCES

1. Young VR, Pellett PL. Plant proteins in relation to human protein and amino acid nutrition. *Am J Clin Nutr.* 1994;59(Suppl):1203S-1212S.

2. Craig WJ, Mangels AR. Position of the American Dietetic Association: vegetarian diets. *J Am Diet Assoc.* 2009;109(7):1266-1282.

3. Drake R, Reddy S, Davies J. Nutrient intake during pregnancy and pregnancy outcome of lacto-ovo-vegetarians, fish-eaters and non-vegetarians. *Veg Nutr.* 1998;2:45-52.

4. Messina V, Mangels AR. Considerations in planning vegan diets: children. *J Am Diet Assoc.* 2001;101:661-669.

5. Whorton JC. Historical development of vegetarianism. *Am J Clin Nutr.* 1994;59(Suppl):103S-109S.

6. Hunt JR. Bioavailability of iron, zinc, and other trace minerals from vegetarian diets. *Am J Clin Nutr.* 2003;78(Suppl): 633S-639S.

7. Mahon AK, Flynn MG, Stewart LK, et al. Protein intake during energy restriction: effects on body composition and markers of metabolic and cardiovascular health in postmenopausal women. *J Am Coll Nutr.* 2007;26:182-189.

8. Appleby PN, Thorogood M, Mann JI, et al. The Oxford Vegetarian study: an overview. *Am J Clin Nutr.* 1999;70:525S-531S.

9. Key TJ, Fraser GE, Thorogood M, et al. Mortality in vegetarians and nonvegetarians: detailed findings from a collaborative analysis of 5 prospective studies. *Am J Clin Nutr.* 1999;70(Suppl):516S-524S.

10. Appleby PN, Davey GK, Key TJ. Hypertension and blood pressure among meat eaters, fish eaters, vegetarians and vegans in EPIC-Oxford. *Public Health Nutr.* 2002;5:645-654.

11. Dewell A, Weidner G, Sumner MD, et al. A very-low-fat vegan diet increases intake of protective dietary factors and decreases intake of pathogenic dietary factors. *J Am Diet Assoc.* 2008;108:347-356.

12. Bernard ND, Katcher HI, Jenkins DJ, et al. Vegetarian and vegan diets in type 2 diabetes management. *Nutr Rev.* 2009;67(5):255-263.

13. Giem P, Beeson WL, Fraser GE. The incidence of dementia and intake of animal products: preliminary findings from the Adventist Health study. *Neuroepidemiology.* 1993;12:28-36.

14. Aldoori WH, Giovannucci EL, Rimm EB, et al. A prospective study of diet and the risk of symptomatic diverticular disease in men. *Am J Clin Nutr.* 1994;60:757-764.

15. Pixley F, Wilson D, McPherson K, et al. Effect of vegetarianism on development of gall stones in women. *Br Med J (Clin Res Ed).* 1985;291:11-12.

16. Muller H, de Toledo FW, Resch KL. Fasting followed by vegetarian diet in patients with rheumatoid arthritis: a systematic review. *Scand J Rheumatol.* 2001;30:1-10.

17. Jenkins DJ, Kendall CW, Marchie A, et al. Direct comparison of a dietary portfolio of cholesterol-lowering foods with a statin in hypercholesterolemic participants. *Am J Clin Nutr.* 2005;81:380-387.

18. Rand WM, Pellett PL, Young VR. Meta-analysis of nitrogen balance studies for estimating protein requirements in healthy adults. *Am J Clin Nutr.* 2003;77:109-127.

19. Tipton KD, Witard OC. Protein requirements and recommendations for athletes: relevance of ivory tower arguments for practical recommendations. *Clin Sports Med.* 2007;26:17-36.

20. Trumbo P, Yates AA, Schlicker S, Poos M. Dietary reference intakes: vitamin A, vitamin K, arsenic, boron, chromium, copper, iodine, iron, manganese, molybdenum, nickel, silicon, vanadium, and zinc. *J Am Diet Assoc.* 2001;101(3):294-301.

21. Marsh AG, Christiansen DK, Sanchez TV, et al. Nutrient similarities and differences of older lacto-ovo-vegetarian and omnivorous women. *Nutr Rep Int.* 1989;39:19-24.

22. Venderley AM, Campbell WW. Vegetarian diets: nutritional considerations for athletes. *Sports Med.* 2006;36:295-305.

Chapter

28 *Yoga*

KEY POINTS

O Health benefits of yoga in a variety of systemic disorders (eg, hypertension and cardiovascular disease) have been proven by RCTs.[1-5]

○ There is limited literature on the use of yoga in GI conditions.

WHAT IS YOGA?[6]

○ Holistic system of medicine that epitomizes self-realization and positive health, attained by fostering a unity of the mind, body, and spirit

○ Not just a system or tool of medicine, but rather a whole lifestyle approach to health and sickness

○ Involves meditation and training of mind, body, and breath, as well as making a spiritual connection with the inner self and the divine power. Chanting may be involved

○ Yoga is available in a variety of approaches, with different combinations and permutations of emphasis on physical, mental, and spiritual exercises. Examples include Raja yoga, Karma yoga, Jnana yoga, Bhakti yoga, and Hatha yoga. The Western concept of yoga involves exercises only, thus it is predominantly Hatha yoga (which is described next)

Rooted in Hindu philosophy, references to yoga are contained in ancient Indian texts, such as Vedas, as well as in Buddhist texts. Knowledge or belief in Hinduism is not a prerequisite in order to practice yoga and reap its benefits.

HATHA YOGA[1]

It is the predominantly physical component of yoga, with the belief that purification of body leads to purification of mind, and involves physical exercises via asanas (or poses). Variations of Hatha yoga include Ashtanga yoga, Bikram yoga, Gentle yoga, Kundalini yoga, and Iyengar yoga.

BENEFITS OF YOGA[2-10]

○ Builds elasticity, endurance, power, concentration, and balance

○ Reduces stress and anxiety

○ Improves sleep

○ Mechanism of action of yoga in providing health benefits is multifactorial[11]

Good to Fair Evidence for Health Benefits for Yoga

- ○ Hypertension
- ○ Cardiovascular disease
- ○ Asthma
- ○ Diabetes mellitus
- ○ Migraine
- ○ Carpal tunnel syndrome
- ○ Psychiatric disorders
- ○ Substance abuse
- ○ Stress management
- ○ Menopausal symptoms

Limited Evidence for Health Benefits for Yoga

- ○ Altitude sickness
- ○ Rheumatoid arthritis
- ○ Epilepsy
- ○ Back pain
- ○ Irritable bowel syndrome[12-14]
- ○ Obesity
- ○ Sexual improvement[7]
- ○ Fibromyalgia[15]
- ○ Improving quality of life in cancer patients

References

1. Dunn KD. A review of the literature examining the physiological processes underlying the therapeutic benefits of Hatha yoga. *Adv Mind Body Med.* 2008;23(3):10-18.

2. Ross A, Thomas S. The health benefits of yoga and exercise: a review of comparison studies. *J Altern Complement Med.* 2010;16:3-12.

3. Brown RP, Gerbarg PL. Yoga breathing, meditation, and longevity. *Ann NY Acad Sci.* 2009;1172:54-62.

4. Mamtani R, Mamtani R. Ayurveda and yoga in cardiovascular diseases. *Cardiol Rev.* 2005;13(3):155-62.

5. Gupta N, Khera S, Vempati RP, Sharma R, Bijlani RL. Effect of yoga based lifestyle intervention on state and trait anxiety. *Indian J Physiol Pharmacol.* 2006;50(1):41-47.

6. Garfinkel M, Schumacher HR Jr. Yoga. *Rheum Dis Clin North Am.* 2000;26(1):125-132.

7.   Brotto LA, Mehak L, Kit C. Yoga and sexual functioning. *J Sex Marital Ther.* 2009;35(5):378-390.

8.   Innes KE, Selfe TK, Vishnu A. Mind-body therapies for menopausal symptoms: a systematic review. *Maturitas.* 2010;66(2):135-149.

9.   Sibbritt D, Adams J, van der Riet P. The prevalence and characteristics of young and mid-age women who use yoga and meditation: results of a nationally representative survey of 19,209 Australian women. *Complement Ther Med.* 2011;19(2):71-77.

10. Saeed SA, Antonacci DJ, Bloch RM. Exercise, yoga, and meditation for depressive and anxiety disorders. *Am Fam Physician.* 2010;81(8):981-986.

11. Kuntsevich V, Bushell WC, Theise ND. Mechanisms of yogic practices in health, aging, and disease. *Mt Sinai J Med.* 2010;77(5):559-569.

12. Kuttner L, Chambers CT, Hardial J, Israel DM, Jacobson K, Evans K. A randomized trial of yoga for adolescents with irritable bowel syndrome. *Pain Res Manag.* 2006;11(4):217-223.

13. Harris LR, Roberts L. Treatments for irritable bowel syndrome: patients' attitudes and acceptability. *BMC Complement Altern Med.* 2008;8:65.

14. Taneja I, Deepak KK, Poojary G, Acharya IN, Pandey RM, Sharma MP. Yogic versus conventional treatment in diarrhea-predominant irritable bowel syndrome: a randomized control study. *Appl Psychophysiol Biofeedback.* 2004;29(1):19-33.

15. Curtis K, Osadchuk A, Katz J. An eight-week yoga intervention is associated with improvements in pain, psychological functioning and mindfulness, and changes in cortisol levels in women with fibromyalgia. *J Pain Res.* 2011;4:189-201.

DIETARY SUPPLEMENTS ARE NOT ALWAYS SAFE

Chapter
29 *Regulation and Safety Concerns*

KEY POINTS

○ Many patients and clinicians are under the false impression that dietary supplement products are at least safe and possibly effective.

○ Medications and dietary supplements are regulated under different laws.

○ Beware of the possibility of not just contaminants, but also the possible spiking of dietary supplements.

○ Clinicians must take it upon themselves to educate themselves about the variety of complementary and alternative therapies so as to meet their patients on a neutral ground.

While as many as 60% of Americans use some form of dietary supplement, about 15% to 20% of Americans consume herbal remedies on a regular basis.[1] The number of people using such therapies has been rising in recent years.[2] Total sales of herbal and dietary supplements in the United States in 2008 was estimated to be $4.8 billion.[3]

The consumer expects—and should get—the correct, affordable, and safe product. However, most of the public is not aware of the regulatory role and authority of the Food and Drug Administration (FDA) as it relates to dietary supplements.[4] The majority believe that these products have been approved by regulatory agencies prior to marketing. At the same time, only 37% believe that these products

Minocha A. *A Guide to Alternative Medicine and the Digestive System* (pp 117-146).
© 2013 Taylor & Francis Group.

have been adequately tested.[4] There is great public support for greater government regulation to ensure accuracy and safety.[5]

Prior to consumption by a person, numerous diverse factors come into play, creating a vast mosaic of variability.

VARIABILITY RELATED TO MANUFACTURING PROCESSES

○ Concentration and potency
○ Lack of standardization
○ Adulteration, substitution, and contamination that may involve toxins, metals, drugs, insecticides, and pesticides, as well as pathogenic organisms
○ Spiking of products

REGULATORY HISTORY IN THE UNITED STATES

Pure Food and Drugs Act of 1906

This law banned interstate commerce in adulterated foods, drinks, and drugs. It created the first federal regulatory agency, which later evolved into the current FDA.

The Food, Drug, and Cosmetic Act (FDCA) Act of 1938

The law required, for the first time, that the manufacturer undertake scientific safety testing prior to approval for marketing.

Dietary Supplement Health and Education Act (DSHEA) of 1994

Dietary supplements are categorized as a special category of foods, rather than as drugs.[6,7] They include vitamins, minerals, herbs or other botanicals, an amino acid, and any dietary product to supplement the diet by increasing the total dietary intake. The definition includes the products in the form of concentrate, metabolite, constituent, extract, or any combination thereof.

The ingredients of supplements sold on market prior to 1994 are grandfathered. The law prohibits making drug-like claims, while structure/function claims are allowed. While a supplement may not be marketed for specific gastrointestinal (GI) disease, it can be sold for "colon health."

Ensuring safety is the manufacturer's responsibility. The FDA can only intervene after the marketing of the product. Unlike pharmaceutical products, the onus of burden of proof that a particular product is unsafe lies on the FDA.[8]

Food and Drug Administration Modernization Act of 1997

The law enhanced regulatory authority regarding health claims for food supplements. Health claims may only be made based on authoritative statements from scientific bodies.

Dietary Supplement and Nonprescription Drug Consumer Protection Act of 2006

The law mandates the reporting of all adverse events to the Secretary of Health and Human Services. The manufacturer is also required to print an address or phone number on the label so that a consumer may promptly report an adverse event to the manufacturer.

Current Good Manufacturing Practices for Dietary Supplements (2007)

The DSHEA authorized the FDA to develop and enforce the good manufacturing practice regulations for dietary supplements. The rule mandates that the manufacturers actually identify the ingredients contained in the product, along with their strength.

SHORTCOMINGS OF CURRENT UNITED STATES REGULATORY STATUS ABOUT DIETARY SUPPLEMENTS

- ○ The bioactive components of most herbal products are not known.
- ○ A dietary supplement is deemed to be adulterated if it can result in a significant or unreasonable risk of illness or injury under normal conditions. However, an action can only be undertaken after the fact.
- ○ The law requires the label to provide the names of each of the constituents, as well as quantity. The supplement must also meet the quality, purity, potency, and compositional standards. However, legal action is undertaken only rarely.
- ○ Reporting of adverse events, although mandated, are rarely detected or diagnosed and are therefore rarely ever reported.

The European Union imposes stricter regulations than the United States. It requires manufacturers of over-the-counter herbal products to register and license the product with the European Agency for the Evaluation of Medicinal Products. It also mandates a premarket evaluation of product quality and safety, as well as postmarketing surveillance, along with reporting of serious adverse events.

Toxic Potential of Supplements

This may occur due to the supplement itself, a contaminant, or be due to an interaction with other medications. The herb-drug interactions may be pharmacokinetic and/or pharmacodynamic. A detailed description of herbal drug interactions and hepatotoxicities is provided in succeeding chapters. Overall, the toxic potential may be enhanced in certain populations, such as children and elderly, or those with chronic liver and kidney disease.

Role of Adulteration and Contamination

Adulteration and contamination continues to be a problem to this day. Some supplements may contain toxic levels of metals (eg, lead, arsenic, and cadmium). Other potential contaminants include pesticides, bacteria, and fungi. Intentional or accidental substitution of plants is also of concern. It is not uncommon for supplements to be adulterated or spiked with biopharmaceuticals.

A Clinician Perspective

There is tremendous public support and hunger for easy access to "natural remedies" with minimal restrictions. Rather than just decry the state of regulatory affairs, clinicians should educate themselves about such products on the market. Patients appreciate and are more likely to follow your advice if they are provided actual information of help versus harm about the herb/product.

References

1. Gershwin ME, Borchers AT, Keen CL, Hendler S, Hagie F, Greenwood M. Public safety and dietary supplementation. *Ann NY Acad Sci.* 2010;1190:104-117.

2. Kelly JP, Kaufman DW, Kelley K, et al. Recent trends in use of herbal and other natural products. *Arch Intern Med.* 2005;165:281-286.

3. American Botanical Council. Herbal supplement sales experience slight increase in 2008. *HerbalGram.* 2009;82:58.

4. Blendon RJ, DesRoches CM, Benson JM, Brodie M, Altman DE. Americans' views on the use and regulation of dietary supplements. *Arch Intern Med.* 2001;161:805-810.

5. Consumers Union. Consumers Union dietary supplements survey: 9 of 10 consumers want dietary supplements to be proven safe before put on store shelves. 2004. Available at: http://www.consumersunion.org/pub/core_product_safety/001171.html. Accessed May 5, 2011.

6. Glisson JK, Walker LA. How physicians should evaluate dietary supplements. *Am J Med.* 2010;123:577-582

7.   McNamara SH. FDA regulation of ingredients in dietary supplements after passage of the Dietary Supplement Health and Education Act of 1994: an update. *Food Drug Law J.* 1996;51:313-318.

8.   Pinco RG, Halpern TH. Guidelines for the promotion of dietary supplements: examining government regulation five years after enactment of the Dietary Supplement Health and Education Act of 1994. *Food Drug Law J.* 1999;54:567-586.

Chapter

30 *Side Effects of Select Supplements*

KEY POINTS

○ Herbal products contain pharmacologically active compounds and, as such, have the potential for toxicity.

○ Toxic manifestations may occur due to the supplement itself or due to additives, contaminants, and drug interactions.

○ Much of the literature about toxic manifestations is based on anecdotal reports and is frequently contradictory.

Dietary supplements, including herbals, are usually considered harmless and devoid of any toxic implications. Let us not forget that these products have pharmacologically active compounds—that is how they exercise their beneficial and even possibly deleterious side effects, as well as potential drug interactions.[1] Some herbal drugs may even be "spiced up."[2]

Table 30-1 lists some of the reported side effects attributed to these products. Much of the data are based on isolated case reports and not rigorously conducted randomized, controlled trials. Frequently, contradictory evidence is seen in the literature, especially related to interactions involving the risk of bleeding (eg, gingko and garlic).[3]

REFERENCES

1.   Ernst E. Risks of herbal medicinal products. *Pharmacoepidemiol Drug Saf.* 2004;13(11):767-771.

2.   Vardakou I, Pistos C, Spiliopoulou CH. Spice drugs as a new trend: mode of action, identification and legislation. *Toxicol Lett.* 2010;197(3):157-162.

3.   Jiang X, Williams KM, Iiauw WS. Effect of ginkgo and ginger on the pharmacokinetics and pharmacodynamics of warfarin in healthy subjects. *Br J Clin Pharmacol.* 2005;59(4):425-432.

Table 30-1. Side Effects

Remedy/Product	Side Effects*
Acacia (*Acacia senegal*)	Allergic rhinitis, GI upset
Aloe vera (*Aloe barbadensis*)	Bloating and cramps, diarrhea, electrolyte abnormalities; topical application may cause rash
Ashwagandha (*Withania somnifera*)	Skin rash, diarrhea, dyspepsia
Astragalus (*Astragalus membranaceous*)	Diarrhea, dyspepsia
Barberry (*Berberis vulgaris*)	Nose bleed and vomiting on high doses; abortifacient
Bilberry (*Vaccinium myrtillus*)	GI upsets
Bitter orange (*Citrus aurantium*)	Hypertension, angina, stroke, tachyarrhythmia, ischemic colitis
Black cohosh (*Actaea racemosa; Cimicifuga racemosa*)	GI upset, skin rash
Borage seed oil (*Borago officinalis*)	Diarrhea, dyspepsia, lowered seizure threshold
Capsaicin (*Capsicum annuum*)	Dyspepsia, abdominal pain, diarrhea; highly irritant to skin or eyes on contact and to lungs on inhalation
Cascara sagrada (*Rhamnus purshiana*)	Bloating, cramps, potassium depletion, arrhythmia
Chamomile (*Matricaria chamomilla*)	Nausea, vomiting, rash, central nervous system depression; may increase risk of bleeding in patients on warfarin
Chaparral (*Larrea tridentata; Luehea divaricata*)	Generally considered unsafe because of serious hepatic and renal toxicity

(continued)

Table 30-1 *(continued)*. Side Effects

Remedy/Product	Side Effects*
Chinese herbal medicine	Hepatotoxicity, interstitial pneumonia, thrombocytopenia
Clove (*Syzygium aromaticum*)	Contact dermatitis
Cowhage (*Mucuna pruriens*)	Altered mental status
Devil's claw (*Harpagophytum procumbens*)	Dyspepsia, diarrhea, anoxia, headache
Echinacea	Allergic reactions
Ephedra or ma huang (*Ephedra sinica*)	Irritability, insomnia, dyspepsia, hypertension, arrhythmia, seizures, stroke and myocardial infarction
Evening primrose oil	Seizures
Flaxseed (*Linum usitatissimum*)	Dyspepsia, diarrhea
Fennel (*Foeniculum vulgare*)	None reported
Fenugreek (*Trigonella foenum-graecum*)	Gas, bloating, dyspepsia, diarrhea, hypoglycemia, galactorrhea
Feverfew (*Tanacetum parthenium*)	Dyspepsia, bowel problems
Garlic (*Allium sativum*)	Dyspepsia, diarrhea, bad breath, increased risk of bleeding via inhibition of platelets; topical use may cause local burns
Ginger (*Zingiber officinale*)	Heartburn, mouth irritation, diarrhea, increased risk of bleeding by interfering with clotting mechanisms

(continued)

Table 30-1 (continued). Side Effects

Remedy/Product	Side Effects*
Ginkgo biloba	Dyspepsia, diarrhea, dizziness, palpitations; skin rash on direct contact; increased risk of bleeding by inhibiting clotting mechanisms
Ginseng (different species)	Skin rash, diarrhea, difficulty sleeping, hypertension, headache, confusion and euphoria, arrhythmia, palpitations, nose bleeds
Greater celandine (*Chelidonium majus*)	Rash, pruritus, dry mouth, insomnia, diarrhea, hepatotoxicity
Green tea (*Camellia sinensis*)	Irritability, insomnia, hepatotoxicity, palpitations, tachyarrhythmias
Guggul (*Commiphora wightii; Commiphora mukul*)	Headache, dyspepsia, diarrhea, hiccups, rash
Hawthorn (*Crataegus laevigata*)	Dyspepsia, tachyarrhythmia, palpitations, headache, fatigue, vertigo, dizziness
Hibiscus (*Hibiscus sabdariffa*)	None reported
Horse chestnut (*Aesculus hippocastanum*)	Dyspepsia, headache, dizziness, hypoglycemia; may worsen kidney dysfunction
Kava (*Piper methysticum*)	Possible hepatotoxicity; lethargy, skin rash, decrease in lymphocyte count, alterations in red blood cells and platelet morphology
Licorice or liquorice (*Glycyrrhiza glabra*)	Hyperaldosteronism (high sodium, low potassium), hypertension, hepatotoxicity, muscle weakness, fatigue, low sperm count

(continued)

Table 30-1 (continued). Side Effects

Remedy/Product	Side Effects*
Marshmallow (*Althaea officinalis*)	Caffeine-like effects; smooth muscle relaxation may slow GI motility
Milk thistle (*Silybum marianum*)	Dyspepsia, diarrhea, headache, anorexia, arthralgias, myalgias, drug rash
Papaya or papaw or pawpaw (*Carica papaya*)	Increased risk of bleeding, hormonal dyshomeostasis in both sexes; very large doses can cause carotenemia; affects sperm motility; high doses demonstrate abortifacient effect in rats
Peppermint	Dyspepsia, diarrhea, urticaria, bronchospasm, gallstones
Picrorhiza	Dyspepsia, diarrhea, skin rash; may cause autoimmune disorders via its immune-stimulant actions
Policosanol	None reported
Red yeast rice (*Monascus purpureus*)	Headache, dizziness, dyspepsia, myalgias, rhabdomyolysis
Rhubarb (*Rheum palmatum*; *Rheum officinale*)	Bloating and spasms, hyperaldosteronism, potassium depletion and arrhythmias, bone damage
S-Adenosylmethionine	Dry mouth, GI upset, dyspepsia, insomnia, restlessness, skin rash
Safflower (*Carthamus tinctorius*)	Diarrhea, palpitations, anorexia, dyspepsia
Saw palmetto (*Serenoa repens*)	Dyspepsia, diarrhea
Senna (*Cassia senna*)	Bloating and spasms, potassium depletion and arrhythmias
Shiitake mushroom (*Lentinula edodes*)	Fever, rash, dyspepsia

(continued)

Table 30-1 (continued). Side Effects

Remedy/Product	Side Effects*
Spirulina	Potential for worsening autoimmune diseases due to its immune-stimulant action
St. John's wort (*Hypericum perforatum*)	Headache, serotonin syndrome (rigidity, fever, altered mental status), photosensitivity reaction, sexual dysfunction
STW 5 (Iberogast)	Increased risk for bleeding, central nervous system depression, hepatotoxicity
Turmeric (*Curcuma longa*)	Dyspepsia, headache
Thymic extracts	Nausea, vomiting
Valerian (*Valeriana officinalis*)	Central nervous system depression, headache, lethargy, drug hangover; may suffer withdrawal upon cessation; some patients get a paradoxical excitatory reaction
Yellow dock (*Rumex crispus*)	Diarrhea, cramps
Yerba mate or erva mate (*Ilex paraguariensis*)	Arrhythmias, increased heart rate

Note: The list in Table 30-1 is based on a low threshold for inclusion, as is seen in *Physicians' Desk Reference*, and should be understood in appropriate context. Hepatotoxicity is discussed in greater detail in the following chapter.

*Allergic reactions may occur due to any and all products.

Chapter

31 *Potential for Hepatotoxicity*

KEY POINTS

○ While many of the reports of herbal-induced hepatotoxicity are very well documented, some have been implicated solely based on occasional case reports—without rigorous medical scrutiny.

○ Best data available from the United States implicate herbal-induced hepatotoxicity in less than 10% of all drug-induced liver toxicity.

Concerns continue to be raised about potential hepatotoxicity from herbal therapies, sometimes bordering on hysteria. While such implications are clearly justified, many times the evidence may not meet the established criteria,[1] however faulted.

The increasing popularity of herbals in the West is in part due to the belief that herbals are natural and thus are not just effective but also safe and superior to the practice of the impersonal nature of modern medicine.[2] With the increasing use of herbals, it is inevitable that reports of the herbal-induced liver injury will continue to rise.

The diagnosis is frequently made based on expert opinion, which usually means the treating physician is not a trained hepatologist or a toxicologist. Scoring systems can help establish a clinical diagnosis and, although considered essential as part of the diagnostic work-up, they are rarely used in cases of herbals.[3,4] Lack of use of a systematic approach of implicating herbals in liver injury makes many of the reports open to challenge. Virtually the entire spectrum of herbal medicines (Tables 31-1 and 31-2) have been implicated in herbal-induced hepatotoxicity, including Chinese and Ayurvedic medicine.[5]

A review of the data from the Drug Induced Liver Injury Network published in 2008 found that, excluding acetaminophen (which is a very common cause), drug-induced liver injury was caused by a single prescription medication in 73% of the cases, while dietary supplements accounted for only in 9% of the cases.[6]

Table 31-1. Select Herbals Implicated in Liver Injury

- ❖ *Atractylis gummifera*
- ❖ Black cohosh
- ❖ Borage (*B officinalis*)
- ❖ Broom corn (*Sorghum vulgare*)
- ❖ *Cascara sagrada*
- ❖ *Centella asiatica* (gotu kola)
- ❖ Copaltra (*Coutarea latiflora* and *Centaurium erythraea*)
- ❖ *Callilepis laureola*
- ❖ Chaparral
- ❖ Comfrey
- ❖ Germander
- ❖ Greater celandine
- ❖ Green tea
- ❖ Herbalife (Herbalife International of America Inc, Torrance, CA)
- ❖ Hydroxycut (Iovate Health Sciences Inc, Oakville, Canada)
- ❖ Kava
- ❖ Kombucha tea
- ❖ LipoKinetix (Syntrax Innovations, Inc, Scott City, MO; a capsule used for weight loss that contains multiple ingredients). (*Note:* In 2009, the FDA issued a warning for consumers to stop using this product because of reports of acute liver injury.)
- ❖ Mistletoe
- ❖ Margosa oil (*Azadirachta indica*)
- ❖ Noni (*Morinda citrifolia*)
- ❖ Pennyroyal
- ❖ Poley (*Teucrium polium*)
- ❖ Sassafras (*Sassafras albidum*)
- ❖ Senna (*Cassia angustifolia*)
- ❖ Skullcap
- ❖ Valerian

Table 31-2. Select Chinese/Ayurvedic Drugs
Implicated in Hepatotoxicity

Chinese Herbal Drugs	Ayurvedic Drugs[5]
❖ Chaso and Onshido	❖ Bakuchi tablets (*Psoralea corylifolia* extract with psoralens)
❖ Dai-Saiko-To, Jin Bu Huan, ma huang	❖ Khadin tablets (*Acacia catechu* extract)
❖ Shen Min, Shou-Wu-Pian	❖ Brahmi tablets (*Eclipta alba* or *Bacopa monnieri*)
	❖ Usheer tea (*Vetiveria zizanioides*)

While herbal medicines are not harmless, it should be noted that many of the implicated herbals actually have been only reported singly or infrequently, and thus may represent a rare hepatotoxic effect occurring in certain predisposed individuals under specific circumstances.[7]

SELECT HERBAL MEDICATIONS IMPLICATED IN LIVER INJURY

Atractylis gummifera

The toxic components include atractyloside and gummifera, which inhibit Krebs cycle.[8] Acute toxicity causes GI distress, including gastroenteritis, headaches, and seizures, along with liver injury that may be fatal. Hepatorenal injury may also occur as a result of cutaneous application.[9] There is no specific therapy. Use of verapamil and dithiothreitol prior to exposure may be of benefit.

Black Cohosh

Several reports, mostly single-case reports, have implicated black cohosh (*A racemosa*/*C racemosa*) in causing acute hepatocellular injury. Autoimmune hepatitis, as well as acute liver failure, has also been reported. However, the causality assessment has been challenged by others.[10,11]

Callilepis laureola

C laureola is a perennial herb from South Africa. It can cause acute fatal hepatocellular necrosis, especially in children, via depletion of cellular glutathione.

Chaparral

Hepatic injury due to chaparral (*L tridentata*) includes hepatocellular damage and cholestatic hepatitis. Severe cases may require liver transplantation. Chaparral is generally considered unsafe for use.

Comfrey (Symphytum officinale)

Comfrey is derived from the roots of *S officinale*. Hepatic injury manifests as venoocclusive disease. The toxic effects are related to its pyrrolizidine alkaloids. Pyrrolizidine alkaloids are also present in other plants (eg, *Heliotropium*, *Senecio*, *Crotalaria*, *Trichodesma*, *Symphytum*, *Eupatorium*, *Leguminosae*, *Teucrium chamaedrys*, Greater Celandine [*C majus*], *Scrophulariaceae* [*Castilleja*], and T'u-san-chi). The FDA recommended withdrawal of comfrey products from the market in 2001.

Germander (Teucrium chamaedrys)

The spectrum of acute and chronic injury includes fulminant hepatitis and cirrhosis, requiring liver transplantation. In France, it was banned in 1992 because of case reports of severe hepatotoxicity. Hepatotoxicity has also been attributed to other similar plants *T polium* and *Teucrium capitatum*.

Greater Celandine (Chelidonium majus)

It is used as a "cleansing" herb. There has been controversy about its hepatoprotective versus hepatotoxic effects.[12] *C majus*, at doses about 50 and 100 times higher than those generally used in humans, does not alter hepatic function in rats.[13] Several case reports have implicated it in causing liver injury, including one confirmed by inadvertent rechallenge. Injury manifests in hepatocellular and cholestatic patterns.

Green Tea (Camellia sinensis)[14,15]

Hepatotoxicity occurs due to epigallocatechin gallate or its metabolites. The US Pharmacopeia Dietary Supplement Information Expert Committee systematically reviewed the safety information for green tea.[15] Only 27 reports pertaining to liver damage were categorized as possible causality, and 7 as probable causality. Considering the widespread use of green tea, the frequency of green tea-induced hepatotoxicity appears to be very rare.

Kava (Piper methysticum)

Reports have implicated Kava in several severe, and even fatal, cases of hepatotoxicity. Immunoallergic mechanisms may be involved.

The regulatory causality evaluation of the reported cases has been mired in debate in the scientific community. The FDA issued a customer advisory regarding the dangers of this agent in 2002. Its use is banned in several European countries.

Many experts have challenged the concept of hepatotoxicity being caused by Kava in many of the reported cases.[16] In vitro data do not support a hepatotoxic potential. Many of the affected patients reported in the literature were also taking other medications.

Teschke concluded in 2010 that Kava may be hepatotoxic in a few individuals due to overdose, prolonged treatment, and comedication and is probably triggered by an unacceptable quality of the Kava raw material.[17]

Mistletoe *(Viscum album)*

Mistletoe protects against carbon tetrachloride-induced hepatotoxicity. However, there are single-case reports of mistletoe-induced hepatotoxicity.[18] Experimental data to support the premise of mistletoe-induced toxicity are lacking.

Pennyroyal *(Mentha pulegium)*

Pennyroyal is a highly toxic agent with potential for both hepatic and neurologic injury. Toxicity occurs due to menthofuran, an oxidative metabolite of the active compound pulegone. N-acetylcysteine has been successfully used for treatment.

Poley *(Teucrium polium)*

Poley belongs to the same genus as germander and has also been implicated in acute liver injury.

Skullcap *(Scutellaria)*

Skullcap is used as a sedative, an antispasmodic, and an anti-inflammatory agent. Hepatic injury has been reported due to products containing skullcap.[19]

Valerian *(Valeriana officinalis)*

Valerian is frequently used as a sleeping aid in addition to its use for headaches. Hepatic injury is rare[20] but has been reported in cases of patients using products with multiple ingredients.

CHINESE HERBAL MEDICINES

Chinese herbal medicine has been used for centuries and continues to be popular. Ascribing a hepatotoxicity to any particular ingredient is challenging. Jin Bu Huan and *Dictamnus dasycarpus* have been the most common herbs that have been implicated.

Chaso and Onshido

These are popular remedies for weight loss in Japan. Hepatotoxicity occurs in the form of hepatocellular injury, including fulminant hepatitis. N-nitroso-fenfluramine, a variant of the appetite-depressant drug fenfluramine, has been documented in the more severe cases and may be the ingredient responsible for hepatotoxicity.[21]

Dai-Saiko-To

There have been isolated case reports of hepatic injury, including autoimmune hepatitis. However, a clear causality remains to be established.[22]

Jin Bu Huan

Hepatic toxicity includes acute and chronic liver injury, and recurs upon rechallenge. Immune mechanisms appear to be involved.[23]

Ma Huang (Ephedra sinica)

Case reports have implicated it in causing liver injury, in addition to fulminant hepatitis. Potential toxic components include ephedrine. A systematic review of herbal medicines, with ma huang, reported only minor side effects that did not include hepatotoxicity.[24]

Shen Min

This is also derived from *Polygonatum multiflorum*, and there are isolated case reports of hepatotoxicity.[25]

Sho-Saiko-To (Xiao Chai Hu Tang)

Sho-Saiko-To (TJ-9) is a popular Chinese herbal concoction used for liver health. It has been shown to be hepatoprotective. However, case reports implicate this mixture in hepatic toxicity.[26]

Shou-Wu-Pian

Shou-Wu-Pian is derived from *P multiflorum*. Case reports have implicated it in causing acute hepatitis. The toxic component is believed to be anthraquinone, which is also contained in some other herbal medications (including He Shou Wu and Jue Ming Zi).[27]

CONCLUSION

Accurate causality assessment in cases of suspected hepatotoxicity is complicated by infrequent documentation of product intake, underreporting of herbal-drug and over-the-counter medications, the complexity of their numerous formulations, and the possibility for product adulteration. A good, objective, reliable, and reproducible means of assessing drug-induced liver injury causality is sorely needed.

REFERENCES

1. Seeff LB. Herbal hepatotoxicity. *Clin Liver Disease*. 2007;11(3):577-596.

2. Kessler RC, Davis RB, Foster DF, et al. Long-term trends in the use of complementary and alternative medical therapies in the United States. *Ann Intern Med*. 2002;135:262-268.

3. Danan G, Benichou C. Causality assessment of adverse reactions to drugs. I. A novel method based on the conclusions of international consensus meetings: application to drug-induced liver injuries. *J Clin Epidemiol*. 1993;46:1323-1330.

4. Maria VA, Victorino RM. Development and validation of a clinical scale for the diagnosis of drug-induced hepatitis. *Hepatology*. 1997;26:664-669.

5. Teschke R, Bahre R. Severe hepatotoxicity by Indian Ayurvedic herbal products: a structured causality assessment. *Ann Hepatol*. 2009;8(3):258-266.

6. Chalasani N, Fontana RJ, Bonkovsky HL, Watkins PB. Causes, clinical features, and outcomes from a prospective study of drug-induced liver injury in the United States. *Gastroenterology*. 2008;135(6):1924-1934.

7. Stickel F, Patsenker E, Schuppan D. Herbal hepatotoxicity. *J Hepatol*. 2005;43:901-910.

8. Larrey D, Stickel F, Daniele C, et al. *Atractylis gummifera L.* poisoning: an ethnopharmacological review. *J Ethnopharmacol*. 2005;28:175-181.

9. Bouziri A, Hamdi A, Menif K, Ben Jaballah N. Hepatorenal injury induced by cutaneous application of *Atractylis gummifera L. Clin Toxicol (Phila)*. 2010;48(7):752-754.

10. Thomsen M. Hepatotoxicity from Cimicifuga racemosa? Recent Australian case report not sufficiently substantiated. *J Altern Complement Med*. 2003;9:337-340.

11. Teschke R, Schwarzenboeck A. Suspected hepatotoxicity by *Cimicifugae racemosae rhizoma* (black cohosh, root): critical analysis and structured causality assessment. *Phytomedicine*. 2009;16(1):72-84.

12. Gilca M, Gaman L, Panait E, Stoian I, Atanasiu V. *Chelidonium majus*—an integrative review: traditional knowledge versus modern findings. *Forsch Komplementmed*. 2010;17(5):241-248.

13. Mazzanti G, Di Sotto A, Franchitto A, et al. *Chelidonium majus* is not hepatotoxic in Wistar rats, in a 4 weeks feeding experiment. *J Ethnopharmacol*. 2009;126(3):518-524.

14. Mazzanti G, Menniti-Ippolito F, Moro PA, et al. Hepatotoxicity from green tea: a review of the literature and two unpublished cases. *Eur J Clin Pharmacol*. 2009;65(4):331-341.

15. Sarma DN, Barrett ML, Chavez ML, et al. Safety of green tea extracts: a systematic review by the US Pharmacopeia. *Drug Saf*. 2008;31(6):469-484.

16. Anke J, Ramzan I. Kava hepatotoxicity: are we any closer to the truth? *Planta Med*. 2004;70(3):193-196.

17. Teschke R. Kava hepatotoxicity—a clinical review. *Ann Hepatol*. 2010;9(3):251-265.

18. Harvey J, Colin-Jones DG. Mistletoe hepatitis. *Br Med J*. 1981;282:186-187.

19. Linnebur SA, Rapacchietta OC, Vejar M. Hepatotoxicity associated with chinese skullcap contained in Move Free Advanced dietary supplement: two case reports and review of the literature. *Pharmacotherapy.* 2010;30(7):750,258e-262e.

20. Cohen DL, Del Toro Y. A case of valerian-associated hepatotoxicity. *J Clin Gastroenterol.* 2008;42(8):961-962.

21. Adachi M, Saito H, Kobayashi H, et al. Hepatic injury in 12 patients taking the herbal weight loss aids Chaso or Onshido. *Ann Intern Med.* 2003;139(6):488-492.

22. Kamiyama T, Nouchi T, Kojima S, Murata N, Ikeda T, Sato C. Autoimmune hepatitis triggered by administration of an herbal medicine. *Am J Gastroenterol.* 1997; 92(4):703-704.

23. Divinsky M. Case report: jin bu huan--not so benign herbal medicine. *Can Fam Physician.* 2002;48:1640-1642.

24. Hasani-Ranjbar S, Nayebi N, Larijani B, et al. A systematic review of the efficacy and safety of herbal medicines used in the treatment of obesity. *World J Gastroenterol.* 2009;15(25): 3073-3085.

25. Cárdenas A, Restrepo JC, Sierra F, Correa G. Acute hepatitis due to shen-min: a herbal product derived from Polygonum multiflorum. *J Clin Gastroenterol.* 2006;40(7):629-632.

26. Chitturi S, Farrell GC. Hepatotoxic slimming aids and other herbal hepatotoxins. *J Gastroenterol Hepatol.* 2008;23(3):366-373.

27. Furukawa M, Kasajima S, Nakamura Y, et al. Toxic hepatitis induced by show-wu-pian, a Chinese herbal preparation. *Intern Med.* 2010;49(15):1537-1540.

Chapter

32 *Herb-Drug Interactions*

KEY POINTS

○ Herbal products have pharmacologically active compounds and have potential for interactions with conventional medications.

○ In many cases of reported interactions, the evidence is weak and contradictory

The potential for interaction between herbal products and conventional products is often overlooked or ignored (Table 32-1).[1]

Table 32-1. Select Listing of Dietary Supplements With Potential for Interaction With Conventional Medications

Dietary Supplement	Potential Drug Interactions
Acacia (*A senegal*)	Impaired absorption of drugs like amoxicillin[2]
Aloe vera (*A barbadensis*)	Potentiates effect of cardiac glycosides, oral hypoglycemics, azidothymidine, and antiplatelet activity of anesthetics sevoflurane
Angelica or Dong quai (*Angelica sinensis*)	Increased effects of anticoagulants, calcium channel blockers
Arnica (*Arnica montana*)	Decreased effects of antihypertensives and anticoagulants; increased analgesic effects of salicylates
Ashwagandha (*W somnifera*)	Enhances effects of paclitaxel
Astragalus (*A membranaceous*)	Potentiates effects of stanozolol
Bilberry (*V myrtillus*)	Enhanced effects of anticoagulants and hypoglycemic agents
Bitter orange (*Aurantii pericarpium*)	Increased levels of dextromethorphan, felodipine, and midazolam; potentiates effects of antidepressants; concomitant use with monoamine oxidase inhibitors may cause hypertensive crisis
Black cohosh (*A racemosa; C racemosa*)	Potentiates effects of antihypertensive and lipid-lowering agents; decreased effects of diuretics; potential for additive effect with estrogens is controversial
Borage seed oil (*B officinalis*)	May potentiate bleeding risk due to anticoagulants and antiplatelet agents
Bromelain (*Ananas comosus*)	Increased absorption of antibiotics, like amoxicillin

(continued)

Table 32-1 (continued). Select Listing of Dietary Supplements With Potential for Interaction With Conventional Medications

Dietary Supplement	Potential Drug Interactions
Chamomile (*Chamomilla recutita*)	Potentiates effects of anticoagulants
Chaste tree (*Vitex agnus castus*)	Enhanced effects of beta-blockers and antihypertensive agents
Chili pepper (*Capsicum spp*)	May counter the effects of antihypertensive agents
Chlorella	Immune-stimulant effect helps boost influenza vaccine; may counteract effects of warfarin
Cowhage (*M pruriens*)	Increased serum levodopa levels; potentiates effects of antihypertensives
Dandelion (*Taraxacum officinale*)	Enhanced effects of antihypertensive drugs and diuretics; may reduce absorption of quinolone antibiotics
Danshen (*Salvia miltiorrhiza*)	Potentiate effects of warfarin and corticosteroids
Devil's claw (*H procumbens*)	Increased risk of bleeding when used with anticoagulants; enhanced effects of antihypertensive drugs
Ephedra, ma huang[3] (*E sinica*)	Increased clearance and reduced efficacy of dexamethasone; potentiates sympathomimetic effect when used with caffeine, theophylline, guanethidine, and monoamine oxidase inhibitors
Fenugreek (*T foenum-graecum*)	Enhanced effects of anticoagulants and lipid-lowering agents
Feverfew (*T parthenium*)	Increased effects of platelet inhibitors and anticoagulant agents
Flaxseed (*L usitatissimum*)	Decreased absorption oral medications, vitamins, minerals, etc

(continued)

Table 32-1 (continued). Select Listing of Dietary Supplements With Potential for Interaction With Conventional Medications

Dietary Supplement	Potential Drug Interactions
Garlic[4,5] (*A sativum*)	Increased effects of anticoagulant, antiplatelet antihypertensives, and anti-lipid agents; reduced plasma concentrations of protease inhibitor saquinavir
Ginger[6] (*Z officinalis*)	May potentiate effects of antiplatelet, anticoagulant, and antihypertensive agents
Ginkgo[4,7] (*G biloba*)	Potentiates effects of anticoagulants and antiplatelet agents; increases concentration of nifedipine
Ginseng[6] (*Panax ginseng, Eleutherococcus senticosus*, and other species)	Synergistic effects with amoxicillin/clavulanic acid and antidiabetic agents; increased antiplatelet activity with NSAIDs; increased international normalized ratio with warfarin; may induce diuretic resistance; increased levels of calcium channel blocker nifedipine; increased digoxin levels; potentiates hepatotoxic potential of imatinib[8]
Goldenseal[9] (*Hydrastis canadensis*), Berberine	Increased effects of antihypertensive agents and calcium channel blockers; may decrease effects of anticoagulants; causes increased levels of cyclosporine A; enhanced antibiotic effect of tetracycline
Grapefruit[10] (*Citrus paradise*)	Inhibits cytochrome p450 system; increases bioavailability of erythromycin, antiepileptic agents, antidepressants, antihistamines, benzodiazepines, scopolamine, estrogenic agents, HMG CoA reductase inhibitors, immunosuppressant cyclosporine, protease inhibitors, and sildenafil; reduces efficacy of ACE-inhibitor losartan, anticancer agent etoposide; potentiates effects of antiplatelet effects of cilostazol

(continued)

Table 32-1 (continued). Select Listing of Dietary Supplements With Potential for Interaction With Conventional Medications

Dietary Supplement	Potential Drug Interactions
Green tea (C sinensis)	Additive antiplatelet activity[11] with antiplatelet agents; decreases anticoagulant effect with warfarin if tea ingested in large amounts[12]
Guggul (C wightii, aka C mukul)	Decreases bioavailability of propranolol and diltiazem
Hawthorn (C laevigata)	May potentiate effect of cardiac glycosides and antihypertensive agents
Horse chestnut (A hippocastanum)	Increased effects of anticoagulants
Licorice[13] (G glabra)	Increased risk for cardiac toxicity with cardiac glycosides, potentiates effects of corticosteroid, pseudohyperaldosteronism with electrolyte abnormalities may potentiate toxicity of diuretics and inhibit effect of antihypertensive agents
Neem (A indica)	Potentiates hepatotoxic potential of acetaminophen
Nettle (Urtica dioica)	Potentiates effects of diuretics and antihypertensive agents
Peppermint oil (Mentha × piperita)	Increases toxicity of cardiac glycosides
Pumpkin seed (Cucurbita pepo)	Enhances effects of diuretics
Red yeast rice (M purpureus)	Potentiates HMG CoA reductase toxicity[14]; avoid use with protease inhibitors and in patients with chronic alcohol abuse
Rhubarb (R palmatum; R officinale)	Potentiates effect of captopril, antipsychotic agents, chlorhexidine, and nifedipine

(continued)

Table 32-1 (continued). Select Listing of Dietary Supplements With Potential for Interaction With Conventional Medications

Dietary Supplement	Potential Drug Interactions
Roman chamomile (*Chamaemelum nobile*)	Enhances effect with anticoagulant agents
Saw palmetto (*S repens*)	May potentiate bleeding risk with anticoagulant/antiplatelet agents
Senna (*C senna*)	Potentiates effects of cardiac glycosides, antiarrhythmic agents, and calcium channel blockers
St. John's wort[9] (*H perforatum*)	Reduces international normalized ratio in patients on warfarin, potentiates effects of antidepressants, reduces benzodiazepine and verapamil concentration; interaction with digoxin varies with St. John's preparation; increases metabolism of certain oral contraceptives, reduces cyclosporine A, simvastatin, protease inhibitors, anti-cancer drug imatinib, irinotecan, methadone, and antiretroviral non-nucleoside reverse transcriptase inhibitor levels
Valerian (*V officinalis*)	Enhances effects of central nervous system depressants

The most common products implicated in supplement-drug interaction include garlic, valerian, Kava, ginkgo, and St. John's wort.[15] Numerous mechanisms are involved.[16]

Contradictory evidence is seen in the literature, especially related to interactions involving bleeding risk with anticoagulants (eg, gingko and garlic).[4] In other cases, the evidence may be weak, and it is difficult to characterize the clinical significance (eg, garlic, ginger, gingko, and ginseng).[6]

REFERENCES

1. Ulbricht C, Chao W, Costa D. Clinical evidence of herb-drug interactions: a systematic review by the Natural Standard Research Collaboration. *Current Drug Metabolism.* 2008;9:1063-1120.

2. Eltayeb IB, Awad AI, Elderbi MA, Shadad SA. Effect of gum arabic on the absorption of a single oral dose of amoxicillin in healthy Sudanese volunteers. *J Antimicrob Chemother.* 2004;54(2):577-578.

3. Holstege CP, Mitchell K, Barlotta K, Furbee RB. Toxicity and drug interactions associated with herbal products: ephedra and St. John's Wort. *Med Clin North Am.* 2005;89(6):1225-1257.

4. Jiang X, Williams KM, Iiauw WS. Effect of ginkgo and ginger on the pharmacokinetics and pharmacodynamics of warfarin in healthy subjects. *Br J Clin Pharmacol.* 2005;59(4):425-432.

5. Berginc K, Žakelj S, Kristl A. In vitro interactions between aged garlic extract and drugs used for the treatment of cardiovascular and diabetic patients. *Eur J Nutr.* 2010;49(6):373-384.

6. Vaes LP, Chyka PA. Interactions of warfarin with garlic, ginger, ginkgo, or ginseng: nature of the evidence. *Ann Pharmacother.* 2000;34(12):1478-1482.

7. Abad MJ, Bedoya LM, Bermejo P. An update on drug interactions with the herbal medicine ginkgo biloba. *Curr Drug Metab.* 2010;11(2):171-181.

8. Bilgi N, Bell K, Ananthakrishnan AN, Atallah E. Imatinib and Panax ginseng: a potential interaction resulting in liver toxicity. *Ann Pharmacother.* 2010 May;44(5):926-8.

9. Gurley BJ, Swain A, Hubbard MA, et al. Clinical assessment of CYP2D6-mediated herb-drug interactions in humans: effects of milk thistle, black cohosh, goldenseal, kava kava, St. John's wort, and Echinacea. *Mol Nutr Food Res.* 2008;52(7):755-763.

10. Hanley MJ, Cancalon P, Widmer WW, Greenblatt DJ. The effect of grapefruit juice on drug disposition. *Expert Opin Drug Metab Toxicol.* 2011;7(3):267-286.

11. Son DJ, Cho MR, Jin YR, et al. Antiplatelet effect of green tea catechins: a possible mechanism through arachidonic acid pathway. *Prostaglandins Leukot Essent Fatty Acids.* 2004;71(1):25-31.

12. Taylor JR, Wilt VM. Probable antagonism of warfarin by green tea. *Ann Pharmacother.* 1999;33(4):426-428.

13. Asl MN, Hosseinzadeh H. Review of pharmacological effects of *Glycyrrhiza sp.* and its bioactive compounds. *Phytother Res.* 2008;22(6):709-724.

14. Hasani-Ranjbar S, Nayebi N, Moradi L, et al. The efficacy and safety of herbal medicines used in the treatment of hyperlipidemia; a systematic review. *Curr Pharm Des.* 2010;16(26):2935-2947.

15. Sood A, Sood R, Brinker FJ, et al. Potential for interactions between dietary supplements and prescription medications. *Am J Med.* 2008;121:207-211.

16.   Colalto C. Herbal interactions on absorption of drugs: mechanisms of action and clinical risk assessment. *Pharmacol Res*. 2010;62(3):207-227.

Chapter 33 *Potential for Interactions With Cancer Treatment*

KEY POINTS

○ Only a few herbal drugs to date have actually been documented to have clinically significant interactions with cancer therapeutic agents. These include St. John's Wort, *G biloba*, and *Echinacea*.

○ The lack of studies on clinically significant interactions may not necessarily mean an absence of such interactions.

○ Antioxidants are best avoided during chemoradiation therapy.

○ It is prudent to avoid imbibing alcohol during chemoradiation therapy.

In addition to the quality control issues, one should be aware of herbal-drug interactions while undergoing cancer therapy. Food, as well as dietary supplements, contain pharmacologically active compounds and may affect cancer chemotherapeutic agents, both via pharmacokinetic and pharmacodynamic interactions (Table 33-1).

It is worth noting that only a few herbal medications have been directly implicated in clinically significant interactions with chemotherapeutic agents. In fact, many of the types of interactions involve already known actions on the cytochrome P450 system.

Even food, routine supplements, and alcohol have a potential for significant effects on cancer chemotherapy.

○ Taking temozolomide with meals can slow and decrease its absorption.

○ Concomitant administration of calcium and vitamin D supplements can decrease plicamycin absorption.

○ Ascorbic acid inhibits antitumor activity of bortezomib in vivo.[1]

○ Use of antioxidant agents during chemoradiation may inhibit the anticancer effects of the therapy.[2]

Table 33-1. Select Herb-Drug Interactions in Cancer Therapy[3-5]

Herb/Dietary Supplement	Drug Involved	Comment
Black cohosh (C racemosa)	Cisplatin	Reduces sensitivity to cisplatin; affects multiple enzymes in cytochrome system but evidence of clinically significant effects is limited
Chaste berry (V agnus-castus)	Letrozole, tamoxifen	Affects cytochrome P450 system, especially CYP2C19 and CYP3A4
Cranberry		No significant interactions
Dong Quai	Letrozole, tamoxifen	Has estrogen-like properties; avoid when taking these anticancer agents
Echinacea	Cyclophosphamide, docetaxel, exemestane, gefitinib, imatinib, irinotecan, letrozole, paclitaxel, tamoxifen, toremifene, vinblastine, vincristine, vinorelbine	Affects cytochrome P450 system, especially CYP3A4 induction; avoid with camptothecins, and EGFR-TK inhibitors
Fenugreek (T foenum-graecum)	Docetaxel, doxorubicin, epirubicin, etoposide, paclitaxel, teniposide, vinblastine, vincristine, vinorelbine	Most studies relate to its constituent quercetin. The bioavailability of quercetin on oral administration of fenugreek remains to be established; caution is advised.

(continued)

Table 33-1 (continued). Select Herb-Drug Interactions in Cancer Therapy[3-5]

Herb/Dietary Supplement	Drug Involved	Comment
Garlic (A sativum)	Docetaxel, dacarbazine	Clinical significance remains to be established
Gingko[6]	Camptothecins, cyclophosphamide, epipodophyllotoxins, taxanes, and vinca alkaloids; alkylating agents, platinum analogues	Affects cytochrome P450 system (especially CYP2C19), but clinical significance is unclear
Ginseng	Cyclophosphamide, docetaxel, doxorubicin, epirubicin, exemestane, gefitinib, ifosfamide, imatinib, paclitaxel, letrozole, tamoxifen, toremifene, vinblastine, vincristine, vinorelbine	Affects cytochrome P450—especially CYP3A4
Grapefruit juice	Bexarotene	Potentiates toxicity
Grapeseed	Camptothecins, cyclophosphamide, EGFR-TK inhibitors, taxanes, vinca alkaloids, alkylating agents, platinum analogues	Antioxidant actions and affects cytochrome P450, especially CYP3A4; paucity of clinical data

(continued)

Table 33-1 (continued). Select Herb-Drug Interactions in Cancer Therapy[3-5]

Herb/Dietary Supplement	Drug Involved	Comment
Green tea (C sinensis)	Bortezomib	May inhibit anticancer activity by competitive interference although there is paucity of clinical data
Guarana (Paullinia cupana)	Cytarabine, ifosfamide	Data on clinically significant interaction are lacking
Kava	Camptothecins, cyclophosphamide, EGFR-TK inhibitors, taxanes, vinca alkaloids	Affects cytochrome P450, especially induction of CYP3A4. Avoid in all patients with chronic liver disease
Liquorice (G glabra)	Letrozole, corticosteroids, tamoxifen	Affects cytochrome P450 system
Milk thistle		No significant interactions
Red clover	Aminoglutethimide, exemestane, goserelin, letrozole, leuprorelin, tamoxifen, toremifene	May induce cellular proliferation; should be used with caution in patients with or at risk for breast cancer
Saw palmetto		No significant interactions
Soy	Letrozole, tamoxifen	Antagonizes tumor growth inhibition

(continued)

Table 33-1 (continued). Select Herb-Drug Interactions in Cancer Therapy[3-5]

Herb/Dietary Supplement	Drug Involved	Comment
St. John's wort[6]	Cyclophosphamide, docetaxel, doxorubicin, epirubicin, etoposide, exemestane, gefitinib, ifosfamide, imatinib, irinotecan, letrozole, paclitaxel, tamoxifen, teniposide, toremifene, vinblastine, vincristine, vinorelbine	Stimulates several cytochrome P450 enzymes while inhibiting others; therapeutic failures upon concomitant use with anticancer agents have been reported
Valerian	Tamoxifen, cyclophosphamide, teniposide	Affects cytochrome P450, especially CYP2C9 and CYP2C19
Wild yam (Dioscorea species)	Letrozole, tamoxifen	Has phytoestrogen activity and has potential to have proliferative effects in estrogen receptor positive breast cancer

○ Fish oil may affect chemotherapeutic agents, but there is a lack of clinical data.

○ Co-enzyme Q10 may reduce the efficacy of chemotherapeutic agents, as well as radiation therapy.

○ It is prudent to avoid imbibing alcohol while undergoing chemotherapy because of a high potential for interactions.

REFERENCES

1.   Perrone G, Hideshima T, Ikeda H, et al. Ascorbic acid inhibits antitumor activity of bortezomib in vivo. *Leukemia.* 2009;23(9):1679-1686.

2.   Lawenda BD, Kelly KM, Ladas EJ, et al. Should supplemental antioxidant administration be avoided during chemotherapy and radiation therapy? *J Natl Cancer Inst.* 2008;100(11):773-783.

3.   Yang AK, He SM, Liu L, et al. Herbal interactions with anticancer drugs: mechanistic and clinical considerations. *Curr Med Chem.* 2010;17(16):1635-1678.

4.   Meijerman I, Beijnen JH, Schellens JH. Herb-drug interactions in oncology: focus on mechanisms of induction. *Oncologist.* 2006;11(7):742-752.

5.   Sparreboom A, Cox MC, Acharya MR, Figg WD. Herbal remedies in the United States: potential adverse interactions with anticancer agents. *J Clin Onc.* 2004;22:2489.

6.   Shord SS, Shah K, Lukose A. Drug-botanical interactions: a review of the laboratory, animal, and human data for 8 common botanicals. *Integr Cancer Ther.* 2009;8(3):208-227.

SOME COMMONLY USED NONHERBAL SUPPLEMENTS

Chapter

34 *Antioxidant-Vitamin Formulations*

KEY POINTS

- ○ Antioxidant supplementation does not protect against cancer, and may even be harmful
- ○ Data from randomized, controlled trial (RCT) results apply to specific supplements or some specific combinations. This does detract from the epidemiological data that have consistently supported the notion of benefit of diets high in antioxidants as the lowering risk of heart disease.

While food contains numerous antioxidants, the vitamins with these properties include vitamin A (including preformed vitamin A or retinol) and the carotenoids (like beta carotene and vitamins C and E).

Antioxidants may theoretically reduce the risk of cancer and cardiovascular disease by multiple mechanisms. A diet rich in vegetables and fruits is associated with a reduced risk of cancer and cardiovascular disease. However, it is unclear whether these effects are related to vitamin content or other constituents of food consumed. Such a diet may also be a marker for healthy lifestyles, which may actually be responsible for the beneficial effects.

Minocha A. *A Guide to Alternative Medicine and the Digestive System* (pp 147-162).

Randomized, Controlled Trials Versus Epidemiological Data

RCTs examining the impact of antioxidant supplements on cancer and cardiovascular disease have not largely confirmed the epidemiologic data.

These results may be due to the unique effects of different antioxidants. Other reasons for discordant results might be that the amount, type, or ratios of antioxidants in foods may be different from what is found in supplements.

Should We Take Antioxidant Supplements?[1,2]

There is no evidence to support the protective effect of antioxidant supplements against cancer; rather, there may be more harm.[2]

Caveat: The potentially harmful effects against cancer relate to the use of antioxidants. Diets rich in antioxidants, on the other hand, have consistently shown to be beneficial.[3,4]

References

1. Bjelakovic G, Nikolova D, Simonetti RG, Gluud C. Antioxidant supplements for preventing gastrointestinal cancers. *Cochrane Database Syst Rev.* 2008;3:CD004183.
2. Myung SK, Kim Y, Ju W, Choi HJ, Bae WK. Effects of antioxidant supplements on cancer prevention: meta-analysis of randomized controlled trials. *Ann Oncol.* 2010;21(1):166-179.
3. Yao H, Xu W, Shi X, Zhang Z. Dietary flavonoids as cancer prevention agents. *J Environ Sci Health C Environ Carcinog Ecotoxicol Rev.* 2011;29(1): 1-31.
4. Pauwels EK. The protective effect of the Mediterranean diet: focus on cancer and cardiovascular risk. *Med Princ Pract.* 2011;20(2):103-111.

Chapter

35 *Vitamins*

Key Points

○ Vitamin E is helpful in nonalcoholic fatty liver disease.
○ Vitamin D deficiency is widely prevalent in the Western world.

○ The effect of folic acid supplementation on colon cancer in average-risk subjects is controversial.

Vitamin A

Vitamin A and Cancer[1]

○ Results of the studies examining effects of vitamin A on cancer risk have been conflicting.

○ While some RCTs have shown no effect, others have actually demonstrated an increased risk of lung and prostate cancer in men receiving vitamin A supplements.

○ There is no effect on the risk for colorectal adenoma.

Vitamin A and Cataracts

Indirect evidence suggests that vitamin A might decrease the risk of cataracts.[2]

Vitamin A in Children

Vitamin A supplementation reduces mortality among children in developing countries by about 30%. The World Health Organization recommends vitamin A supplementation in developing countries. The magnitude of benefit may not be the same in developed countries where diet is adequate.

Vitamin A Supplements and Toxicity

Higher vitamin A levels have been linked to an increased risk for fractures in multiple studies. Vitamin A supplements thus should be avoided in the absence of deficiency.

Vitamin D

Vitamin D, or calciferol, refers to a group of lipid soluble compounds with a 4-ringed cholesterol backbone.

Sources of Vitamin D

Food

Few foods contain adequate amounts of vitamin D. In addition to vitamin D-fortified milk, the dietary sources rich in vitamin D include fatty fish, cod-liver oil, and eggs. Vitamin D_2, or ergocalciferol, is a plant steroid used for milk fortification.

SKIN

Because of the paucity of vitamin D in foods, the human body depends on skin exposure to sun, which leads to indigenous production of vitamin D in body.

> While some argue that vitamin D insufficiency is a growing epidemic across the world, the Institute of Medicine opines that the majority are doing well and the deficiency mostly involves select populations, such as adolescents and the elderly.

Consequences of Vitamin D Deficiency[3]

Although rickets is rare these days, subclinical vitamin D deficiency is common. Pathologic states linked to vitamin D deficiency include osteoporosis, impaired immune function, and increased risk of various malignancies, including colon cancer, cardiovascular disease, falls, and fractures.

Low levels of vitamin D are associated with an increased risk of all-cause mortality. The role of vitamin D supplementation in reducing mortality is controversial.

Vitamin D Requirements

A minimum of 200 IU per day is needed in healthy adults.

○ Pregnant and lactating mothers: 600 IU/d
○ Infants who are exclusively breastfed: 400 IU/d
○ Elderly: 800 IU/d plus 1.2 g of calcium per day
○ Patients noncompliant with daily vitamin D therapy may benefit from high-dose intermittent therapy (100,000 units every 4 months)
○ Dose of vitamin D is 800 IU per day in postmenopausal women with osteoporosis, whereas premenopausal women and men with osteoporosis may benefit from 400 to 600 IU per day
○ Toxic dose: greater than 2000 IU per day

> The role of vitamin D supplementation is mired in debate, and routine vitamin D supplementation for disease prevention is not recommended. Many experts argue that the normal daily dose of vitamin D in at-risk subjects should be 1000 to 2000 IU per day. Vitamin D toxicity includes altered mental status, polyuria, polydipsia, anorexia, vomiting, muscle weakness, bone demineralization with pain, hypercalcemia, and hypercalciuria.

VITAMIN E

Vitamin E and Cancer

○ In contrast to observational studies, evidence from RCTs does not support the beneficial effect of vitamin E supplements in preventing cancer. [4]

○ Randomized, controlled data do not show an effect in breast, lung, or colon cancer. [5]

○ The above notwithstanding, there may be some beneficial effect in prostate cancer.

Vitamin E and Cardiovascular Disease

Vitamin E supplementation may actually increase the risk of heart failure. One exception may be that hemodialysis patients with heart disease may benefit from vitamin E supplementation.

Vitamin E and Stroke

○ Results of the studies on the effect of vitamin E in cerebrovascular accidents have yielded conflicting results.[6]

○ Vitamin E supplementation does not confer any benefit in stroke.

Vitamin E and Dementia

Vitamin E is of no benefit in dementia.

Immunity and Vitamin E

Some but not all trials in the elderly have documented beneficial effect on reduction of infections.[7]

Vitamin E and Nonalcoholic Fatty Liver Disease

Sanyal and colleagues[3] demonstrated that vitamin E supplementation results in greater improvement when compared to placebo.

Vitamin E is effective in nonalcoholic fatty liver disease.[8]

Vitamin E and Venous Thrombosis

Vitamin E appears to have a weak anticoagulant effect, and one study showed that supplementation reduces the risk of deep venous thrombosis.[9]

A meta-analysis determined that vitamin E supplementation does not lower mortality but may in fact increase it.

VITAMIN B$_2$ (RIBOFLAVIN)

Riboflavin is a source for flavin redox cofactors.[10] It plays a critical role in maintaining the integrity of mucous membranes. Only about 25% of ingested riboflavin is absorbed.

Deficiency

Riboflavin deficiency usually occurs in conjunction with a deficiency of other nutrients. Mild cases of deficiency frequently go undetected because of nonspecific manifestations. It may be seen in developing countries[11] or in patients with anorexia nervosa, celiac sprue, short bowel syndrome, diabetes mellitus, and chronic alcoholism. Manifestations include pharyngitis, cheilitis, angular stomatitis, glossitis, magenta tongue, and fatigue.[12] Complete blood count shows normocytic normochromic anemia.

Therapeutic Benefits

Riboflavin administration results in a significant decrease in migraine attacks.[13] Certain anti-HIV medications cause lactic acidosis, which may be reversed by riboflavin administration.

VITAMIN B$_6$ (PYRIDOXINE)

- ❍ There is a lack of benefits of vitamin B$_6$ supplementation in coronary artery disease.
- ❍ Higher plasma B$_6$ levels are associated with a reduced risk of breast cancer.
- ❍ A multicenter, double-blind clinical RCT of high-dose vitamin supplements (5 mg/d of folate, 25 mg/d of vitamin B$_6$, 1 mg/d of vitamin B$_{12}$) in patients with Alzheimer's disease found that this regimen does not have any impact on the cognitive decline in Alzheimer's disease.[14]

VITAMIN B$_{12}$

Subtle B$_{12}$ deficiency may occur, even in the absence of anemia, and cause problems, especially in the elderly. Routine vitamin B$_{12}$ supplementation is recommended in the elderly, vegans, alcoholics, atrophic gastritis, and postgastric bypass surgery.

VITAMIN C

While vitamin C does not have a benefit in cancer and stroke, the results of studies examining its effect in coronary heart disease have yielded conflicting results.[15,16,17] It may have a beneficial effect in diseases such as cataract and macular degeneration. Whether high doses of vitamin C increase risk of renal stones remains to be established.

> Supplemental vitamin C over a 10-year period is associated with small decreases in the risk of total mortality, although there was no effect on cardiovascular mortality.[18]

FOLIC ACID

Foods rich in folic acid include green leafy vegetables, fresh fruit, grains, nuts, and meats.

Folic Acid in Pregnancy

○ Folic acid supplementation during pregnancy decreases the risk of neural tube defects in newborns.

○ It is important to take folic acid supplements as soon as possible after conception in order to maximize the benefits since the neural tube develops in the first 4 weeks of pregnancy.

Folic Acid and Cancer

○ Folate is involved in numerous critical metabolic reactions involved in DNA metabolism.

○ Folic acid supplementation lowers the risk of colon cancer in ulcerative colitis.

○ Data on folic acid supplementation and colon cancer are conflicting with some studies showing a decreased risk, while others actually document an increased risk of colon cancer.[19]

Folate and Other Disease States

○ High folic acid consumption is inversely proportional to the risk of hypertension.

○ The jury is still out on the role of folic acid supplementation in reducing age-related hearing loss.

○ Since high homocysteine levels correlate with fractures and dementia due to aging, folic acid supplementation may lower the risk.

Multivitamin Formulations

Multivitamin formulations contain 100% to 150% of recommended daily allowance. They may not help subjects that consume a healthy diet every day. Subjects likely to benefit from multivitamin supplements include those with unhealthy eating habits, inflammatory bowel disease (IBD), or hemodialysis; vegans; alcoholics; and those postgastroduodenal surgery.

Health Benefits of Multivitamin Supplementation

- ○ Lower all-cause mortality
- ○ Prospective study of Swedish women showed that multivitamin supplementation increased the risk for breast cancer[20]
- ○ Regular intake of multivitamins does not reduce the risk for prostate cancer

References

1. Mamede AC, Tavares SD, Abrantes AM, et al. The role of vitamins in cancer: a review. *Nutr Cancer.* 2011;2:1-16.
2. Agte V, Tarwadi K. The importance of nutrition in the prevention of ocular disease with special reference to cataract. *Ophthalmic Res.* 2010;44(3):166-172.
3. Rosen CJ. Clinical practice. Vitamin D insufficiency. *N Engl J Med.* 2011;364(3):248-254.
4. Goodman M, Bostick RM, Kucuk O, Jones DP. Clinical trials of antioxidants as cancer prevention agents: past, present, and future. *Free Radic Biol Med.* 2011;51(5):1068-1084.
5. Lee IM, Cook NR, Gaziano JM, et al. Vitamin E in the primary prevention of cardiovascular disease and cancer: the Women's Health Study: a randomized controlled trial. *JAMA.* 2005;294(1):56-68.
6. Schürks M, Glynn RJ, Rist PM, Tzourio C, Kurth T. Effects of vitamin E on stroke subtypes: meta-analysis of randomised controlled trials. *BMJ* 2010;341:c5702.
7. Meydani SN, Han SN, Jamer DH. Vitamin E and respiratory infection in the elderly. *Ann N Y Acad Sci.* 2004;1031:214-222.
8. Sanyal AJ, Chalasani N, Kowdley KV, et al. Pioglitazone, vitamin E, or placebo for nonalcoholic steatohepatitis. *N Engl J Med.* 2010;362:1675-1685.
9. Glynn RJ, Ridker PM, Goldhaber SZ, Zee RY, Buring JE. Effects of random allocation to vitamin E supplementation on the occurrence of venous thromboembolism: report from the Women's Health Study. *Circulation.* 2007;116(13):1497-503.
10. Henriques BJ, Olsen RK, Bross P, Gomes CM. Emerging roles for riboflavin in functional rescue of mitochondrial β-oxidation flavoenzymes. *Curr Med Chem.* 2010;17(32):3842-3854.

11. Torheim LE, Ferguson EL, Penrose K, Arimond M. Women in resource-poor settings are at risk of inadequate intakes of multiple micronutrients. *J Nutr.* 2010;140(11):2051S-2058S.

12. Reamy BV, Derby R, Bunt CW. Common tongue conditions in primary care. *Am Fam Physician.* 2010;81(5):627-634.

13. Airola G, Allais G, Castagnoli GI, et al. Non-pharmacological management of migraine during pregnancy. *Neurol Sci.* 2010;31(Suppl 1):S63-S65.

14. Aisen PS, Schneider LS, Sano M, et al. Alzheimer Disease Cooperative Study. High-dose B vitamin supplementation and cognitive decline in Alzheimer disease: a randomized controlled trial. *JAMA.* 2008;300(15):1774-1783.

15. Coulter ID, Hardy ML, Morton SC, Hilton LG, Tu W, Valentine D, Shekelle PG. Antioxidants vitamin C and vitamin E for the prevention and treatment of cancer. *J Gen Intern Med.* 2006;21(7):735-744.

16. Enstrom JE, Kanim LE, Klein MA. Vitamin C intake and mortality among a sample of the United States population. *Epidemiology.* 1992;3(3):194-202.

17. Sesso HD, Buring JE, Christen WG, et al. Vitamins E and C in the prevention of cardiovascular disease in men: the Physicians' Health Study II randomized control trial. *JAMA.* 2008;300(18):2123-2133.

18. Pocobelli G, Peters U, Kristal AR, White E. Use of supplements of multivitamins, vitamin C, and vitamin E in relation to mortality. *Am J Epidemiol.* 2009;170(4):472-483.

19. Duthie SJ. Folate and cancer: how DNA damage, repair and methylation impact on colon carcinogenesis. *J Inherit Metab Dis.* 2011;34(1):101-109.

20. Larsson SC, Akesson A, Bergkvist L, Wolk A. Multivitamin use and breast cancer incidence in a prospective cohort of Swedish women. *Am J Clin Nutr.* 2010;91(5):1268-1272.

Chapter

36 *Minerals*

KEY POINTS

○ Multiple studies have documented the beneficial role of zinc in reducing infection in respiratory and gastrointestinal (GI) infection-related morbidity and mortality in children and the elderly.[1]

○ Epidemiological data notwithstanding, studies on the role of selenium supplementation for preventing cancer have largely yielded disappointing results.[2]

○ Moderate to high doses of calcium may actually increase the risk of cardiovascular disease.

ZINC[3]

○ Present throughout the body, mostly inside skeletal muscles and bones

○ Plays an important role in immunity[4]

Zinc Deficiency

Serum zinc levels can be misleading. Risk factors for zinc deficiency include chronic pancreatic disorders, pregnancy, malabsorption syndrome, long-term parenteral nutrition support, chronic diarrhea, and irritable bowel disease (IBD).

The role of zinc in diabetes mellitus is like a double-edged sword. Zinc excretion is increased in diabetes mellitus, leading to impaired immune function; however, supplementation may worsen the glycemic control.

Role of Zinc Supplementation

○ Zinc supplementation can enhance growth, especially in children with zinc deficiency.

○ Multiple studies have documented the beneficial role in reducing infection in both respiratory and GI infection-related morbidity and mortality in children and the elderly.[5]

○ It is frequently used as part of the treatment for the common cold.[6]

○ Reduces risks of premature or prolonged labor, premature birth, etc.

○ Improves fetal bone growth and sperm counts.

○ May protect against cancer.[7]

○ Chronic high-dose zinc supplementation can lead to copper deficiency.

Preventative zinc supplementation improves morbidity and mortality due to diarrhea, pneumonia, and malaria in developing countries.[8]

CALCIUM[9]

Calcium plays an important role in bone health and has benefits in hypertension as well as breast cancer. Mixed results have been seen for its role in colorectal cancer, prostate cancer, and pregnancy-related disorders. A 2010 meta-analysis suggested that calcium supplementation has a minimal effect on the risk of cardiovascular disease.[10] Recent data, however, indicate that while increased dietary calcium may not decrease cardiovascular risk, use of cardiovascular supplements may actually increase the risk.[11]

SELENIUM

It is involved in numerous metabolic functions, such as DNA and protein synthesis, as well as membrane stabilization. Patients on long-term total parenteral nutrition are at an increased risk for selenium deficiency.

Results of Selenium Deficiency

○ Cardiomyopathy[12]
○ Skeletal muscle dysfunction
○ Impaired cell-mediated immunity
○ Psychological (mood) dysfunction

Selenium Supplementation

○ Potentiates antiviral activity
○ Low doses in animals improve glycemic control
○ Improves outcomes in critically ill patientsParadoxically, selenium can increase the risk of diabetes in humans
○ Reduces risk of postpartum thyroiditis and the severity of auto-immune thyroiditis

While epidemiological data are consistent with a beneficial role of selenium in reducing cancer mortality, meta-analysis has found no evidence to support the protective effect of selenium supplementation against cancer.[13] Results of studies examining the effect of supplementation for reducing atherosclerotic disease have yielded mixed results.

IODINE

○ Introduction of iodized salt has helped prevent goiter and reduced growth retardation due to hypothyroidism.

○ Iodine deficiency is widespread in developing countries but rare in the developed countries due to iodine fortification in salt, water, and bread.

○ Excess iodine intake may manifest as hypothyroidism associated with goiter or hyperthyroidism.

COPPER

Copper deficiency is not rare. Risk factors for copper deficiency include premature babies, gastroduodenal surgery, chronic diarrhea, and peritoneal dialysis. Manifestations of copper deficiency include anemia (which may be normocytic or microcytic), leukopenia, osteoporosis, and neurological derangements mimicking vitamin B_{12} deficiency.

High copper levels may be seen in chronic inflammatory diseases, Wilson's disease, pregnancy, diabetes mellitus, renal failure, accidental ingestion, and contaminated water supply.

Manifestations of copper toxicity include GI distress, liver failure, and renal failure. Shock and death may occur in severe cases.

CHROMIUM

○ Initially characterized as "glucose tolerance factor," chromium is part of metalloenzymes involved in numerous metabolic reactions.

○ Absorption may be reduced in cases of antacid and nonsteroidal anti-inflammatory drug use, whereas it is increased by vitamin C.

○ There is a paucity of evidence to support the use of chromium supplementation for muscle building or weight loss.

○ Toxicity is rare except in cases of industrial exposure (eg, tannery workers). Dermatitis, ulcers, and lung cancer may occur.

Chromium deficiency is associated with glucose intolerance. Supplementation may improve glycemic control in select patients.

REFERENCES

1. Yakoob MY, Theodoratou E, Jabeen A, et al. Preventive zinc supplementation in developing countries: impact on mortality and morbidity due to diarrhea, pneumonia and malaria. *BMC Public Health.* 2011; 11(Suppl. 3):S23.

2. Myung SK, Kim Y, Ju W, Choi HJ, Bae WK. Effects of antioxidant supplements on cancer prevention: meta-analysis of randomized controlled trials. *Ann Oncol.* 2010;21(1):166-179.

3. Prasad AS. Impact of the discovery of human zinc deficiency on health. *J Am Coll Nutr.* 2009;28(3):257-265.

4. Maggini S, Wenzlaff S, Hornig D. Essential role of vitamin C and zinc in child immunity and health. *J Int Med Res.* 2010;38(2):386-414.

5. Barnett JB, Hamer DH, Meydani SN. Low zinc status: a new risk factor for pneumonia in the elderly? *Nutr Rev.* 2010;68(1):30-37.

6. Singh M, Das RR. Zinc for the common cold. *Cochrane Database Syst Rev.* 2011;2:CD001364.

7. Prasad AS, Beck FW, Snell DC, Kucuk O. Zinc in cancer prevention. *Nutr Cancer.* 2009;61(6):879-887.

8. Yakoob MY, Theodoratou E, Jabeen A, et al. Preventive zinc supplementation in developing countries: impact on mortality and morbidity due to diarrhea, pneumonia and malaria. *BMC Public Health.* 2011;11 (Suppl 3):S23.

9. Souberbielle JC, Body JJ, Lappe JM, et al. Vitamin D and musculoskeletal health, cardiovascular disease, autoimmunity and cancer: recommendations for clinical practice. *Autoimmun Rev.* 2010;9(11):709-715.

10. Wang L, Manson JE, Song Y, Sesso HD. Systematic review: vitamin D and calcium supplementation in prevention of cardiovascular events. *Ann Intern Med.* 2010;152(5):315-323.

11. Lin K, Kaaks R, Linseisen J, Rohrmann S. Associations of dietary calcium intake and calcium supplementation with myocardial infarction and stroke risk and overall cardiovascular mortality in the Heidelberg cohort of the European Prospective Investigation into Cancer and Nutrition study (EPIC-Heidelberg). *Heart.* 2012;98(12):920-925.

12. Steinnes E. Soils and geomedicine. *Environ Geochem Health.* 2009;31(5):523-535.

13. Novotny L, Rauko P, Kombian SB, Edafiogho IO. Selenium as a chemoprotective anti-cancer agent: reality or wishful thinking? *Neoplasma.* 2010;57(5):383-391.

37 *Melatonin is not Just for Sleep*

KEY POINTS

○ Melatonin is an important regulator of both inflammation and motility in the GI tract.

○ Preliminary data indicate a potential benefit in ulcerative colitis and irritable bowel syndrome (IBS).[1,2,3]

Melatonin is one of the most versatile and ubiquitous hormonal molecules in the body and is associated with numerous metabolic functions, circadian rhythm, and wake-sleep cycle.[4,5]

ACTIONS OF MELATONIN FOR HEALTHY GUT

○ Melatonin is an important regulator of both inflammation and motility in the GI tract.

○ Melatonin acts as an autocrine and paracrine hormone, directly or indirectly influencing the epithelium, the immune system, and the intestinal smooth muscle.

○ Melatonin usually opposes the actions of serotonin in the gut.

The amount of melatonin in the gut is 400-fold greater than the pineal gland. Evidence indicates a potentially beneficial role in irritable bowel syndrome (IBS) and irritable bowel disease (IBD).[1,2,3]

ANIMAL STUDIES

○ Melatonin improves colitis in animal models of colitis.

○ Studies of trinitrobenzene sulfonic acid-induced colitis suggest that while short-term administration of melatonin is protective, it may have negative consequences on the evolution of the disease in the long run.[6]

○ Melatonin has beneficial effects on colitis-related colon carcinogenesis by modulating the mitotic and apoptotic indices in a dextran sodium sulfate-induced model of colitis in rats.[7]

Human Data

○ Preliminary reports document the beneficial role of melatonin in ulcerative colitis and IBS.[8-10]

○ Paradoxically, melatonin administration may trigger Crohn's disease symptoms in some cases.

References

1. Mozaffari S, Rahimi R, Abdollahi M. Implications of melatonin therapy in irritable bowel syndrome: a systematic review. *Curr Pharm Des.* 2010;16(33):3646-3655.

2. Terry PD, Villinger F, Bubenik GA, Sitaraman SV. Melatonin and ulcerative colitis: evidence, biological mechanisms, and future research. Inflamm Bowel Dis. 2006;15(1):134-140.

3. Chojnacki C, Wisniewska-Jarosinksa M, Walecka-Kapica E, Klupinska G, Jaworek J, Chojnacki J. Evaluation of melatonin effectiveness in the adjuvant treatment of ulcerative colitis. *J Physiol Pharmacol.* 2011;62(3):327-334.

4. Hardeland R. Melatonin, hormone of darkness and more: occurrence, control mechanisms, actions and bioactive metabolites. *Cell Mol Life Sci.* 2008;65(13):2001-2018.

5. Hardeland R, Cardinali DP, Srinivasan V, et al. Melatonin—a pleiotropic, orchestrating regulator molecule. *Prog Neurobiol.* 2011;93(3):350-384.

6. Marquez E, Sánchez-Fidalgo S, Calvo JR, la de Lastra CA, Motilva V. Acutely administered melatonin is beneficial while chronic melatonin treatment aggravates the evolution of TNBS-induced colitis. *J Pineal Res.* 2006;40(1):48-55.

7. Tanaka T, Yasui Y, Tanaka M, Tanaka T, Oyama T, Rahman KM. Melatonin suppresses AOM/DSS-induced large bowel oncogenesis in rats. *Chem Biol Interact.* 2009;177(2):128-136.

8. Swanson GR, Burgess HJ, Keshavarzian A. Sleep disturbances and inflammatory bowel disease: a potential trigger for disease flare? *Expert Rev Clin Immunol.* 2011;7(1):29-36.

9. Terry PD, Villinger F, Bubenik GA, Sitaraman SV. Melatonin and ulcerative colitis: evidence, biological mechanisms, and future research. *Inflamm Bowel Dis.* 2009;15(1):134-140.

10. Mozaffari S, Rahimi R, Abdollahi M. Implications of melatonin therapy in irritable bowel syndrome; a systematic review. *Curr Pharm Des.* 2010;16(33):3646-3655.

UPPER GASTROINTESTINAL DISORDERS

Chapter

38 *Esophageal Disorders*

KEY POINTS

○ Lifestyle modifications help ameliorate esophageal symptoms in a vast number of cases.

○ In addition to general diet recommendations for gastroesophageal reflux disease (GERD), they can also be made patient-specific, depending upon the patient's symptom triggers.

○ Psychological therapies may be of benefit for patients with GERD and noncardiac chest pain.

HISTORICAL PERSPECTIVE

Until the late 18th and early 19th centuries, most symptoms of possible GERD and peptic ulcer disease (PUD) were lumped into the entity of dyspepsia or indigestion. Some of these treatments have stood the test of time and are still preferred over modern medicine by millions of people.

PHYTOBOTANICALS

Peppermint Oil (Mentha Piperita L)

The administration of peppermint oil eliminates chest pain, as well as simultaneous esophageal contractions in patients with diffuse esophageal spasm.[1,2]

163

Minocha A. *A Guide to Alternative Medicine and the Digestive System* (pp 163-198). © 2013 Taylor & Francis Group.

Patients with GERD have long been warned to avoid peppermint oil. However, this recommendation appears to be based predominantly on theoretical grounds and lacks data from randomized, controlled trials (RCTs) to support it. This recommendation also flies in the face of centuries-old use of peppermint after meals, with perceived beneficial effects against indigestion.

Chili Powder

Capsaicin enhances noxious postprandial heartburn.[3-5] The mechanisms include direct effects on sensory neurons. While chili pepper may cause symptoms in susceptible subjects in the short term, it may be helpful in patients with functional heartburn and noncardiac chest pain acting via capsaicin-induced desensitization of the selective nociceptive C fibers.

Hange-Koboku-To (Ban Xia Hou Po Tang)

Hange-koboku-to accelerates gastric emptying in patients with dyspepsia, as well as in healthy controls. Based on its gastrokinetic effects, it is likely to play a beneficial role in GERD.

Liu-Jun-Zi-Tang (TJ-43)

Liu-Jun-Zi-Tang, also known as *Rikkunshito* and TJ-43, is a Chinese herbal medicine that contains spray-dried aqueous extracts of *Atractylodis lanceae rhizoma*, *Radix Ginseng*, *Pinelliae tuber*, *Hoelen*, *Zizyphi fructus*, *Aurantii nobilis pericarpium*, *Radix Glycyrrhizae*, and *Zingiberis rhizoma*. It increases gastric emptying. Compared to placebo, TJ-43 (2.5 g 3 times a day) improves gastric emptying as well as heartburn.[6]

STW 5

It lowers gastric acidity, inhibits secondary hyperacidity, and protects against esophagitis.[7,8] STW 5-induced stimulation of gastric relaxation and antral motility may help against GERD.[9]

Tangweikang

Tangweikang hastens gastric emptying in diabetic gastroparesis[10] and may be useful as an anti-GERD agent.

Terminalia

Terminalia chebula is commonly advocated in Ayurveda to improve gastrointestinal (GI) motility. It reduces gastric emptying time in rats.[11] As such, it has the potential to be helpful in GERD as a prokinetic agent.

*Turmeric (*Curcuma longa*)*

SCIENCE BEHIND IT

It blocks H2 histamine receptors[12] as well as proton potassium ATPase activity.[13] These acid inhibitory effects may play a role against GERD.

ACUPUNCTURE

The gastrokinetic effects of acupuncture are well documented.[14,15] The mechanism may be related to the content of brain-gut peptides, thus supporting its role in functional heartburn and noncardiac chest pain in addition to GERD.[16] Acupuncture reduces both the mean basal acid output, as well as maximal acid output, and may help in GERD. There is a lack of clinical studies documenting or refuting efficacy of acupuncture in esophageal disorders.

PROBIOTICS

Certain probiotics enhance gastric motility.[17] As such, the prokinetic probiotics may have a role in GERD.

PSYCHOLOGICAL THERAPIES

Psychological factors are involved in both noncardiac chest pain and functional heartburn. Relaxation exercises ameliorate gastroesophageal reflux symptoms by reducing esophageal acid exposure.[18] Successful treatment of refractory diffuse esophageal spasm by biofeedback and self-regulation, resulting in weight gain and reduction in chest pain, has been described.

Use of psychological therapies for noncardiac chest pain appears promising.[19-21] An RCT of cognitive behavioral therapy for the treatment of persistent noncardiac chest pain demonstrated significant reductions in chest pain and psychological morbidity.[19]

Treatment involving a psychological treatment package (education, relaxation, breathing training, graded exposure to activity and exercise, and challenging automatic thoughts about heart disease) reduces chest pain episodes from a median 6.5 to 2.5 per week and is accompanied by improvements in exercise tolerance.[22]

The role of psychological therapies for GERD and noncardiac chest pain is promising.

Homeopathy

There is a lack of data confirming or refuting the effect of homeopathy in esophageal disorders. A case of esophageal ulcer due to a homeopathic pill has been described.[23]

Minerals

Most of the data in this category pertain to the use of zinc. Zinc reduces gastric acid secretion in animals and humans.[24] The use of zinc in esophageal disorders is supported by evidence of local tissue healing properties, as well as the ability to reduce gastric acid.

Preventive Strategies

Aside from pharmacotherapeutics for esophageal illness, patients may be advised to follow some lifestyle modification. Many of these factors produce alterations in gastroesophageal physiology; their role in affecting disease itself is mired in controversy. The affect may be patient specific.

- ❍ Quit smoking. Smoking increases gastric acidity and also increases the risk for esophageal cancer.
- ❍ Raise the head end of the bed by about 4 to 6 inches.
- ❍ Avoid alcohol.
- ❍ Eat small frequent meals, and avoid large fatty meals, especially at dinner. Do not eat within 3 hours of bedtime.
- ❍ Attempt weight reduction if overweight.
- ❍ Dietary modifications should also be individualized based on the patient's symptom triggers. (The role of carbonated beverages remains to be established.)
- ❍ Wear loose fitting clothes, especially at home.
- ❍ An education program for GERD improves self-management.
- ❍ Improve stress coping mechanisms and avoid potentially harmful environmental contaminants.

REFERENCES

1. Pimentel M, Bonorris GG, Chow EJ, et al. Peppermint oil improves the manometric findings in diffuse esophageal spasm. *J Clin Gastroenterol.* 2001;33(1):27-31.

2. Mizuno S, Kato K, Ono Y, et al. Oral peppermint oil is a useful antispasmodic for double-contrast barium meal examination. *J Gastroenterol Hepatol.* 2006;21(8):1297-1301.

3. Herrera-López JA, Mejía-Rivas MA, Vargas-Vorackova F, Valdovinos-Díaz MA. Capsaicin induction of esophageal symptoms in different phenotypes of gastroesophageal reflux disease. *Rev Gastroenterol Mex.* 2010;75(4):396-404.

4. Kindt S, Vos R, Blondeau K, Tack J. Influence of intra-oesophageal capsaicin instillation on heartburn induction and oesophageal sensitivity in man. *Neurogastroenterol Motil.* 2009;21(10):1032-e1082.

5. Rodriguez-Stanley S, Collings KL, Robinson M, Owen W, Miner PB Jr. The effects of capsaicin on reflux, gastric emptying and dyspepsia. *Aliment Pharmacol Ther.* 2000;14(1):129-134.

6. Tatsuta M, Iishi H. Effect of treatment with liu-jun-zi-tang (TJ-43) on gastric emptying and gastrointestinal symptoms in dyspeptic patients. *Aliment Pharmacol Ther.* 1993;7(4):459-462.

7. Khayyal MT, Seif-El-Nasr M, El-Ghazaly MA, et al. Mechanisms involved in the gastro-protective effect of STW 5 (Iberogast) and its components against ulcers and rebound acidity. *Phytomedicine.* 2006;13(Suppl 5):56-66.

8. Abdel-Aziz H, Zaki HF, Neuhuber W, et al. Effect of an herbal preparation, STW 5, in an acute model of reflux oesophagitis in rats. *J Pharmacol Sci.* 2010;113(2):134-142.

9. Pilichiewicz AN, Horowitz M, Russo A, et al. Effects of Iberogast on proximal gastric volume, antropyloroduodenal motility and gastric emptying in healthy men. *Am J Gastroenterol.* 2007;102(6):1276-1283.

10. Jiang RQ, Zhang DX, Bai CY. Clinical study on Tangweikang in treating diabetic gastroparesis. *Zhongguo Zhong Xi Yi Jie He Za Zhi.* 2007;27(2):114-116.

11. Tamhane MD, Thorat SP, Rege NN, Dahanukar SA. Effect of oral administration of *Terminalia chebula* on gastric emptying: an experimental study. *J Postgrad Med.* 1997;43(1):12-13.

12. Kim DC, Kim SH, Choi BH, et al. *Curcuma longa* extract protects against gastric ulcers by blocking H2 histamine receptors. *Biol Pharm Bull.* 2005;28(12):2220-2224.

13. Siddaraju MN, Dharmesh SM. Inhibition of gastric H(+),K(+)-ATPase and *H. pylori* growth by phenolic antioxidants of *Curcuma amada.* *J Agric Food Chem.* 2007;55(18):7377-7786.

14. Shiotani A, Tatewaki M, Hoshino E, Takahashi T. Effects of electroacupuncture on gastric myoelectrical activity in healthy humans. *Neurogastroenterol Motil.* 2004;16(3):293-298.

15. Tatewaki M, Harris M, Uemura K, et al. Dual effects of acupuncture on gastric motility in conscious rats. *Am J Physiol Regul Integr Comp Physiol.* 2003;285(4):R862-872.

16. Lin YP, Yi SX, Yan J, Chang XR. Effect of acupuncture at Foot-Yangming Meridian on gastric mucosal blood flow, gastric motility and brain-gut peptide. *World J Gastroenterol.* 2007;13(15):2229-2233.

17. Indrio F, Riezzo G, Raimondi F, Bisceglia M, Cavallo L, Francavilla R. The effects of probiotics on feeding tolerance, bowel habits, and gastrointestinal motility in preterm newborns. *J Pediatr.* 2008;152(6):801-806.

18. McDonald-Haile J, Bradley LA, Bailey MA, et al. Relaxation training reduces symptom reports and acid exposure in patients with gastroesophageal reflux disease. *Gastroenterology*. 1994;107(1):61-69.

19. Klimes I, Mayou RA, Pearce MJ, Coles L, Fagg JR. Psychological treatment for atypical non-cardiac chest pain: a controlled evaluation. *Psychol Med*. 1990;20:605-611.

20. Mayou RA, Bryant BM, Sanders D, et al. A controlled trial of cognitive behavioural therapy for non-cardiac chest pain. *Psychol Med*. 1997;27(5):1021-1031.

21. van Peski-Oosterbaan AS, Spinhoven P, van Rood Y, et al. Cognitive-behavioral therapy for noncardiac chest pain: a randomized trial. *Am J Med*. 1999;106:424-429.

22. Potts SG, Lewin R, Fox KA, Johnstone EC. Group psychological treatment for chest pain with normal coronary arteries. *QJM*. 1999;92(2):81-86.

23. Corleto VD, D'Alonzo L, Zykaj E, et al. A case of oesophageal ulcer developed after taking homeopathic pill in a young woman. *World J Gastroenterol*. 2007;13(14):2132-2134.

24. Kirchhoff P, Socrates T, Sidani S, et al. Zinc salts provide a novel, pro-longed and rapid inhibition of gastric acid secretion. *Am J Gastroenterol*. 2011;106(1):62-70.

Chapter 39
Nausea and Vomiting of Pregnancy

KEY POINTS

○ Dietary modification and avoidance of triggers plays an important role in prevention.

○ Expert reviews on the role of acupressure/acupuncture have come to conflicting conclusions.[1,2]

○ Studies on the role of hypnotherapy have shown encouraging positive results.[3]

○ Most data indicate ginger is effective and superior to vitamin B_6.[4,5]

○ The data on the efficacy of complimentary therapies should be taken in the context that there is a lack of good efficacy data to recommend the use of commonly used antiemetics and acid blockers.[6]

Pregnant women frequently suffer from nausea and vomiting during pregnancy (Table 39-1).[7] Hyperemesis gravidarum represents the most severe form of the spectrum.

Table 39-1. Triggers to Avoid

- Small crowded rooms
- Bright light
- Smells including foods and perfume
- Smoke
- Noise
- Heat
- Motion due to driving, flying
- Medications like nonsteroidal anti-inflammatory drugs (NSAIDs), oral iron

TREATMENT[8,9]

General Measures

Usual management is supportive, including adequate hydration. Patients are requested to minimize contact with family members. Patients with a severe form usually respond to bowel rest and intravenous hydration. Pharmacotherapy involves antiemetics and acid suppressive agents, although there is a lack of good efficacy data. Enteral and/or parenteral nutrition support may be needed in refractory cases.

Nutrition

- Small, frequent, low-fat, high-carbohydrate meals. Cold food is better since food aroma may trigger symptoms.
- Protein-predominant meals allow for better control of symptoms.
- Frequent snacks in small amounts, like nuts and crackers.
- Spicy/salty foods are triggers for symptoms in some, while others are helped by eating such foods.
- Drink cold, clear drinks like ginger ale and mint tea. Consume electrolyte-replacement drinks and oral nutritional supplements, again in small amounts.
- Avoid having an empty stomach and eat as soon as hungry.
- Avoid brushing teeth immediately after eating.

Paradoxically, women who suffer from nausea and/or vomiting during pregnancy have a reduced risk of miscarriage.[10]

ACUPRESSURE/ACUPUNCTURE

RCTs have shown that acupressure at P6 and vitamin B_6 relieve nausea and vomiting in pregnancy to a similar degree.[9,11] No pregnancy-related adverse events have been reported with P6 acupuncture or acupressure.

Ginger

An RCT compared the effect of a ginger (0.5 g bid) capsule with dimenhydrinate (50 mg bid). The treatments were equally effective, but the ginger group experienced fewer side effects, especially drowsiness.[12] It is at least equal in efficacy to vitamin B_6. Evidence suggests efficacy of powdered ginger (dose 1 to 1.5 g/d in 3 to 4 divided doses).[13,14] Ginger lollipops may be used. Another option is to chew on a thin slice of fresh ginger root 2 to 4 times a day as needed.

Pyridoxine

RCTs suggest the effectiveness of pyridoxine for the management of nausea and vomiting in pregnancy.[15,16] The recommended dose is 75 mg/d.

Diclectin

A large double-blind, multicenter, placebo-controlled RCT examined the effect of Diclectin (doxylamine succinate 10 mg, pyridoxine hydrochloride 10 mg).[17] The Diclectin group demonstrated a significantly greater improvement in symptoms of nausea and vomiting of pregnancy compared to placebo. *Note:* Doxylamine was withdrawn from the US market for concerns of toxicity.

Hypnosis

Hypnotherapy has been successfully used for the treatment of nausea and vomiting of pregnancy.[18]

Psychotherapy

Psychotherapy may be of benefit, especially as an adjunctive therapy, in select patients with a predominant anxiety/stress component.

REFERENCES

1.   Xu J, MacKenzie IZ. The current use of acupuncture during pregnancy and childbirth. *Curr Opin Obstet Gynecol.* 2012;24(2):65-71.

2.   Matthews A, Dowswell T, Haas DM, Doyle M, OMathúna DP. Interventions for nausea and vomiting in early pregnancy. *Cochrane Database Syst Rev.* 2010;Sep 8(9):CD007575.

3.   McCormack D. Hypnosis for hyperemesis gravidarum. *J Obstet Gynaecol.* 2010;30(7):647-653.

4. Ensiyeh J, Sakineh MA. Comparing ginger and vitamin B6 for the treatment of nausea and vomiting in pregnancy: a randomised controlled trial. *Midwifery.* 2009;25(6):649-653.

5. Smith C, Crowther C, Willson K, Hotham N, McMillian V. A randomized controlled trial of ginger to treat nausea and vomiting in pregnancy. *Obstet Gynecol.* 2004;103(4):639-645.

6. Bottomley C, Bourne T. Management strategies for hyperemesis. *Best Pract Res Clin Obstet Gynaecol.* 2009;23(4):549-564.

7. Niebyl JR. Clinical practice. Nausea and vomiting in pregnancy. *N Engl J Med.* 2010;363(16):1544-1550.

8. Matthews A, Dowswell T, Haas DM, Doyle M, O'Mathúna DP. Interventions for nausea and vomiting in early pregnancy. *Cochrane Database Syst Rev.* 2010;(9):CD007575.

9. Jueckstock JK, Kaestner R, Mylonas I. Managing hyperemesis gravidarum: a multimodal challenge. *BMC Med.* 2010;8:46.

10. Weigel RM, Weigel MM. Nausea and vomiting of early pregnancy and pregnancy outcome. A meta-analytical review. *Br J Obstet Gynaecol.* 1989;96(11):1312-1318.

11. Lee EJ, Frazier SK. The efficacy of acupressure for symptom management: a systematic review. *J Pain Symptom Manage.* 2011;42(4):589-603.

12. Pongrojpaw D, Somprasit C, Chanthasenanont A. A randomized comparison of ginger and dimenhydrinate in the treatment of nausea and vomiting in pregnancy. *J Med Assoc Thai.* 2007;90(9):1703-1709.

13. Ozgoli G, Goli M, Simbar M. Effects of ginger capsules on pregnancy, nausea, and vomiting. *J Altern Complement Med.* 2009;15(3):243-246.

14. Tan PC, Omar SZ. Contemporary approaches to hyperemesis during pregnancy. *Curr Opin Obstet Gynecol.* 2011;23(2):87-93.

15. Vutyavanich T, Wongtra-ngan S, Ruangsri R. Pyridoxine for nausea and vomiting of pregnancy: a randomized, double-blind, placebo-controlled trial. *Am J Obstet Gynecol.* 1995;173(3 Pt 1):881-884.

16. Sahakian V, Rouse D, Sipes S, Rose N, Niebyl J. Vitamin B6 is effective therapy for nausea and vomiting of pregnancy: a randomized, double-blind placebo-controlled study. *Obstet Gynecol.* 1991;78(1):33-36.

17. Koren G, Clark S, Hankins GD, et al. Effectiveness of delayed-release doxylamine and pyridoxine for nausea and vomiting of pregnancy: a randomized placebo controlled trial. *Am J Obstet Gynecol.* 2010;203(6):571.e1-7.

18. McCormack D. Hypnosis for hyperemesis gravidarum. *J Obstet Gynaecol.* 2010;30(7):647-653.

Chapter

40 *Peptic Ulcer Disease*

KEY POINTS

○ Patients should avoid nonsteroidal anti-inflammatory drugs (NSAIDs) as much as possible, including over-the-counter varieties. If NSAIDs are needed, use the lowest possible dose and avoid multiple NSAIDs.

○ Smoking and alcohol increase gastric acidity and adversely affect gastroprotective mechanisms.

○ Zinc-based medications are effective in peptic ulcers.

○ Psychological interventions may be helpful in select patients.

HISTORICAL PERSPECTIVE

The ancient description of the use of powdered coral, chalk, and sea shells for relief of dyspepsia provides clues to the occurrence of this problem long before the modern descriptions of GERD and PUD. Hunter, in 1784, advocated the use of milk as a natural antacid.[1]

Illogical treatments of the past (eg, use of antimony, arsenic, mercury, alcohol, glucose rectal enemas and complete bowel rest, as well as application of leeches to the abdomen) were in vogue in the 18th century. Other treatments used in the past include synthetic resins, cabbage, pectin, pituitary extract, insulin, and histamine.

Surgeons like Billroth, Dean, and Codvilla made the first advances in modern treatment of peptic ulcer and gastric cancer by performing gastroduodenal surgery in the late 1880s.[2] *H pylori* was rediscovered by Warren and Marshall in the 1980s, which earned them the Nobel prize.[3]

PHYTOBOTANICAL THERAPIES (TABLE 40-1)

Amalaki

Amalaki is an Ayurvedic herbal remedy derived from pericarp of the dried fruit of *Emblica officinalis*. It is as effective as antacids for peptic ulcer.[4] Compared to the baseline, symptoms improved in both

Table 40-1. Miscellaneous Phytobotanical Therapies
Used for Gastroduodenal Ulceration

Phytobotanical Therapy	Comment
Berberine	An alkaloid from a variety of plants, it has gastroprotective effects in animal models
C majus (Greater Celandine)	Roots and juice are used in GI distress
Cnicus benedictus (Blessed Thistle)	Traditionally used for digestive problems; scientific data are lacking
Cranberry juice	Inhibits *H pylori* and may be useful in PUD
Galipea longiflora Krause	Protects against NSAID-, ethanol-, and stress-induced ulcers in animals
Ginger root	Helps with nausea and vomiting; data in PUD are lacking
Grape seed extract	Proanthocyanidin-rich grape seed extract protects against gastric injury in animals
Landolphia owariensis	Inhibits gastric acid and increases gastric mucus
Lemon balm	Traditionally used for dyspepsia
Maytenus robusta and *Maytenus ilicifolia*	Inhibits gastric acid and protects against experimental gastric ulcers in animals
Ocimum suave	Protects against ulcers in animals
Panax notoginseng	Protects against stress ulceration by up-regulating melatonin receptor expression
Tea catechins	Protects against acute gastric mucosal injury; promotes healing of chronic gastric ulcers via antioxidant properties and increasing gastric mucus
Virola surinamensis (epicatechin is the main active component)	Resin protects against gastric injury induced by NSAIDs and pylorus ligation

treatment groups. Side effects during Amalaki treatment included diarrhea and vomiting in some patients.

Artichoke Leaf Extract

Oral administration of artichoke leaf extract reduces gastric injury induced in animal models of experimental gastric mucosal ulceration, without altering the basal acid secretion. Although the artichoke leaf extract helps in patients with functional dyspepsia, its efficacy in human PUD has not been explored.

Asparagus racemosus (Shatavari)

Asparagus racemosus (Shatavari) inhibits gastric acid secretion and protects against indomethacin-induced gastric mucosal damage.[5]

Azadirachta indica (Neem)

It inhibits $H(+)$-$K(+)$-ATPase activity and prevents gastric ulcers in animals. Neem bark extract (30 mg bid) reduces gastric acid secretion by 77% in humans. The bark extract at the dose of 30 to 60 mg bid for 10 weeks heals duodenal ulcers.

Banana Powder (Plantain Banana)

The natural flavonoid present in unripe plantain banana pulp protects the gastric mucosa from aspirin-induced erosions.[6]

Bilberry (Vaccinium myrtillus)

Anthocyanidin from *V myrtillus* protects against experimental gastric ulcerations in animals by strengthening the gastric barrier.

Brahmi

Fresh juice from the whole plant of *B monnieri* Wettst, commonly known as *Brahmi*, promotes mucosal defenses via enhanced mucin secretion and decreased cell shedding in experimental models of ulcer.[7]

Chili Powder (Capsaicin)

Epidemiologic surveys in Singapore have shown that gastric ulcers are 3 times more common in people of Chinese descent than in those of Malaysian and Indian descent, who tend to consume more chili peppers.[8] Capsaicin administered orally also protects against aspirin-induced gastroduodenal injury in healthy human subjects.[9]

Liquorice (Licorice)

Licorice protects against *H pylori*. Numerous studies in experimental models have documented the gastroprotective effects of licorice. Clinical trials using licorice in PUD have yielded conflicting results.[10] However, the ingestion of licorice, and/or its active metabolites, can lead to an acquired form of apparent mineralocorticoid excess syndrome.

Mastic

Mastic, a concrete resinous exudate obtained from *Pistacia lentiscus,* reduces the intensity of experimentally induced gastric mucosal damage. A double-blind, placebo-controlled trial of mastic for the treatment of duodenal ulcer demonstrated endoscopically proven healing in 70% of patients on mastic compared to 22% patients on placebo.[11]

Terminalia arjuna

T arjuna bark suppresses the release of nitric oxide and superoxide from macrophages and protects against damage by *H pylori*. It protects against diclofenac-induced gastric ulcer in rats.

Turmeric (Curcuma longa)

Turmeric inhibits histamine type-2 receptors, proton potassium ATPase activity, as well as *H pylori* growth.[12] One study found that turmeric (*C longa Linn* 600 mg x 5/d x 4 weeks) resulted in the healing of 48% of cases of peptic ulcer. Seventy-six percent of patients did not have ulcers at the end of 12 weeks. A controlled clinical trial found liquid antacid and *C longa Linn* to be equivalent in the treatment of gastric ulcers.[13]

Withania somnifera Dunal

Also known as *ashwagandha* in Ayurvedic medicine, it protects against stress-induced ulceration in animals. Its efficacy is comparable to that of ranitidine.[14]

Herbal Combinations

Gorei-San (TJ-17)

Gorei-san (TJ-17) is a Japanese herbal medicine composed of 5 herbs (*Alismatis rhizoma, A lanceae rhizoma, Polyporus, Hoelen,* and *Cinnamomi cortex*). While it has been shown to be helpful for dyspeptic symptoms, there is a lack of studies examining its role in PUD.

Hange-Koboku-To (Banxia-Houpo-Tang)

Hange-koboku-to improves dyspeptic symptoms in patients with functional dyspepsia; however, its role in PUD has not been examined.

STW 5

STW 5 is a fixed combination of 9 herbs: bitter candytuft plant (aka, clown's mustard), German chamomile flower, peppermint leaves, caraway fruit, licorice, lemon balm leaves, celandine, angelica root and rhizome, and milk thistle. It lowers gastric acidity.[15] It has not been studied for the treatment of peptic ulcers.

MISCELLANEOUS HERBAL COMBINATIONS

Pepticaire (Ayurlab Herbals Pvt Ltd, Gujarat, India) is an Ayurvedic herbomineral formulation that includes *G glabra*, *E officinalis*, and *Tinospora cordifolia*. In an experimental rat model, it results in the reduction of gastric ulcer index, the reduction in total gastric acid, and an increase in the pH of gastric fluid.[16]

Rats with ulceration treated with a mixture of an Ayurvedic medicine mixture of *G glabra*, *T chebula*, *Piper longum*, and *Shankha bhasma* recover faster, with concomitant increase in beta-glucuronidase activity in the Brunner's glands.

ACUPUNCTURE AND ELECTROMAGNETIC THERAPIES

Acupuncture reduces both the mean basal acid output, as well as the maximal acid output in duodenal ulcer patients. A multi-center RCT of acupuncture at Zhongwan (CV 12) in patients with peptic ulcer found that the acupuncture group experienced less stomachache and improved appetite faster than the control group, although the total effective rate was similar in the 2 groups.[17] The addition of transcutaneous and reflex magnetolaser impact to anti-*H pylori* treatment shortens the time of ulcer healing and promotes eradication of *H pylori* in patients with duodenal ulcer exacerbation.[18]

PROBIOTICS

Probiotics suppress *H pylori*,[19] inhibit experimental gastric ulceration, and accelerate healing.[20]

PSYCHOLOGICAL THERAPIES

War and stress are risk factors for PUD.[21] PUD is common during wars and among war survivors.[22]

Colgan et al conducted a controlled trial of hypnotherapy in relapse prevention of duodenal ulcers healed with ranitidine.[23] After a follow-up of 12 months, 100% of the control subjects had relapsed, in contrast to only 53% of the hypnotherapy group. A case of hypnotic control of upper GI hemorrhage has also been described.[24]

HOMEOPATHY

There is a lack of good studies establishing its role in PUD.

NUTRITIONAL SUPPLEMENTS

Colostrum

Colostrum has antibodies protective against *H pylori*. It may have potential for use in PUD.

Melatonin

It protects against both stress and indomethacin-induced gastric injury in animals. Melatonin (5 mg before aspirin) and its precursor L-tryptophan (0.5 g before aspirin) prevent acute gastric mucosal damage induced by aspirin in humans.[25] It accelerates omeprazole-induced healing of gastroduodenal ulcers in humans.[26]

Free Radical Scavengers

The effect of the free radical scavengers allopurinol and dimethyl sulfoxide taken orally was examined in a randomized, placebo-controlled trial of patients with hematemesis due to NSAID-induced ulcerations. A follow-up endoscopy 2 days later found that gastric erosions were present in 50% of the control group compared to 9% in the allopurinol group and 7% in the dimethyl sulfoxide group. The study patients also required significantly fewer blood transfusions.[27]

Zinc

It reduces basal gastric acid secretion in duodenal ulcer patients by almost 60%. It lowers the risk of experimental duodenal lesions in a dose-dependent manner. A meta-analysis found zinc acexamate to be superior to placebo and as effective as H2 receptor antagonists for the treatment of PUD.[28]

REFERENCES

1. Chen TS, Chen PS, eds. *The History of Gastroenterology: Essays on Its Development and Accomplishments*. New York, NY: Parthenon Publishing Group; 1995.

2. Hirschowitz BI. History of acid-peptic diseases: from Bismuth to Billroth to Black to Bismuth. In: Kirsner JB, ed. *The Growth of Gastroenterologic Knowledge During the Twentieth Century*. Philadelphia, PA: Lea & Febiger; 1994:54-88.

3. Pincock S. Nobel Prize winners Robin Warren and Barry Marshall. *Lancet*. 2005;366(9495):1429.

4. Chawla YK, Dubey P, Singh R, Nundy S, Tandon BN. Treatment of dyspepsia with Amalaki (*Emblica officinalis Linn.*)—an Ayurvedic drug. *Indian J Med Res*. 1982;76(Suppl):95-98.

5. Bhatnagar M, Sisodia SS. Antisecretory and antiulcer activity of *Asparagus racemosus Willd.* against indomethacin plus phyloric ligation-induced gastric ulcer in rats. *J Herb Pharmacother*. 2006;6(1):13-20.

6.   Mohan Kumar M, Joshi MC, Prabha T, Dorababu M, Goel RK. Effect of plantain banana on gastric ulceration in NIDDM rats: role of gastric mucosal glycoproteins, cell proliferation, antioxidants and free radicals. *Indian J Exp Biol.* 2006;44(4):292-299.

7.   Rao CV, Sairam K, Goel RK. Experimental evaluation of *Bocopa monniera* on rat gastric ulceration and secretion. *Indian J Physiol Pharmacol.* 2000;44(4):435-441.

8.   Kang JY, Yeoh KG, Chia HP, et al. Chili—protective factor against peptic ulcer? *Dig Dis Sci.* 1995;40(3):576-579.

9.   Yeoh KG, Kang JY, Yap I, et al. Chili protects against aspirin-induced gastroduodenal mucosal injury in humans. *Dig Dis Sci.* 1995;40(3):580-583.

10. Engqvist A, von Feilitzen F, Pyk E, Reichard H. Double-blind trial of deglycyrrhizinated liquorice in gastric ulcer. *Gut.* 1973;14(9):711-715.

11. Al-Habbal MJ, Al-Habbal Z, Huwez FU. A double-blind controlled clinical trial of mastic and placebo in the treatment of duodenal ulcer. *Clin Exp Pharmacol Physiol.* 1984;11(5):541-544.

12. Siddaraju MN, Dharmesh SM. Inhibition of gastric H(+),K(+)-ATPase and *Helicobacter pylori* growth by phenolic antioxidants of *Curcuma amada. J Agric Food Chem.* 2007;55(18):7377-7386.

13. Kositchaiwat C, Kositchaiwat S, Havanondha J. *Curcuma longa Linn.* in the treatment of gastric ulcer comparison to liquid antacid: a controlled clinical trial. *J Med Assoc Thai.* 1993;76(11):601-605.

14. Bhatnagar M, Sisodia SS, Bhatnagar R. Antiulcer and antioxidant activity of *Asparagus racemosus Willd* and *Withania somnifera Dunal* in rats. *Ann NY Acad Sci.* 2005;1056:261-278.

15. Khayyal MT, Seif-El-Nasr M, El-Ghazaly MA, et al. Mechanisms involved in the gastro-protective effect of STW 5 (Iberogast) and its components against ulcers and rebound acidity. *Phytomedicine.* 2006;13(Suppl 5):56-66.

16. Bafna PA, Balaraman R. Anti-ulcer and anti-oxidant activity of pepticare, a herbomineral formulation. *Phytomedicine.* 2005;12(4):264-270.

17. Niu HY, Yang M, Qiang BQ, et al. Multicentral randomized controlled trials of acupuncture at Zhongwan (CV 12) for treatment of peptic ulcer. *Zhongguo Zhen Jiu.* 2007;27(2):89-92.

18. Minakov EV, Romanova MM, Khimina IN. Polymagnetolaser correction of vegetative and bioelectric imbalance in patients with duodenal ulcer. *Klin Med (Mosk).* 1999;77(12):33-37.

19. Tamura A, Kumai H, Nakamichi N, et al. Suppression of *Helicobacter pylori*-induced interleukin-8 production in vitro and within the gastric mucosa by a live *Lactobacillus* strain. *J Gastroenterol Hepatol.* 2006;21(9):1399-1406.

20. Uchida M, Shimizu K, Kurakazu K. Yogurt containing *Lactobacillus gasseri OLL 2716* (LG21 yogurt) accelerated the healing of acetic acid-induced gastric ulcer in rats. *Biosci Biotechnol Biochem.* 2010;74(9):1891-1894.

21.   Levenstein S. Peptic ulcer at the end of the 20th century: biological and psychological risk factors. *Can J Gastroenterol.* 1999;13(9):753-759.

22.   Jhun HJ, Ju YS, Kim JB, Kim JK. Present status and self-reported diseases of the Korean atomic bomb survivors: a mail questionnaire survey. *Med Confl Surviv.* 2005;21(3):230-236.

23.   Colgan SM, Faragher EB, Whorwell PJ. Controlled trial of hypnotherapy in relapse prevention of duodenal ulceration. *Lancet.* 1988;1(8598):1299-1300.

24.   Bishay EG, Stevens G, Lee C. Hypnotic control of upper gastrointestinal hemorrhage: a case report. *Am J Clin Hypn.* 1984;27(1):22-25.

25.   Konturek PC, Konturek SJ, Celinski K, et al. Role of melatonin in mucosal gastroprotection against aspirin-induced gastric lesions in humans. *J Pineal Res.* 2010;48(4):318-323.

26.   Celinski K, Konturek SJ, Konturek PC, et al. Melatonin or l-tryptophan accelerates healing of gastroduodenal ulcers in patients treated with omeprazole. *J Pineal Res.* 2011;50(4):389-394.

27.   Salim AS. A new approach to the treatment of nonsteroidal anti-inflammatory drugs induced gastric bleeding by free radical scavengers. *Surg Gynecol Obstet.* 1993;176(5):484-490.

28.   Jiménez E, Bosch F, Galmés JL, Baños JE. Meta-analysis of efficacy of zinc acexamate in peptic ulcer. *Digestion.* 1992;51(1):18-26.

Chapter

41 Helicobacter pylori

KEY POINTS

○   The addition of probiotics to standard antibiotic treatment may increase *H pylori* eradication, while reducing the therapy-associated side effects.

○   Vitamin C and E supplements may reduce the efficacy of *H pylori* eradication therapy.

○   Cranberry juice has potential as an adjunctive therapy for eradication of *H pylori*.

In addition to conventional anti-*H pylori* treatment, using combinations of antibiotics and proton pump inhibitors following complementary treatments have been used and cited in literature and may be useful—especially as adjunctive treatments.

PHYTOBOTANICAL TREATMENTS

Berberine

Berberine 300 mg tid is superior to ranitidine 150 mg bid for *H pylori* clearance in patients with a duodenal ulcer.[1]

Cranberry

Cranberry constituents have antiadhesion activity against *H pylori* in vitro. Cranberry juice beverages twice daily for 90 days results in an eradication rate of 14% compared to 5% for placebo (p<0.05).[2] The addition of cranberry juice to omeprazole-amoxicillin-clarithromycin triple therapy improves the rate of *H pylori* eradication in females to 95% compared to 87% with omeprazole-amoxicillin-clarithromycin alone.[3]

Curcuma longa *(Turmeric)*

Turmeric inhibits *H pylori* growth in animals. Curcumin alone does not have any effect on *H pylori* infection in humans.

Hydrastis canadensis

The crude extract of *H canadensis* rhizomes possesses anti-*H pylori* activity in vitro.

Mastic

Mastic resinous exudate from the tree *P lentiscus* kills *H pylori*, although the effect is modest.[4]

Peppermint Oil

Peppermint inhibits the in vitro proliferation of *H pylori* in a dose-dependent manner. There are no human data examining its role for *H pylori* eradication.

Sanguinaria canadensis

S canadensis inhibits the growth of *H pylori* in vitro.

Terminalia

Terminalia ameliorates severe cellular damage and pathological changes caused by *H pylori* lipopolysaccharide.[5]

ACUPUNCTURE AND ELECTROMAGNETIC THERAPIES

The addition of transcutaneous and reflex magnetolaser impact to anti-*H pylori* treatment shortens the time of ulcer healing and promotes eradication of *H pylori* in patients with duodenal ulcer.[6]

PROBIOTICS

Probiotics suppress *H pylori* and reduce *H pylori*-induced inflammation. Many but not all clinical and epidemiologic studies have documented their efficacy in humans.[7-17]

AB-yogurt (President Enterprise Corp, Tainan, Taiwan) is fermented milk containing sugar, high-fructose corn syrup, pectin, galactoolipogosaccharide, and a mixture of *L acidophilus La5, B lactis Bb12, L bulgaricus*, and *S thermophilus*. Regular intake of AB-yogurt significantly decreases the urease activity of *H pylori* after 6 weeks of therapy in asymptomatic *H pylori*-positive subjects.[7]

An epidemiologic study documented a protective effect of yogurt consumption on the prevalence of *H pylori*.[8] A review of literature regarding *H pylori* and probiotics concluded that probiotics are effective in reducing *H pylori*-associated gastric inflammation.[15] Meta-analyses have concluded that *Lactobacilli* have anti-*H pylori* activity, and *S boulardii* reduces side effects associated with anti-*H pylori* treatment.[16,17]

NUTRITIONAL THERAPIES

Colostrum

Colostrum containing IgA directed against *H pylori* inhibits the adhesion of *H pylori* in vitro. Supplementation of bovine colostrum is of benefit in relieving NSAID-induced GI disturbances.

Minerals

Most of the data in this category pertain to the use of bismuth. In fact, evidence for the role of bismuth is so strong that its use is no longer considered to be part of complementary and alternative medicine.

Vitamins

Limited data support the use of vitamins in *H pylori* infection.[18] Adding vitamin C to 1-week triple therapy for *H pylori* can allow reduction of the clarithromycin dose, while preserving the eradication of clarithromycin-susceptible *H pylori*. Paradoxically, vitamin C and E supplementation to lansoprazole-amoxicillin-metronidazole triple therapy may reduce the eradication rate of metronidazole-susceptible *H pylori* infection.[19]

A NOTE OF CAUTION

H pylori has existed for over 58,000 years during the course of evolution and human migration from east Africa. Was it always "bad" or is it a recent phenomenon? The following is some food for thought:

○ Presence of *H pylori* is associated with reduced risk of Barrett's esophagus as well as adenocarcinoma of esophagus.[20]

○ The stomach produces 5% to 10% of the body's leptin and 60% to 80% of the body's ghrelin. Leptin has anorexic effects, while ghrelin is the opposite. Presence of *H pylori* in the stomach is associated with alteration in ghrelin and leptin levels. A decrease in *H pylori* infection due to improved sanitary conditions as well as widespread eradication over the last couple of decades may have played a role in the rising epidemic of obesity, although it is unclear to what degree.[21] However, data on the prevalence of *H pylori* in obese versus nonobese individuals are controversial.

○ Similarly, the decreasing prevalence of *H pylori* has been linked to increasing incidence of bronchial asthma and allergies.[22] A cause-effect relationship remains to be established.

References

1. Hu FL. Comparison of acid and *Helicobacter pylori* in ulcerogenesis of duodenal ulcer disease. *Zhonghua Yi Xue Za Zhi.* 1993;73(4):217-219,253.

2. Zhang L, Ma J, Pan K, Go VL, Chen J, You WC. Efficacy of cranberry juice on *Helicobacter pylori* infection: a double-blind, randomized placebo-controlled trial. *Helicobacter.* 2005;10(2):139-145.

3. Shmuely H, Yahav J, Samra Z, et al. Effect of cranberry juice on eradication of *Helicobacter pylori* in patients treated with antibiotics and a proton pump inhibitor. *Mol Nutr Food Res.* 2007;51(6):746-751.

4. Huwez FU, Thirlwell D, Cockayne A. Mastic gum kills *Helicobacter pylori. N Engl J Med.* 1998;339(26):1946.

5. Devi RS, Kist M, Vani G, Devi CS. Effect of methanolic extract of *Terminalia arjuna* against *Helicobacter pylori* 26695 lipopolysaccharide-induced gastric ulcer in rats. *J Pharm Pharmacol.* 2008;60(4):505-514.

6. Minakov EV, Romanova MM, Khimina IN. Polymagnetolaser correction of vegetative and bioelectric imbalance in patients with duodenal ulcer. *Klin Med (Mosk).* 1999;77(12):33-37.

7. Wang KY, Li SN, Liu CS, et al. Effects of ingesting *Lactobacillus*- and *Bifidobacterium*-containing yogurt in subjects with colonized *Helicobacter pylori. Am J Clin Nutr.* 2004;80(3):737-741.

8. Ornelas IJ, Galvan-Potrillo M, López-Carrillo L. Protective effect of yoghurt consumption on *Helicobacter pylori* seropositivity in a Mexican population. *Public Health Nutr.* 2007;10(11):1283-1287.

9. Sheu BS, Wu JJ, Lo CY, et al. Impact of supplement with *Lactobacillus*- and *Bifidobacterium*-containing yogurt on triple therapy for *Helicobacter pylori* eradication. *Aliment Pharmacol Ther.* 2002;16(9):1669-1675.

10. Sheu BS, Cheng HC, Kao AW, et al. Pretreatment with *Lactobacillus-* and *Bifidobacterium*-containing yogurt can improve the efficacy of quadruple therapy in eradicating residual *Helicobacter pylori* infection after failed triple therapy. *Am J Clin Nutr.* 2006;83(4):864-869.

11. Gotteland M, Andrews M, Toledo M, et al. Modulation of *Helicobacter pylori* colonization with cranberry juice and *Lactobacillus johnsonii La1* in children. *Nutrition.* 2008;24(5):421-426.

12. Cindoruk M, Erkan G, Karakan T, Dursun A, Unal S. Efficacy and safety of *Saccharomyces boulardii* in the 14-day triple anti-*Helicobacter pylori* therapy: a prospective randomized placebo-controlled double-blind study. *Helicobacter.* 2007;12(4):309-316.

13. Cremonini F, Di Caro S, Covino M, et al. Effect of different probiotic preparations on anti-*Helicobacter pylori* therapy-related side effects: a parallel group, triple blind, placebo-controlled study. *Am J Gastroenterol.* 2002;97(11):2744-2749.

14. Armuzzi A, Cremonini F, Bartolozzi F, et al. The effect of oral adminis-tration of *Lactobacillus GG* on antibiotic-associated gastrointestinal side-effects during *Helicobacter pylori* eradication therapy. *Aliment Pharmacol Ther.* 2001;15(2):163-169.

15. Lesbros-Pantoflickova D, Corthésy-Theulaz I, Blum AL. *Helicobacter pylori* and probiotics. *J Nutr.* 2007;137(3 Suppl 2):812S-818S.

16. Zou J, Dong J, Yu X. Meta-analysis: *Lactobacillus* containing quadruple therapy versus standard triple first-line therapy for *Helicobacter pylori* eradication. *Helicobacter.* 2009;14(5):97-107.

17. McFarland LV. Systematic review and meta-analysis of *Saccharomyces boulardii* in adult patients. *World J Gastroenterol.* 2010;16(18):2202-2222.

18. Chuang CH, Sheu BS, Kao AW, et al. Adjuvant effect of vitamin C on omeprazole-amoxicillin-clarithromycin triple therapy for *Helicobacter pylori* eradication. *Hepatogastroenterology.* 2007;54(73):320-324.

19. Chuang CH, Sheu BS, Huang AH, Yang HB, Wu JJ. Vitamin C and E supplements to lansoprazole-amoxicillin-metronidazole triple therapy may reduce the eradication rate of metronidazole-susceptible *Helicobacter pylori* infection. *Helicobacter.* 2002;7(5):310-316.

20. Islami F, Kamangar F. *Helicobacter pylori* and esophageal cancer risk: a meta-analysis. *Cancer Prev Res (Phila).* 2008;1(5):329-338.

21. Jang EJ, Park SW, Park JS, et al. The influence of the eradication of *Helicobacter pylori* on gastric ghrelin, appetite, and body mass index in patients with peptic ulcer disease. *J Gastroenterol Hepatol.* 2008;23(Suppl 2):S278-285.

22. Chen Y, Blaser MJ. Inverse associations of *Helicobacter pylori* with asth-ma and allergy. *Arch Intern Med.* 2007;167(8):821-827.

Chapter

42 *Functional Dyspepsia*

KEY POINTS

○ Therapies based on Chinese medicine (eg, STW 5 and acupuncture) are effective in functional dyspepsia.[1,2]

○ Use of psychological interventions can improve outcomes in functional GI disorders.

○ The role of diet in the management of patients with functional dyspepsia is patient specific.

Modern treatment of functional dyspepsia has been mostly disappointing. Most diagnoses made by practitioners of complementary and alternative medicine are based on symptoms and follow the holistic treatment pattern. Similar patients may receive different treatment plans, however, based on a variety of other factors.

HERBAL THERAPIES

Table 42-1 lists some common phytobotanical treatments in vogue for dyspepsia.

Amalaki

Amalaki is derived from pericarp of the dried fruit of *E officinalis*. It is comparable to antacids for the treatment of nonulcer dyspepsia.[3]

Artichoke Leaf Extract

Artichoke leaf extract (2 x 320 mg plant extract 3 tid) demonstrates superior efficacy in alleviating symptoms and improving quality of life in functional dyspepsia compared to placebo.[4]

Asparagus racemosus *(Shatavari)*

Asparagus racemosus (Shatavari) is used in Ayurveda for dyspepsia. It reduces gastric acidity and emptying time.[5]

Azadirachta indica *(Neem)*

Its extract protects against gastric ulceration by inhibiting the proton pump and reducing acidity in animals. It may have the potential for treatment of functional dyspepsia.

Banana Powder (Plantain Banana)

Treatment (8 capsules per day for 8 weeks) results in marked improvement (partial or complete relief) of patients with nonulcer dyspepsia compared to controls.[6]

Berberine

Berberine is an alkaloid found in plants as Berberis, or goldenseal (*H canadensis* and *Coptis chinensis*). Its role in dyspepsia remains to be established.

Bilberry (Vaccinium myrtillus)

OptiBerry (InterHealth Nutraceuticals Inc, Benicia, CA), a combination of berries including wild bilberry, is a potent antioxidant with antimicrobial activity against *H pylori*. As such, bilberry may be effective in *H pylori*-induced dyspepsia.

Blessed Thistle (Cnicus benedictus)

It has antimicrobial and cytotoxic properties. Traditionally, it has been used to treat dyspeptic symptoms.

Table 42-1. Phytobotanical Therapies of Benefit in Functional Dyspepsia

- ❖ Amalaki
- ❖ Artichoke leaf extract
- ❖ Banana powder
- ❖ Hot chili powder
- ❖ Turmeric powder (curcumin)
- ❖ Mastic gum
- ❖ Peppermint oil
- ❖ Liu-Jun-Zi-Tang (TJ-43)
- ❖ Hange-koboku-to (Ban Xia Hou Po Tang)
- ❖ STW 5
- ❖ Shenxia hewining
- ❖ Xiao Yao San
- ❖ Herbal combination of boldo (*P boldus*), cascara (*R purshiana*), gentian (*G lutea*), and rhubarb (*Rheum spp*)

Brahmi

Fresh juice from the plant *B monnieri Wettst*, commonly known as *Brahmi*, is used in Ayurveda for dyspepsia. Although used for centuries for dyspepsia, studies for its use in functional dyspepsia are lacking.

Carob (Ceratonia siliqua)

HL-350, a formula thickened with locust bean gum from carob seeds, reduces regurgitation episodes in infants. Studies in dyspepsia are lacking.

Chili Powder (Capsaicin)

Red pepper improves overall symptom score, as well as the epigastric pain, fullness, and nausea scores, compared to placebo.[7] It relieves functional dyspepsia by capsaicin-induced desensitization of the selective nociceptive fibers.

Cranberry

It inhibits *H pylori*. Studies for its use in dyspepsia are lacking.

Curcumin (Turmeric)

It blocks gastric acid secretion and promotes gallbladder contraction, in addition to its antispasmodic activity. An RCT found that 87% of patients with dyspepsia responded to turmeric capsules, compared to 53% to placebo.[8]

Ginger Root

Ginger accelerates gastric emptying in healthy volunteers. Consumption of 1 g of ginger results in rapid gastric emptying without changes in fundic dimensions or change in symptoms of patients with functional dyspepsia. While it hastens gastric emptying in patients, its effect on relieving dyspeptic symptoms is controversial.[9]

Greater Celandine (Chelidonium majus)

Greater celandine or tetterwort is derived from celandine plant, a member of the poppy family. It is reputed to have calming effects and is widely used for intestinal spasms.

Lemon Balm (Melissa officinalis)

It is contained in many herbal combinations like STW 5 that are useful in dyspepsia. Studies on this phytobotanical alone are lacking.

Liquorice (Licorice)

Efficacy of licorice in functional dyspepsia remains to be established.

Mastic

Mastic is a concrete resinous exudate obtained from the stem of the tree *P lentiscus*. Mastic gum (350 mg tid for 3 weeks) results in significant improvement in symptoms of dyspepsia.[10]

Peppermint Oil (Mentha × piperita L)

In addition to relaxing pylorus, peppermint oil enhances gastric emptying, thus affecting gastroduodenal motility. A double-blind, double-dummy RCT showed that peppermint oil reduces gastric spasm during upper endoscopy. Peppermint oil plus caraway oil is superior to placebo for the treatment of functional dyspepsia.[11] Another multi-center, double-blind equivalence study found peppermint/caraway oil preparation and cisapride to be equivalent for the treatment of functional dyspepsia.[12]

Terminalia

T chebula is commonly advocated in Ayurveda to improve GI motility and dyspeptic symptoms. It protects against noxious stimuli like NSAIDs and accelerates gastric emptying in rats.

HERBAL COMBINATIONS

Gorei-San (TJ-17)

Gorei-san (TJ-17) is a Japanese herbal medicine composed of 5 herbs (*A rhizoma, A lanceae rhizoma, Polyporus, Hoelen*, and *C cortex*). Yamada et al examined the efficacy of TJ-17 for treatment of SSRI-induced nausea or dyspepsia.[13] TJ-17 was added to the previous regimen in 20 such patients. Symptoms disappeared completely in 9 patients and were decreased in 4 patients.

Hange-Koboku-To (Banxia-Houpo-Tang)

Hange-koboku-to accelerates gastric emptying in patients with dyspepsia, as well as in healthy controls. The improved gastric emptying is accompanied by improvement in dyspeptic symptoms.[14]

Liu-Jun-Zi-Tang (TJ-43)

Liu-Jun-Zi-Tang, also known as *Rikkunshito* and TJ-43, is a Chinese herbal medicine that contains spray-dried aqueous extracts of *A lanceae rhizoma, R Ginseng, P tuber, Hoelen, Z fructus, A nobilis pericarpium, R Glycyrrhizae*, and *Z rhizoma*.

It promotes gastric adaptive relaxation. Compared to placebo, TJ-43 improves gastric emptying as well as GI symptoms of epigastric fullness, heartburn, belching, and nausea.[15]

Shenxia Hewining

Shenxia hewining is a Chinese herbal medicine that contains *R Ginseng, P tuber, Coptidis rhizoma, Z rhizoma exsiccata,* and *R Glycyrrhizae.* Shenxia hewining (15 capsules/d; 0.42 g/capsule) improves symptoms of dyspepsia in 92% of the patients compared to only 20% in the controls.[16]

STW 5

STW 5[1] is a fixed combination of the 9 herbs described previously. It lowers gastric acidity and stimulates gastric relaxation and antral motility.

Multiple studies have documented the efficacy of STW 5 and STW 5-II in the treatment of functional dyspepsia.[17,18] Meta-analysis of double-blind RCTs conclude that STW 5 demonstrates a clear and highly significant overall therapeutic effect.[19]

> Based on efficacy and safety, STW 5 is a valid therapeutic option for patients seeking phytotherapy for symptoms of functional dyspepsia.

Tangweikang

Tangweikang, a Chinese herbal preparation, hastens gastric emptying in diabetic gastroparesis. The prokinetic effect may help patients with functional dyspepsia.

Xiao Yao San

Qin et al conducted a systematic review to examine the use of modified Xiao Yao San for functional dyspepsia, and concluded that Xiao Yao San is more effective than prokinetic agents—without serious adverse events.[20]

> The therapeutic efficacy of herbal combinations challenges the current trend of highly targeted drug molecules that usually focus on one single target or mechanism for disorders with redundancies in the pathogenic pathways wherein no single receptor group may play a critical role for the control of symptoms.

Miscellaneous Herbal Combinations

○ Borgia et al conducted a double-blind, multi-center controlled trial on the therapeutic activity of a combination of medicinal herbs, including boldo (*Peumus boldus*), cascara (*R purshiana*), gentian (*Gentiana lutea*), and rhubarb (*Rheum spp*).[21] This combination produced significant improvements in appetite, dyspepsia, and constipation.

○ Pepticare is an Ayurvedic formulation that includes *G glabra*, *E officinalis*, and *T cordifolia*. It inhibits gastric acidity. There are no studies documenting its use in dyspepsia.

○ Thamlikitkul et al conducted a randomized, double-blind, placebo-controlled study of *Curcuma domestica Val* for dyspepsia in a multi-center study (n = 116).[8] Patients received turmeric (2 g/day), placebo, or a combination treatment known as Flatulence (which includes cascara dry extract, nux vomica extract, asafoetida tincture, capsicum powder, ginger powder, and diastase). Eighty-three percent of people in the Flatulence formula group and 87% of patients receiving *Curcuma* responded to treatment compared to only 53% in the placebo group (p<0.05).

○ Niederau and Göpfert[22] studied the effect of *Chelidonium* and turmeric root extract on upper abdominal pain due to functional disorders of the biliary system in a placebo-controlled double-blind trial. The reduction of colicky pain was faster in the treatment group.

○ A hydro-alcoholic solution of phytocompound based on *Gentianae*, *Cinchona*, *Absinthii*, and *Cinnamomi* accelerates gastric emptying in dyspeptic patients and, thus, may be helpful in functional dyspepsia.

ACUPUNCTURE

Although acupuncture reduces gastric acid, its beneficial effects in dyspepsia appear to be mediated via modification of gastroduodenal motility patterns.

Multiple studies have documented its efficacy for treatment of functional dyspepsia.[23-27] An RCT of acupuncture and cisapride in patients with functional dyspepsia demonstrated a significant symptomatic improvement in both groups, accompanied by an improvement in gastric emptying.[24]

PROBIOTICS

Studies on the use of probiotics for dyspepsia have yielded mixed results.[28-30] An open-label trial found that *L acidophilus* improves symptoms of bloating, abdominal pain and pressure, and flatulence in patients with dysbiosis/maldigestion. A double-blind RCT of *L rhamnosus GG* for functional abdominal pain in children found that it improves symptoms in subjects with irritable bowel syndrome, but not in those with functional dyspepsia.[29]

PSYCHOLOGICAL THERAPIES[31]

War and stress are risk factors for functional bowel disorders. Multiple studies have documented the positive effects of psychological therapies for functional dyspepsia.

Hypnotherapy

Gut-oriented hypnosis accelerates gastric emptying in dyspeptic as well as healthy subjects. A randomized, placebo-controlled trial of hypnotherapy for functional dyspepsia found that both the short- and long-term symptom scores improved in the hypnotherapy group compared to the controls.[32]

Cognitive Behavioral Therapy

A randomized, placebo-controlled comparison concluded that cognitive behavioral therapy is better than education alone for the treatment of functional bowel disorders.[33]

Biofeedback

Biofeedback has the potential to allow patients to manipulate the pathogenic gastroduodenal alterations implicated in dyspepsia. Gastric myoelectric activity can be modified using biofeedback and relaxation techniques through imagery, while watching electroglottograph activity on the screen.

Relaxation Exercise

Breathing exercises with vagal biofeedback can increase drinking capacity and improve the quality of life for patients with functional dyspepsia, without altering the vagal tone.[34,35]

Music Therapy

Listening to enjoyable music increases the amplitude of gastric myoelectrical activity in healthy humans. Music therapy may improve gastric motility and may be used to stimulate gastric emptying.[36]

HOMEOPATHY

The role of homeopathy in dyspepsia has not been critically examined. A large university hospital outpatient observational study of homeopathic treatment for chronic diseases (n = 6544), including GI diseases, found it to be beneficial.

SUPPLEMENTS

Bovine Colostrum

Bovine colostrum has activity against *H pylori.* These actions could potentially help in relieving dyspeptic symptoms.

Minerals and Vitamins

Most of the data in this category pertain to the use of zinc. Zinc reduces gastric acid secretion. There are no studies examining the effects of zinc in functional dyspepsia.

Preventive Strategies

Aside from pharmacotherapeutics for functional dyspepsia, patients may be advised to follow some lifestyle modifications and to take care when using medications, including over-the-counter medicines.

- ○ Avoid NSAIDs as much as medically possible.
- ○ Avoid smoking and alcohol since they disrupt gastroprotective mechanisms.
- ○ The role of diet is patient specific.
- ○ Dietary modifications must be individualized based on the patient's symptom triggers.

REFERENCES

1. Rösch W, Liebregts T, Gundermann KJ, Vinson B, Holtmann G. Phytotherapy for functional dyspepsia: a review of the clinical evidence for the herbal preparation STW 5. *Phytomedicine.* 2006;13(Suppl 5):114-121.

2. Takahashi T. Acupuncture for functional gastrointestinal disorders. *J Gastroenterol.* 2006;41(5):408-417.

3. Chawla YK, Dubey P, Singh R, Nundy S, Tandon BN. Treatment of dyspepsia with Amalaki (*Emblica officinalis Linn.*)—an Ayurvedic drug. *Indian J Med Res.* 1982;76(Suppl):95-98.

4. Holtmann G, Adam B, Haag S, Collet W, Grünewald E, Windeck T. Efficacy of artichoke leaf extract in the treatment of patients with functional dyspepsia: a six-week placebo-controlled, double-blind, multicentre trial. *Aliment Pharmacol Ther.* 2003;18(11-12):1099-1105.

5. Dalvi SS, Nadkarni PM, Gupta KC. Effect of *Asparagus racemosus* (Shatavari) on gastric emptying time in normal healthy volunteers. *J Postgrad Med.* 1990;36(2):91-94.

6. Arora A, Sharma MP. Use of banana in non-ulcer dyspepsia. *Lancet.* 1990;335(8689):612-613.

7. Bortolotti M, Coccia G, Grossi G, Miglioli M. The treatment of functional dyspepsia with red pepper. *Aliment Pharmacol Ther.* 2002;16(6):1075-1082.

8. Thamlikitkul V, Bunyapraphatsara N, Dechatiwongse T, et al. Randomized double blind study of *Curcuma domestica Val.* for dyspepsia. *J Med Assoc Thai.* 1989;72(11):613-620.

9. Hu ML, Rayner CK, Wu KL, et al. Effect of ginger on gastric motility and symptoms of functional dyspepsia. *World J Gastroenterol.* 2011;17(1):105-110.

10. Dabos KJ, Sfika E, Vlatta LJ, et al. Is Chios mastic gum effective in the treatment of functional dyspepsia? A prospective randomised double-blind placebo controlled trial. *J Ethnopharmacol.* 2010;127(2):205-209.

11. May B, Köhler S, Schneider B. Efficacy and tolerability of a fixed combination of peppermint oil and caraway oil in patients suffering from functional dyspepsia. *Aliment Pharmacol Ther.* 2000;14(12):1671-1677.

12. Madisch A, Heydenreich CJ, Wieland V, Hufnagel R, Hotz J. Treatment of functional dyspepsia with a fixed peppermint oil and caraway oil combination preparation as compared to cisapride. A multicenter, reference-controlled double-blind equivalence study. *Arzneimittelforschung.* 1999;49(11):925-932.

13. Yamada K, Yagi G, Kanba S. Effectiveness of Gorei-san (TJ-17) for treatment of SSRI-induced nausea and dyspepsia: preliminary observations. *Clin Neuropharmacol.* 2003;26(3):112-114.

14. Oikawa T, Ito G, Hoshino T, Koyama H, Hanawa T. Hangekobokuto (Banxia-houpo-tang), a kampo medicine that treats functional dyspepsia. *Evid Based Complement Altern Med.* 2009;6(3):375-378.

15. Tatsuta M, Iishi H. Effect of treatment with liu-jun-zi-tang (TJ-43) on gastric emptying and gastrointestinal symptoms in dyspeptic patients. *Aliment Pharmacol Ther.* 1993;7(4):459-462.

16. Chen Z. Clinical and experimental study on non-ulceratic dyspepsia treated with shenxia hewining *Zhongguo Zhong Xi Yi Jie He Za Zhi.* 1994;14(2):83-85.

17. Madisch A, Holtmann G, Mayr G, Vinson B, Hotz J. Treatment of functional dyspepsia with a herbal preparation. A double-blind, randomized, placebo-controlled, multicenter trial. *Digestion.* 2004;69(1):45-52.

18. von Arnim U, Peitz U, Vinson B, Gundermann KJ, Malfertheiner P. STW 5, a phytopharmacon for patients with functional dyspepsia: results of a multicenter, placebo-controlled double-blind study. *Am J Gastroenterol.* 2007;102(6):1268-1275.

19. Melzer J, Rösch W, Reichling J, Brignoli R, Saller R. Meta-analysis: phytotherapy of functional dyspepsia with the herbal drug preparation STW 5 (Iberogast). *Aliment Pharmacol Ther.* 2004;20(11-12):1279-1287.

20. Qin F, Huang X, Ren P. Chinese herbal medicine modified xiaoyao san for functional dyspepsia: meta-analysis of randomized controlled trials. *J Gastroenterol Hepatol.* 2009;24(8):1320-1325.

21. Borgia M, Camarri E, Cataldi V, et al. Double-blind double-controlled polycenter study on the therapeutic activity of a well-known combination of medicinal herbs. *Clin Ter.* 1985;114(5):401-409

22. Niederau C, Göpfert E. [The effect of chelidonium- and turmeric root extract on upper abdominal pain due to functional disorders of the biliary system. Results from a placebo-controlled double-blind study]. *Med Klin (Munich)*. 1999;94(8):425-430.

23. Xu S, Hou X, Zha H, Gao Z, Zhang Y, Chen JD. Electroacupuncture accelerates solid gastric emptying and improves dyspeptic symptoms in patients with functional dyspepsia. *Dig Dis Sci*. 2006;51(12):2154-2159.

24. Chen JY, Pan F, Xu JJ. Effects of acupuncture on the gastric motility in patients with functional dyspepsia. *Zhongguo Zhong Xi Yi Jie He Za Zhi*. 2005;25(10):880-882.

25. Park YC, Kang W, Choi SM, Son CG. Evaluation of manual acupuncture at classical and nondefined points for treatment of functional dyspepsia: a randomized-controlled trial. *J Altern Complement Med*. 2009;15(8):879-884.

26. Wang YG, Yao SK. Study on effects of low frequency pulse plus auricular point magnetic therapy on electrogastrogram and clinical therapeutic effect in the patient of functional dyspepsia. *Zhongguo Zhen Jiu*. 2007;27(4):245-248.

27. da Silva JB, Nakamura MU, Cordeiro JA, Kulay L Jr, Saidah R. Acupuncture for dyspepsia in pregnancy: a prospective, randomised, controlled study. *Acupunct Med*. 2009;27(2):50-53.

28. S Kim L, Hilli L, Orlowski J, Kupperman JL, Baral MF, Waters R. Efficacy of probiotics and nutrients in functional gastrointestinal disorders: a preliminary clinical trial. *Dig Dis Sci*. 2006;51(12):2134-2144.

29. Gawronska A, Dziechciarz P, Horvath A, Szajewska H. A randomized double-blind placebo-controlled trial of *Lactobacillus GG* for abdominal pain disorders in children. *Aliment Pharmacol Ther*. 2007;25(2):177-184.

30. Kalman DS, Schwartz HI, Alvarez P, et al. A prospective, randomized, double-blind, placebo-controlled parallel-group dual site trial to evaluate the effects of a *Bacillus coagulans*-based product on functional intestinal gas symptoms. *BMC Gastroenterol*. 2009;9:85.

31. Miller V, Whorwell PJ. Hypnotherapy for functional gastrointestinal disorders: a review. *Int J Clin Exp Hypn*. 2009;57(3):279-292.

32. Calvert EL, Houghton LA, Cooper P, Morris J, Whorwell PJ. Long-term improvement in functional dyspepsia using hypnotherapy. *Gastroenterology*. 2002;123(6):1778-1785.

33. Drossman DA, Toner BB, Whitehead WE, et al. Cognitive-behavioral therapy versus education and desipramine versus placebo for moderate to severe functional bowel disorders. *Gastroenterology*. 2003;125(1):19-31.

34. Hjelland IE, Svebak S, Berstad A, Flatabø G, Hausken T. Breathing exercises with vagal biofeedback may benefit patients with functional dyspepsia. *Scand J Gastroenterol*. 2007;42(9):1054-1062.

35. Haag S, Senf W, Tagay S, et al. Is there a benefit from intensified medical and psychological interventions in patients with functional dyspepsia not responding to conventional therapy? *Aliment Pharmacol Ther*. 2007;25(8):973-986.

36. Lin HH, Chang WK, Chu HC, et al. Effects of music on gastric myoelectrical activity in healthy humans. *Int J Clin Pract*. 2007;61(7):1126-1130.

Chapter

43 *Gastroparesis*

KEY POINTS

- ○ Therapies based on Chinese medicine (eg, STW 5 and acupuncture) are effective.
- ○ Dietary lifestyle modifications like small, frequent, low-fiber meals may help symptoms.
- ○ Mind-body therapies have a beneficial effect.

INTRODUCTION

There is paucity of prokinetic medications in mainstream medicine. Metoclopramide, or Reglan, is full of side effects mediated by its effects on the nervous system, is the target of many lawsuits, and is avoided by many physicians. Cisapride had to be withdrawn from the market a few years ago because of serious side effects. Benefit from erythromycin is limited at best. Domperidone is not available in the United States.

Many patients just use over-the-counter medications, but complementary and alternative treatments are gaining in popularity (Table 43-1). There is a lack of good correlation between severity of gastroparesis and the symptoms.

HERBAL THERAPIES

Asparagus racemosus *(Shatavari)*

A racemosus (Shatavari) is an Ayurvedic remedy that reduces gastric emptying time in normal healthy volunteers.[1]

Ginger root

Administration of 3 ginger capsules (total 1200 mg 1 hour before a meal) accelerates gastric emptying and stimulates antral contractions in healthy volunteers.[2]

Peppermint Oil (Mentha × piperita L)

It enhances the early phase of gastric emptying,[3] and the effect of peppermint and caraway oils on gastric emptying is similar to that of the drug cisapride. A multi-center, reference-controlled, double-blind

Table 43-1. Strategies of Benefit in Gastroparesis[4]

- ❖ Lifestyle strategies
- ❖ Smoking cessation
- ❖ Alcohol cessation
- ❖ Avoid carbonated beverages
- ❖ Weight control, if overweight
- ❖ Small frequent (5 to 6 meals)
- ❖ Avoid fried foods
- ❖ Low fiber diet
- ❖ Short slow-paced walk after meals
- ❖ Relaxation exercises
- ❖ Avoid stressful situations as much as possible

- ❖ CAM therapies
- ❖ Asparagus racemosus (Shatavari)
- ❖ Ginger
- ❖ Tangweikang (TWK)
- ❖ Liu-Jun-Zi-Tang (TJ-43)
- ❖ Hange-koboku-to
- ❖ Terminalia chebula
- ❖ Peppermint oil
- ❖ Probiotics
- ❖ Acupuncture
- ❖ Hypnosis
- ❖ Music therapy

equivalence study using a peppermint/caraway oil preparation or cisapride found them to be equivalent for the treatment of functional dyspepsia.[5]

Terminalia

T chebula is advocated in Ayurveda to improve GI motility.[6]

HERBAL COMBINATIONS

Both functional and organic disorders have multiple underlying pathogenic mechanisms. The use of herbal combinations has the potential to affect a disease process at multiple levels in its pathogenesis.

Hange-Koboku-To (Banxia-Houpo-Tang)

Hange-koboku-to accelerates gastric emptying in patients with dyspepsia, as well as in healthy controls. This improvement in gastric emptying is accompanied by improvement in dyspeptic symptoms in patients with dyspepsia.[7]

Liu-Jun-Zi-Tang (TJ-43)

Liu-Jun-Zi-Tang, also known as *Rikkunshito*, contains extracts of *A lanceae rhizoma, R Ginseng, P tuber, Hoelen, Z fructus, A nobilis pericarpium,*

R Glycyrrhizae, and *Z rhizoma*. Compared to placebo, TJ-43 (2.5 g 3 tid) improves gastric emptying, as well as GI symptoms of epigastric fullness, heartburn, belching, and nausea.[8]

STW 5

STW 5 is a fixed combination of 9 herbs and stimulates antral motility. A double-blind, double-dummy study demonstrated that the effects of STW 5 and STW 5-II administered for 4 weeks are equivalent to those of cisapride, a promotility agent, for the treatment of patients with functional dyspepsia of dysmotility type.[9]

Tangweikang

Tangweikang is a Chinese herbal preparation that hastens gastric emptying in diabetic gastroparesis.[10]

ACUPUNCTURE AND OTHER ELECTROMAGNETIC TREATMENTS

Acupuncture accelerates gastric emptying in several animal models and humans.[11-15] Electroacupuncture not only improves gastric emptying in subjects with gastroparesis, but it also improves symptoms of functional dyspepsia in patients with normal, as well as delayed, gastric emptying.[11] Acupuncture also improves gastric emptying in critically ill patients.[15]

Acupuncture administered by an expert may be a reasonable option for patients with refractory gastroparesis that is refractory to standard management.

Probiotics

The gastric emptying rate is significantly faster in the newborns receiving *L reuteri* compared to formula with placebo. *L reuteri*-supplemented babies have a motility pattern resembling that of newborns fed with breast milk.[16]

MIND-BODY THERAPIES

Gut-oriented hypnosis accelerates gastric emptying.[17] Music therapy may improve gastric motility and may be used to stimulate gastric emptying.[18] Biofeedback and relaxation techniques can be helpful since they can modulate gastric myoelectric activity through imagery while watching electroglottograph activity on the screen. Breathing exercises with vagal biofeedback can increase drinking capacity.[19]

Homeopathy

Homeopathy, while extremely popular outside of the United States, continues to defy biological plausibility and baffles scientists. The debate on its effectiveness continues. There is a lack of data examining the effect of homeopathy in gastroparesis.

REFERENCES

1. Dalvi SS, Nadkarni PM, Gupta KC. Effect of *Asparagus racemosus* (Shatavari) on gastric emptying time in normal healthy volunteers. *J Postgrad Med.* 1990;36(2):91-94.

2. Wu KL, Rayner CK, Chuah SK, et al. Effects of ginger on gastric emptying and motility in healthy humans. *Eur J Gastroenterol Hepatol.* 2008;20(5):436-440.

3. Inamori M, Akiyama T, Akimoto K, et al. Early effects of peppermint oil on gastric emptying: a crossover study using a continuous real-time 13C breath test (BreathID system). *J Gastroenterol.* 2007;42(7):539-542.

4. Abell TL, Malinowski S, Minocha A. Nutrition aspects of gastroparesis and therapies for drug-refractory patients. *Nutr Clin Pract.* 2006;21(1):23-33.

5. Madisch A, Heydenreich CJ, Wieland V, Hufnagel R, Hotz J. Treatment of functional dyspepsia with a fixed peppermint oil and caraway oil combination preparation as compared to cisapride. A multicenter, reference-controlled double-blind equivalence study. *Arzneimittelforschung.* 1999;49(11):925-932.

6. Tamhane MD, Thorat SP, Rege NN, Dahanukar SA. Effect of oral administration of *Terminalia chebula* on gastric emptying: an experimental study. *J Postgrad Med.* 1997;43(1):12-13.

7. Oikawa T, Ito G, Hoshino T, Koyama H, Hanawa T. Hangekobokuto (Banxia-houpo-tang), a Kampo medicine that treats functional dyspepsia. *Evid Based Complement Alternat Med.* 2009;6(3):375-378.

8. Tatsuta M, Iishi H. Effect of treatment with liu-jun-zi-tang (TJ-43) on gastric emptying and gastrointestinal symptoms in dyspeptic patients. *Aliment Pharmacol Ther.* 1993;7(4):459-462.

9. Rösch W, Vinson B, Sassin I. A randomised clinical trial comparing the efficacy of a herbal preparation STW 5 with the prokinetic drug cisapride in patients with dysmotility type of functional dyspepsia. *Z Gastroenterol.* 2002;40(6):401-408.

10. Jiang RQ, Zhang DX, Bai CY. Clinical study on Tangweikang in treating diabetic gastroparesis. *Zhongguo Zhong Xi Yi Jie He Za Zhi.* 2007;27(2):114-116.

11. Xu S, Hou X, Zha H, et al. Electroacupuncture accelerates solid gastric emptying and improves dyspeptic symptoms in patients with functional dyspepsia. *Dig Dis Sci.* 2006;51(12):2154-2159.

12. Chen JY, Pan F, Xu JJ. Effects of acupuncture on the gastric motility in patients with functional dyspepsia. *Zhongguo Zhong Xi Yi Jie He Za Zhi.* 2005;25(10):880-882.

13. Wang CP, Kao CH, Chen WK, Lo WY, Hsieh CL. A single-blinded, randomized pilot study evaluating effects of electroacupuncture in diabetic patients with symptoms suggestive of gastroparesis. *J Altern Complement Med.* 2008;14(7):833-839.

14. Sun BM, Luo M, Wu SB, Chen XX, Wu MC. Acupuncture versus metoclopramide in treatment of postoperative gastroparesis syndrome in abdominal surgical patients: a randomized controlled trial. *Zhong Xi Yi Jie He Xue Bao.* 2010;8(7):641-644.

15. Pfab F, Winhard M, Nowak-Machen M, et al. Acupuncture in critically ill patients improves delayed gastric emptying: a randomized controlled trial. *Anesth Analg.* 2011;112(1):150-155.

16. Indrio F, Riezzo G, Raimondi F, et al. The effects of probiotics on feeding tolerance, bowel habits, and gastrointestinal motility in preterm newborns. *J Pediatr.* 2008;152(6):801-806.

17. Chiarioni G, Vantini I, De Iorio F, et al. Prokinetic effect of gut-oriented hypnosis on gastric emptying. *Aliment Pharmacol Ther.* 2006;23(8):1241-1249.

18. Lin HH, Chang WK, Chu HC, et al. Effects of music on gastric myoelectrical activity in healthy humans. *Int J Clin Pract.* 2007;61(7):1126-1130.

19. Hjelland IE, Svebak S, Berstad A, Flatabø G, Hausken T. Breathing exercises with vagal biofeedback may benefit patients with functional dyspepsia. *Scand J Gastroenterol.* 2007;42(9):1054-1062.

LOWER GASTROINTESTINAL DISORDERS

Chapter

44 *Irritable Bowel Syndrome*

KEY POINTS

○ Fiber and peppermint oil are part of the recommendations of the American College of Gastroenterology for the treatment of irritable bowel syndrome (IBS).

○ Several phytobotanicals, including Chinese herbal medicine, have been shown to be effective.

○ Effects of probiotics in IBS are strain specific.

○ Cognitive behavioral therapy (CBT) is at least as effective as drugs acting on 5HT receptors.

○ Gut-directed hypnotherapy benefits IBS patients.

○ Yoga-based interventions are of benefit.

○ An appropriately targeted elimination diet may help a significant number of patients.

WHY IS IRRITABLE BOWEL SYNDROME SO COMMON IN MODERN SOCIETY?

There have been numerous and complex changes in the human environment (eg, in diet and other lifestyle conditions). These started with the introduction of agriculture and animal husbandry and living in jungles or countryside approximately several millennia ago, all the way to current living in large cities with a fast-paced life and emphasis on industrialization and the use of processed foods. Dietary changes

Minocha A. *A Guide to Alternative Medicine and the Digestive System* (pp 199-290). © 2013 Taylor & Francis Group.

have resulted in alterations in glycemic load, fatty acid composition, macronutrient composition, micronutrient density, acid-base balance, sodium-potassium ratio, and fiber content.[1]

The etiopathogenesis of IBS involves an interaction between diet, environment, antibiotics, and psychosocial factors. Infection may be involved in etiopathogenesis in 5% to 32% of IBS patients. Food hypersensitivity is a common perception among IBS patients.[2] An ideal treatment of IBS has been elusive.

PHYTOBOTANICALS, INCLUDING AYURVEDA

Aegle marmelos

A marmelos has antidiarrheal effects, as measured by the gastrointestinal (GI) transit of charcoal markers. Ayurvedic formulation composed of *A marmelos* (bael fruit) and *B monnieri* has been used for GI upsets and may be helpful in IBS.

Agrimony

Labeled at one time as "all-heal," it has been used widely for diarrhea, wound healing, asthma, etc across different cultures. Data on specific GI effects are lacking.

Artichoke Leaf Extract

While the hydrophilic extract of artichoke increases contractions in rat ileum, the lipophilic extracts actually relax the intestine. Artichoke leaf extract reduces symptoms of IBS and improves the quality of life in otherwise healthy volunteers suffering from concomitant dyspepsia.[3] Walker et al showed that 96% of patients rated artichoke leaf extract as better than or at least equal to previous therapies administered for their IBS symptoms.[4]

Bacopa monnieri

Bacopa has mast cell stabilizing activity and has been used in a variety of herbal combinations for IBS.

Belladonna

Belladonna, because of its antispasmodic properties, has long been used for IBS. No good studies have examined its efficacy.

Boswellia

Ayurvedic plant *Boswellia serrata* reduces diarrhea by normalizing intestinal motility in disease states, without slowing the rate of transit in control animals.

Chamomile

Long known for its spasmolytic and soothing/calming properties, chamomile has been used by patients suffering from IBS. However, there is a lack of literature examining this herb in IBS.

Fennel (Foeniculum vulgare)

Fennel seed oil has been shown to reduce intestinal spasms and increase motility. A randomized placebo-controlled trial found that treatment with fennel oil emulsion eliminates colic in 65% of infants compared to only 24% with placebo.[5] Another randomized, double-blind, placebo-controlled trial demonstrated that neither fumitory nor *Curcuma* have any therapeutic benefit over placebo in patients with IBS.[6]

Marrubiin

Marrubium vulgare is a medicinal plant employed in Brazil and other countries. Marrubiin is the main bioactive analgesic compound. Marrubiin has potent antispasmodic and antinociceptive properties and is superior to some well-known analgesic drugs.[7]

Nutmeg

Nutmeg may be useful in IBS on account of its antidiarrheal, antihistamine, and sedative properties.

Peppermint Oil

Clinical trials have documented the efficacy of peppermint in IBS.[8-10] Patients on peppermint-oil formulation (Colpermin) experience a significantly greater alleviation of the abdominal pain, abdominal distension, stool frequency, abdominal gas, and flatulence compared to controls.[8] Another randomized, double-blind, placebo-controlled trial of peppermint oil in outpatients with IBS yielded similar results.[10]

> In contrast to the past, the current evidence-based American College of Gastroenterology guidelines recommend use of peppermint oil in patients with IBS.

Rhubarb

Rhubarb has been used in intestinal disorders, including IBS. It has been used as a prokinetic drug since ancient times. Rhubarb can positively modulate the acute inflammatory response, promote restoration of postoperative GI motility, and promote enteral nutrition support in patients who have undergone major operations for gastric cancer. Clinical studies examining it alone in IBS are lacking.

Turmeric

Bundy concluded that turmeric may help reduce IBS symptomology.[11] Another randomized, placebo-controlled, double-blind clinical trial failed to confirm its efficacy in IBS.[6]

Tibetan Medicine

PADMA LAX

Padma Lax, a Tibetan medicine, is superior to placebo in relieving symptoms in patients with constipation-predominant IBS.[12] This herbal combination contains ginger root, rhubarb root, frangula bark, *C sagrada*, gentian root, *T chebula*, *Inula helenium*, *Aloe vera*, *Aloe ferox*, *Jateorhiza calumba* (Calumba bark), *Gonolobus condurango*, *P longum* (long pepper), and *Strychnos nux-vomica* (nux vomica seed).

Miscellaneous Herbal Combinations

❍ A randomized, double-blind, placebo-controlled trial of a standardized extract of *Matricaria recutita*, *F vulgare*, and *M officinalis* in the treatment of breastfed, colicky infants found that the colic improved within 1 week of treatment.[13]

❍ Phytotherapy using Cinarepa containing artichoke leaf (*Cynara scolymus*), chlorogenic acid, dandelion radix (*T officinalis*), inulin, turmeric, and rosemary bud essential oil microencapsulated (*Rosmarinus officinalis*) has been shown to be effective in functional dyspepsia, and appears promising in IBS.

❍ Smooth Move tea (Traditional Medicinals, Sebastopol, CA) contains organic licorice root, bitter fennel fruit, sweet orange peel, cinnamon bark, coriander fruit, ginger rhizome, and orange peel oil on gum arabic. It is effective in constipation and may be of benefit in constipation-predominant IBS.

❍ Yadav et al compared "standard therapy" (containing clidinium bromide, chlordiazepoxide, and ispaghula) with a compound Ayurvedic preparation (*A marmelos Correa* plus *B monnieri Linn*), along with a matching placebo in patients with IBS.[14] The Ayurvedic preparation was effective in 65%, while standard therapy was beneficial in 78%, as opposed to 33% in the placebo group.

Chinese Herbal Therapy

SHUGAN JIANPI GRANULE

Shugan Jianpi granule reduces the number of intestinal 5HT-positive cells in patients with IBS.[15]

STW 5

STW 5, or Iberogast, is a complex herbal preparation (9 constituents) including *Iberis amara*, *Chelidonii herba*, *Cardui mariae fructus*, *Melissae folium*, *Carvi fructus*, *Liquiritiae radix*, *Radix Angelicae*, *Matricariae flos*, and *M × piperita folium*. STW 5 modulates excitatory and inhibitory neurotransmission and slow wave rhythmicity of intestines. It has a prosecretory effect in the intestine, and this may be the mechanism of action for its benefit in IBS constipation. It reduces the sensitivity of intestinal afferents in rats, and may affect pain by affecting neuronal hypersensitivity.

Madisch et al conducted a double-blind, randomized, placebo-controlled, multicenter trial and found that STW 5 is effective in alleviating IBS symptoms.[16]

Shi et al conducted a systematic review of herbal medicine in IBS.[17] In addition to STW 5, they found that superior improvement in global IBS symptoms (compared to conventional treatment) occurs as a result of treatment with Lizhong huoxie decoction, Huatan Liqi Tiaofu decoction, Geqin Shujiang Saocao decoction, Huanchang decoction, Congpi Lunzhi Formula, Xiangsha Liujunzi decoction, and Shunji mixture. In contrast, ineffective therapies included individualized Chinese herbal medicine, bitter candytuft, *Curcuma*, fumitory, Changkang capsule, and Jiejing Yiji decoction.

MISCELLANEOUS CHINESE HERBAL FORMULA

○ Bensoussan, in a randomized, controlled trial (RCT), demonstrated that 42% of the IBS patients receiving Chinese herbal formula had relief of symptoms compared to only 16% in the placebo group.[18]

○ Tong Xie Yao Fang-modified decoction and Tong Xie Yao Fang plus Si Ni San decoction, when compared to conventional medicine, have antidiarrheal effects in patients with IBS. Their effects are similar to Liyiting decoction and Tongxie yihao capsule.

○ Gegan Qinlian pellet is also effective. Wuma Simo decoction is similar in efficacy to conventional medicine in patients with constipation-predominant IBS.

A Cochrane database review of herbal therapies in IBS concluded that, when compared with placebo, standard Chinese herbal formula, individualized Chinese herbal medicine, STW 5 and STW 5-II, Tibetan herbal medicine Padma Lax, traditional Chinese formula Tong Xie Yao Fang, and Ayurvedic preparation demonstrate significant improvement of global symptoms in IBS.[19]

MIND-BODY THERAPIES

Psychological stress causes GI distress through alteration of intestinal function, via alterations in neuroimmune humoral system. Numerous studies have examined the role of antidepressants and psychological treatments in IBS. However, the pathophysiological basis of such interventions remains unclear.

Cognitive Behavioral Therapy

CBT appears to have a direct effect on global IBS manifestations without any correlation to psychological distress. Improvement in IBS symptoms[20-23] is associated with improvements in the quality of life, and the improvement in psychological distress may be a reason for, effect of, or part of it.

Drossman et al conducted a randomized, comparator-controlled, multicenter trial to examine the effect of CBT versus education, and tricyclic antidepressant (desipramine) versus placebo in female patients with moderate to severe functional bowel disorders, including IBS.[20] A significantly higher number of patients responded in the CBT group compared to education (70% versus 37%), while antidepressants had effects similar to placebo in an intent to treat analysis.

The addition of nurse-administered CBT to standard general practice management of IBS (antispasmodic agent mebeverine) in primary care is significantly superior to the mebeverine-only group at 3 months.[21] CBT-based self management, in the form of a structured manual without much contact with the therapist, is superior to controls for the treatment of patients with IBS in primary care.[23] In contrast, there are a few negative studies as well reporting that CBT and relaxation therapy seem not to be superior to standard care alone in IBS.[24]

Hypnotherapy

Gut-directed hypnotherapy is most beneficial in patients with predominant abdominal pain and distension. The GI nurses can administer hypnotherapy and have a potential role in the management of IBS.[25]

In addition to relieving the symptoms of IBS, hypnotherapy significantly improves the quality of life and reduces absenteeism from work. As such, despite being relatively expensive, it may be a good long-term investment.[26,27]

Multiple studies have documented beneficial effects.[28-31] Whorwell et al conducted a controlled trial of hypnotherapy versus psychotherapy in the treatment of severe refractory IBS.[28] While the psychotherapy patients showed a small but significant improvement, there was a dramatic improvement in the hypnosis group.

The use of a specially devised audiotape for gut-directed hypnotherapy may be equally effective.[29] The beneficial effects of hypnotherapy appear to last at least 5 years.[30] Whitehead concludes that hypnosis is effective even for patients refractory to standard therapies.[31]

A Cochrane database review concluded that hypnotherapy is superior to waiting list controls, as well as the usual management of IBS.[32] The use of hypnotherapy in IBS qualifies for the highest level of acceptance as being both efficacious and specific.

Relaxation Therapy and Meditation

Most studies indicate that relaxation response meditation as well as meditation are beneficial over the short and long term in patients with IBS.[33-37] Voirol and Hipolito investigated the effect of relaxation therapy for 6 months in patients with IBS.[33] The control group received conventional treatment. The number of consultations in the control group was 53 before and 41 after conventional treatment, and the consultations in the relaxation group fell from 74 before to 6 after relaxation therapy. The improvement was statistically significant.

Multicomponent Therapies

Mostly positive results have been obtained from multicomponent therapy use.[38-40] Guthrie et al studied patients with medically refractory IBS in a controlled trial of psychological treatment involving psychotherapy, relaxation, and standard medical treatment compared with standard medical treatment alone over a 3-month period.[39] The investigators documented a significantly greater improvement on gastroenterologists' as well as the patients' ratings of diarrhea and abdominal pain. Another study, however, reported that the results of multicomponent treatment were similar to the attention-placebo condition.[41]

Stress Management

Shaw et al assigned IBS patients to either a stress management program or usual treatment including antispasmodics. The stress management program was effective in relieving symptoms of two-thirds of the patients compared to few in the conventional group.[42]

Ford et al conducted a meta-analysis and concluded that both antidepressants and psychological therapies are equally effective, with the number needed to treat being 4 for both strategies.[43]

PROBIOTICS

Data from numerous animal studies suggest that consumption of probiotics can restore gut function back to baseline.[44]

Probiotic Benefits Are Strain Specific

Not all species of probiotics have the same therapeutic potential in any particular condition. Particular strains of probiotic may target different manifestations of IBS like diarrhea, constipation, bloating, etc.

Why Literature Appears Contradictory[45-52]

Many investigators tend to lump all potential probiotics in one group, and then analyze the effects as if they were one and the same. A clear definition and understanding of probiotic strain selection, dose, and method of delivery are important. This presents a plausible explanation for the variability in the evidence documented by the various published trials.

A 5-month trial of multispecies probiotic supplementation (*L rhamnosus GG, L rhamnosus Lc705, P freudenreichii ssp shermanii JS,* and *B animalis ssp lactis Bb12)* results in a significant improvement of the composite IBS score.[45] Treatment with *B infantis 35624* is significantly superior to placebo for relief of abdominal pain, bloating, bowel dysfunction, incomplete evacuation, straining, and the passage of gas.[47]

Negative results have been reported by some authors, including Niv et al, who found that *L reuteri ATCC 55730* was similar in efficacy to placebo in patients with IBS.[51]

Caution: L plantarum MF1298 may worsen symptoms in patients with IBS.

Preclinical and clinical data suggest that probiotics offer a rational therapeutic approach to IBS.[53] A systematic review concluded that probiotics are significantly better than placebo with a number needed to treat (NNT) of 4.[54]

PREBIOTICS

Oligofructose

Hunter et al[55] conducted a double-blind crossover trial of oligofructose (Raftilose P95) against sucrose daily for 4 weeks in patients with IBS. The authors found that oligofructose was of no benefit.

Partially Hydrolyzed Guar Gum

Partially hydrolyzed guar gum is a water-soluble, non-gelling fiber. It increases colonic short-chain fatty acids (SCFAs), *lactobacilli*, and *bifidobacteria*. Ingestion of partially hydrolyzed guar gum decreases symptoms in constipation-predominant and diarrhea-predominant forms of IBS that are associated with improvement of quality of life.

Inulin

Inulin significantly increases *bifidobacteria* and may increase GI symptoms, such as flatulence and bloatedness in some healthy adults. The consumption of Jerusalem artichoke inulin or chicory inulin increases counts of *bifidobacteria* and reduces the pathogenic bacteria associated with a slight increase in stool frequency.

Konjac

Konjac glucomannan is used for constipation. Konjac supplementation significantly increases the defecation frequency and stool weight along with promoting the daily output of *bifidobacteria*, *lactobacilli*, and fecal short-chain fatty acids (SCFAs).

Effect of Fiber in Irritable Bowel Syndrome May Be Fiber Specific

A meta-analysis conducted by Ford et al sums up the data well on use of fiber in IBS.[56] The number needed to treat to prevent one patient with persistent symptoms was 11. Subgroup analysis revealed that bran had no significant effect on IBS. In contrast, ispaghula was effective in treating IBS, and the number needed to treat for ispaghula was 6.

GUIDING PRINCIPLES OF FIBER MANAGEMENT OF IRRITABLE BOWEL SYNDROME

○ Fiber is especially effective in constipation-predominant IBS.

○ There is a high placebo response rate.

○ At the worst, fiber supplementation serves as a healthy, cheap, and effective placebo.

○ Fiber is probably more effective in the primary care setting than secondary care.

○ Soluble fiber should be the fiber of choice.[57]

○ Excessive intake of insoluble cereal fibers can worsen IBS symptoms, especially abdominal pain, in up to 50% of patients.

○ It may be prudent to first recommend a trial of exclusion of cereal fiber in some IBS patients, especially those with significant gas and bloating.

In an evidence-based position statement, the American College of Gastroenterology IBS task force concluded that psyllium (ispaghula husk) is moderately effective.[58] Wheat bran or corn bran is no more effective than placebo in the relief of global IBS symptoms, and they did not recommend its routine use. Optimal dose of ispaghula husk in IBS is 20 g per day.

ACUPUNCTURE AND RELATED THERAPIES

Electroacupuncture modulates visceral hyperalgesia by down-regulating central serotonergic activities in the rat brain-gut axis.[59] Clinical evidence on the use of acupuncture in IBS has yielded mixed results.[60-64]

Transcutaneous electrical acustimulation at the acupoints ST36 and P6 increases the threshold of rectal sensation of gas, desire to defecate, and pain compared to the control in IBS patients. However, a prospective, blinded, sham-controlled trial of acupuncture in IBS found that both groups improved equally at the end of treatment.[61] Acupuncture combined with massage therapy shows a better therapeutic effect than acupuncture alone in IBS.[62] It is unclear if acupuncture is more effective than sham acupuncture or other interventions in patients with IBS.[63,64]

EXCLUSION DIETS

Elevated serum antibodies to various foods have been found in IBS, although a cause-effect relationship remains to be established.[65] Adults with atopic symptoms report a high incidence of IBS, suggesting a possible link between atopy and IBS. Food hypersensitivity is a common perception among IBS patients. The majority of IBS patients identify 2 to 5 foods that upset them, with overall range being 1 to 14 foods.[2] More than 50% of IBS patients show evidence of sensitization to some food or inhalant without any typical clinical signs.[66]

Foods Implicated

Patients are usually unable to identify potentially offending foods. Skin prick tests and food-specific serum IgG4 and IgE antibodies may help in identifying the offending foods. However, there is lack of a correlation between skin prick test results and reported food allergies.

There is higher reactivity to food antigens in diarrhea-predominant IBS—compared to the constipation-predominant IBS and controls—and implicates the role of leaky gut. Zar et al found that IBS patients had significantly higher IgG4 titers to wheat, beef, pork, and lamb compared to controls.[67] However, the antibody titers to potatoes, rice, fish, chicken, yeast, tomato, and shrimp were similar to controls. There was no correlation between the pattern of antibody titers and the patients' symptoms.

The order of frequency of food allergens in IBS is as follows: milk protein, soybean, tomato, peanut, and egg white (Table 44-1).

Food is often a forgotten factor in IBS.[68]

Patients with diarrhea-predominant IBS suffer from more adverse food reactions compared to healthy controls. Interventions like a low or no fiber polymeric diet and antibiotic therapy, which reduce colonic bacterial fermentation, improve symptoms of IBS.[69]

Although carbohydrate malabsorption can provoke symptoms in some IBS patients, there is no consistent association between such a phenomenon and the presence of either jejunal hypersensitivity or dysmotility. Fructose-sorbitol malabsorption is frequently seen in patients with IBS. However, symptomatic patients do not differ from asymptomatic patients regarding the presence or absence of fructose-sorbitol malabsorption.

Several studies have documented the benefit of elimination diets in IBS.[70-74] An antibody-guided experimental exclusion diet showed a 10% greater reduction in symptom score than the sham diet at 12 weeks, with this value increasing to 26% in fully compliant patients.[70] Body-guided exclusion diet improves IBS symptoms and is associated with improvement in rectal compliance.[71] Appropriate dietary exclusions based on food-specific IgG antibodies in patients led to decrease in levels of serum food-specific IgG antibodies, as well

Table 44-1. Avoiding These Foods Helps Many Patients

- ❖ Soybean
- ❖ Tomatoes
- ❖ Peppers
- ❖ Nuts
- ❖ Eggs, especially egg whites
- ❖ Wheat
- ❖ Red meat
- ❖ Seafood
- ❖ Dairy products
- ❖ Juicy fruits

as frequency and severity of symptoms and improvement of the quality of life.[73]

Different elimination strategies, including a low FODMAP (fermentable oligo-, di- and monosaccharides, and polyols) diet (see Chapter 10), have been shown to ameliorate symptoms in many patients.

SUPPLEMENTS

Beidellitic Montmorillonite

Beidellitic montmorillonite is purified clay containing a double aluminum and magnesium silicate. Ducrotte et al assessed its efficacy and the safety (3 g tid for 8 weeks) in IBS patients in a multicenter, double-blind, placebo-controlled study with parallel groups.[75] Significant improvement was seen for patients with constipation-predominant IBS.

Clay

Dioctahedral smectite is a natural adsorbent clay used for the management of acute diarrhea. Chang et al studied the efficacy of dioctahedral smectite in patients with diarrhea-predominant IBS over 8 weeks in a randomized, double-blind, placebo-controlled fashion.[76] Both treatments were equally effective, with respect to primary efficacy.

L-Glutamine

Its role in strengthening the intestinal barrier provides an attractive therapeutic target for intervention in IBS.

Zinc

Zinc carnosine stabilizes small bowel integrity and stimulates gut repair processes. The role of zinc supplementation in IBS remains to be established.

MISCELLANEOUS THERAPIES FOR IRRITABLE BOWEL SYNDROME

Yogic Intervention or Yoga

Taneja et al conducted an RCT to evaluate the effect of yogic and conventional treatment in diarrhea-predominant IBS.[77] Two months of both conventional and yogic intervention showed a significant decrease of bowel symptoms and state anxiety. Another comparative study reported that the yoga group suffered fewer GI symptoms, lower levels of functional disability, and lower anxiety.[78]

Chiropractic

There is a lack of studies on the use of chiropractic techniques in classic IBS. Chiropractic distractive decompression is effective in treating pelvic pain and pelvic organic dysfunction, including bowel problems.[79] Many experts think of infantile colic as an infantile version of IBS. Conflicting results have been reported on the use of spinal manipulation for infantile colic.[80,81]

Reflexology

Reflexology has not been shown to be of benefit in IBS.

Osteopathic Treatment

Riot et al[82] studied patients with levator ani syndrome prospectively over 1 year. Forty-seven of them also had IBS. Massages were given with a patient lying on the left side. Physical treatment of the pelvic joint disorders was given at the end of each massage session. The symptoms were ameliorated in 72% of the patients; most of the IBS patients also benefited from this treatment.

Table 44-2 reviews the therapies of benefit for IBS.

REFERENCES

1. Cordain L, Eaton SB, Sebastian A, et al. Origins and evolution of the Western diet: health implications for the 21st century. *Am J Clin Nutr.* 2005;81(2):341-354.
2. Nanda R, James R, Smith H, Dudley CR, Jewell DP. Food intolerance and the IBS. *Gut.* 1989;30(8):1099-1104.

Table 44-2. Therapies of Benefit in
Irritable Bowel Syndrome

Herbal Therapies	Nonherbal Therapies
❖ Artichoke leaf extract ❖ Padma lax ❖ Peppermint oil ❖ Turmeric (mixed results) ❖ Ayurveda combination of *A marmelos correa* plus *B monnieri Linn* ❖ Lizhong huoxie decoction ❖ Huatan Liqi Tiaofu decoction ❖ STW 5 or iberogast ❖ Geqin Shujiang Saocao decoction ❖ Huanchang decoction ❖ Congpi Lunzhi Formula ❖ Xiangsha Liujunzi decoction ❖ Shunji mixture ❖ Tong Xie Yao Fang (TXYF and TXYF-A) formula ❖ Gegan Qinlian pellet	❖ Elimination/exclusion diets (see Chapter 10, Tables 10-3 and 10-4) ❖ High fiber (effects may be fiber specific [eg, ispaghula works and bran may not]) ❖ Pre- and probiotics ❖ Cognitive behavioral therapy ❖ Hypnotherapy ❖ Relaxation meditation ❖ Meditation ❖ Stress management ❖ Yoga ❖ Acupuncture (controversial) ❖ Beidellitic montmorillonite

3. Bundy R, Walker AF, Middleton RW, Marakis G, Booth JC. Artichoke leaf extract reduces symptoms of irritable bowel syndrome and improves quality of life in otherwise healthy volunteers suffering from concomitant dyspepsia: a subset analysis. *J Altern Complement Med.* 2004;10(4):667-669.

4. Walker AF, Middleton RW, Petrowicz O. Artichoke leaf extract reduces symptoms of irritable bowel syndrome in a post-marketing surveillance study. *Phytother Res.* 2001;15(1):58-61.

5. Alexandrovich I, Rakovitskaya O, Kolmo E, Sidorova T, Shushunov S. The effect of fennel (*Foeniculum vulgare*) seed oil emulsion in infantile colic: a randomized, placebo-controlled study. *Altern Ther Health Med.* 2003;9(4):58-61.

6. Brinkhaus B, Hentschel C, Von Keudell C, et al. Herbal medicine with curcuma and fumitory in the treatment of irritable bowel syndrome: a randomized, placebo-controlled, double-blind clinical trial. *Scand J Gastroenterol.* 2005;40(8):936-943.

7. De Jesus RA, Cechinel-Filho V, Oliveira AE, Schlemper V. Analysis of the antinociceptive properties of marrubiin isolated from *Marrubium vulgare*. *Phytomedicine.* 2000;7(2):111-115.

8. Liu JH, Chen GH, Yeh HZ, Huang CK, Poon SK. Enteric-coated peppermint-oil capsules in the treatment of irritable bowel syndrome: a prospective, randomized trial. *J Gastroenterol.* 1997;32(6):765-768.

9. Grigoleit HG, Grigoleit P. Peppermint oil in irritable bowel syndrome. *Phytomedicine.* 2005;12(8):601-606.

10. Merat S, Khalili S, Mostajabi P, et al. The effect of enteric-coated, delayed-release peppermint oil on irritable bowel syndrome. *Dig Dis Sci.* 2010;55(5):1385-1390.

11. Bundy R, Walker AF, Middleton RW, Booth J. Turmeric extract may improve irritable bowel syndrome symptomology in otherwise healthy adults: a pilot study. *J Altern Complement Med.* 2004;10(6):1015-1018.

12. Sallon S, Ben-Arye E, Davidson R, et al. A novel treatment for constipation-predominant irritable bowel syndrome using Padma Lax, a Tibetan herbal formula. *Digestion.* 2002;65(3):161-171.

13. Savino F, Cresi F, Castagno E, Silvestro L, Oggero R. A randomized double-blind placebo-controlled trial of a standardized extract of *Matricariae recutita*, *Foeniculum vulgare* and *Melissa officinalis* (ColiMil) in the treatment of breastfed colicky infants. *Phytother Res.* 2005;19(4):335-340.

14. Yadav SK, Jain AK, Tripathi SN, Gupta JP. Irritable bowel syndrome: therapeutic evaluation of indigenous drugs. *Indian J Med Res.* 1989;90:496-503.

15. Wang ZJ, Li HX, Wang JH, Zhang F. Effect of Shugan Jianpi granule () on gut mucosal serotonin-positive cells in patients with irritable bowel syndrome of stagnated Gan-qi attacking Pi syndrome type. *Chin J Integr Med.* 2008;14(3):185-189.

16. Madisch A, Holtmann G, Plein K, Hotz J. Treatment of irritable bowel syndrome with herbal preparations: results of a double-blind, randomized, placebo-controlled, multi-centre trial. *Aliment Pharmacol Ther.* 2004;19(3):271-279.

17. Shi J, Tong Y, Shen JG, Li HX. Effectiveness and safety of herbal medicines in the treatment of irritable bowel syndrome: a systematic review. *World J Gastroenterol.* 2008;14(3):454-462.

18. Bensoussan A, Talley NJ, Hing M, et al. Treatment of irritable bowel syndrome with Chinese herbal medicine: a randomized controlled trial. *JAMA.* 1998;280(18):1585-1589.

19. Liu JP, Yang M, Liu YX, Wei ML, Grimsgaard S. Herbal medicines for treatment of irritable bowel syndrome. *Cochrane Database Syst Rev.* 2006;(1):CD004116.

20. Drossman DA, Toner BB, Whitehead WE, et al. Cognitive-behavioral therapy versus education and desipramine versus placebo for moderate to severe functional bowel disorders. *Gastroenterology.* 2003;125(1):19-31.

21. Kennedy T, Jones R, Darnley S, Seed P, Wessely S, Chalder T. Cognitive behaviour therapy in addition to antispasmodic treatment for irritable bowel syndrome in primary care: randomised controlled trial. *BMJ.* 2005;331(7514):435.

22. Ljótsson B, Falk L, Vesterlund AW, et al. Internet-delivered exposure and mindfulness based therapy for irritable bowel syndrome—a randomized controlled trial. *Behav Res Ther.* 2010;48(6):531-539.

23. Moss-Morris R, McAlpine L, Didsbury LP, Spence MJ. A randomized controlled trial of a cognitive behavioural therapy-based self-management intervention for irritable bowel syndrome in primary care. *Psychol Med.* 2010;40(1):85-94.

24. Boyce PM, Talley NJ, Balaam B, Koloski NA, Truman G. A randomized controlled trial of cognitive behavior therapy, relaxation training, and routine clinical care for the irritable bowel syndrome. *Am J Gastroenterol.* 2003;98(10):2209-2218.

25. Smith GD. Effect of nurse-led gut-directed hypnotherapy upon health-related quality of life in patients with irritable bowel syndrome. *J Clin Nurs.* 2006;15(6):678-684.

26. Houghton LA, Heyman DJ, Whorwell PJ. Symptomatology, quality of life and economic features of irritable bowel syndrome—the effect of hypnotherapy. *Aliment Pharmacol Ther.* 1996;10(1):91-95.

27. Lea R, Houghton LA, Calvert EL, et al. Gut-focused hypnotherapy normalizes disordered rectal sensitivity in patients with irritable bowel syndrome. *Aliment Pharmacol Ther.* 2003;17(5):635-642.

28. Whorwell PJ, Prior A, Faragher EB. Controlled trial of hypnotherapy in the treatment of severe refractory irritable-bowel syndrome. *Lancet.* 1984;2(8414):1232-1234.

29. Forbes A, MacAuley S, Chiotakakou-Faliakou E. Hypnotherapy and therapeutic audiotape: effective in previously unsuccessfully treated irritable bowel syndrome? *Int J Colorectal Dis.* 2000;15(5-6):328-334.

30. Gonsalkorale WM, Miller V, Afzal A, Whorwell PJ. Long term benefits of hypnotherapy for irritable bowel syndrome. *Gut.* 2003;52(11):1623-1629.

31. Whitehead WE. Hypnosis for irritable bowel syndrome: the empirical evidence of therapeutic effects. *Int J Clin Exp Hypn.* 2006;54(1):7-20.

32. Webb AN, Kukuruzovic RH, Catto-Smith AG, Sawyer SM. Hypnotherapy for treatment of irritable bowel syndrome. *Cochrane Database Syst Rev.* 2007;(4):CD005110.

33. Voirol MW, Hipolito J. Anthropo-analytical relaxation in irritable bowel syndrome: results 40 months later. *Schweiz Med Wochenschr.* 1987;117(29):1117-1119.

34. Blanchard EB, Greene B, Scharff L, Schwarz-McMorris SP. Relaxation training as a treatment for irritable bowel syndrome. *Biofeedback Self Regul.* 1993;18(3):125-132.

35. Keefer L, Blanchard EB. The effects of relaxation response meditation on the symptoms of irritable bowel syndrome: results of a controlled treatment study. *Behav Res Ther.* 2001;39(7):801-811.

36. Keefer L, Blanchard EB. A one year follow-up of relaxation response meditation as a treatment for irritable bowel syndrome. *Behav Res Ther.* 2002;40(5):541-546.

37. van der Veek PP, van Rood YR, Masclee AA. Clinical trial: short- and long-term benefit of relaxation training for irritable bowel syndrome. *Aliment Pharmacol Ther.* 2007;26(6):943-952.

38. Schwarz SP, Taylor AE, Scharff L, Blanchard EB. Behaviorally treated irritable bowel syndrome patients: a four-year follow-up. *Behav Res Ther.* 1990;28(4):331-335.

39. Guthrie E, Creed F, Dawson D, Tomenson B. A controlled trial of psychological treatment for the irritable bowel syndrome. *Gastroenterology.* 1991;100(2):450-457.

40. Heymann-Mönnikes I, Arnold R, Florin I, Herda C, Melfsen S, Mönnikes H. The combination of medical treatment plus multicomponent behavioral therapy is superior to medical treatment alone in the therapy of irritable bowel syndrome. *Am J Gastroenterol.* 2000;95(4):981-994.

41. Blanchard EB, Schwarz SP, Suls JM, et al. Two controlled evaluations of multicomponent psychological treatment of irritable bowel syndrome. *Behav Res Ther.* 1992;30(2):175-189.

42. Shaw G, Srivastava ED, Sadlier M, Swann P, James JY, Rhodes J. Stress management for irritable bowel syndrome: a controlled trial. *Digestion.* 1991;50(1):36-42.

43. Ford AC, Talley NJ, Schoenfeld PS, Quigley EM, Moayyedi P. Efficacy of antidepressants and psychological therapies in irritable bowel syndrome: systematic review and meta-analysis. *Gut.* 2009;58(3):367-378.

44. McKernan DP, Fitzgerald P, Dinan TG, Cryan JF. The probiotic *Bifidobacterium infantis* 35624 displays visceral antinociceptive effects in the rat. *Neurogastroenterol Motil.* 2010;22(9):1029-1035, e268.

45. Kajander K, Myllyluoma E, Rajilic-Stojanovic M, et al. Clinical trial: multispecies probiotic supplementation alleviates the symptoms of irritable bowel syndrome and stabilizes intestinal microbiota. *Aliment Pharmacol Ther.* 2008;27(1):48-57.

46. Kajander K, Krogius-Kurikka L, Rinttilä T, et al. Effects of multispecies probiotic supplementation on intestinal microbiota in irritable bowel syndrome. *Aliment Pharmacol Ther.* 2007;26(3):463-473.

47. Whorwell PJ, Altringer L, Morel J, et al. Efficacy of an encapsulated probiotic *Bifidobacterium infantis* 35624 in women with irritable bowel syndrome. *Am J Gastroenterol.* 2006;101(7):1581-1590.

48. O'Mahony L, McCarthy J, Kelly P, et al. *Lactobacillus* and *Bifidobacterium* in irritable bowel syndrome: symptom responses and relationship to cytokine profiles. *Gastroenterology.* 2005;128(3):541-551.

49. Guyonnet D, Chassany O, Ducrotte P, et al. Effect of a fermented milk containing *Bifidobacterium animalis* DN-173 010 on the health-related quality of life and symptoms in irritable bowel syndrome in adults in primary care: a multicentre, randomized, double-blind, controlled trial. *Aliment Pharmacol Ther*. 2007;26(3):475-486.

50. Drouault-Holowacz S, Bieuvelet S, Burckel A, Cazaubiel M, Dray X, Marteau P. A double blind randomized controlled trial of a probiotic combination in 100 patients with irritable bowel syndrome. *Gastroenterol Clin Biol*. 2008;32(2):147-152.

51. Niv E, Naftali T, Hallak R, Vaisman N. The efficacy of *Lactobacillus reuteri* ATCC 55730 in the treatment of patients with irritable bowel syndrome--a double blind, placebo-controlled, randomized study. *Clin Nutr*. 2005;24(6):925-931.

52. Guandalini S, Magazzù G, Chiaro A, et al. VSL#3 improves symptoms in children with irritable bowel syndrome: a multicenter, randomized, placebo-controlled, double-blind, crossover study. *J Pediatr Gastroenterol Nutr*. 2010;51(1):24-30.

53. Quigley EM. The efficacy of probiotics in IBS. *J Clin Gastroenterol*. 2008;42(Suppl 2):S85-S90.

54. Moayyedi P, Ford AC, Talley NJ, et al. The efficacy of probiotics in the treatment of irritable bowel syndrome: a systematic review. *Gut*. 2010;59(3):325-332.

55. Hunter JO, Tuffnell Q, Lee AJ. Controlled trial of oligofructose in the management of irritable bowel syndrome. *J Nutr*. 1999;129(7 Suppl):1451S-3S.

56. Ford AC, Talley NJ, Spiegel BM, et al. Effect of fibre, antispasmodics, and peppermint oil in the treatment of irritable bowel syndrome: systematic review and meta-analysis. *BMJ*. 2008;337:a2313.

57. Bijkerk CJ, Muris JW, Knottnerus JA, Hoes AW, de Wit NJ. Systematic review: the role of different types of fibre in the treatment of irritable bowel syndrome. *Aliment Pharmacol Ther*. 2004;19(3):245-251.

58. American College of Gastroenterology Task Force on Irritable Bowel Syndrome, Brandt LJ, Chey WD, et al. An evidence-based position statement on the management of irritable bowel syndrome. *Am J Gastroenterol*. 2009;104(Supp 1):S1-S35.

59. Wu JC, Ziea ET, Lao L, et al. Effect of electroacupuncture on visceral hyperalgesia, serotonin and fos expression in an animal model of irritable bowel syndrome. *J Neurogastroenterol Motil*. 2010;16(3):306-314.

60. Chan J, Carr I, Mayberry JF. The role of acupuncture in the treatment of irritable bowel syndrome: a pilot study. *Hepatogastroenterology*. 1997;44(17):1328-1330.

61. Forbes A, Jackson S, Walter C, Quraishi S, Jacyna M, Pitcher M. Acupuncture for irritable bowel syndrome: a blinded placebo-controlled trial. *World J Gastroenterol*. 2005;11(26):4040-4044.

62. Huang ZD, Liang LA, Zhang WX. Acupuncture combined with massage for treatment of irritable bowel syndrome. *Zhongguo Zhen Jiu*. 2006;26(10):717-718.

63. Lim B, Manheimer E, Lao L, Ziea E, Wisniewski J, Liu J, Berman B. Acupuncture for treatment of irritable bowel syndrome. *Cochrane Database Syst Rev.* 2006;(4):CD005111.

64. Maneerattanaporn M, Chey WD. Acupuncture for irritable bowel syndrome: sham or the real deal? *Gastroenterology.* 2010;139(1):348-350, discussion 350-351.

65. Zuo XL, Li YQ, Li WJ, Guo YT, Lu XF, Li JM, Desmond PV. Alterations of food antigen-specific serum immunoglobulins G and E antibodies in patients with irritable bowel syndrome and functional dyspepsia. *Clin Exp Allergy.* 2007;37(6):823-830.

66. Dainese R, Galliani EA, De Lazzari F, Di Leo V, Naccarato R. Discrepancies between reported food intolerance and sensitization test findings in irritable bowel syndrome patients. *Am J Gastroenterol.* 1999;94(7):1892-1897.

67. Zar S, Benson MJ, Kumar D. Food-specific serum IgG4 and IgE titers to common food antigens in irritable bowel syndrome. *Am J Gastroenterol.* 2005;100(7):1550-1557.

68. Eswaran S, Tack J, Chey WD. Food: the forgotten factor in the irritable bowel syndrome. *Gastroenterol Clin North Am.* 2011;40(1):141-162.

69. Dear KL, Elia M, Hunter JO. Do interventions which reduce colonic bacterial fermentation improve symptoms of irritable bowel syndrome? *Dig Dis Sci.* 2005;50(4):758-766.

70. Atkinson W, Sheldon TA, Shaath N, Whorwell PJ. Food elimination based on IgG antibodies in irritable bowel syndrome: a randomised controlled trial. *Gut.* 2004;53(10):1459-1464.

71. Zar S, Mincher L, Benson MJ, Kumar D. Food-specific IgG4 antibody-guided exclusion diet improves symptoms and rectal compliance in irritable bowel syndrome. *Scand J Gastroenterol.* 2005;40(7):800-807.

72. Drisko J, Bischoff B, Hall M, McCallum R. Treating irritable bowel syndrome with a food elimination diet followed by food challenge and probiotics. *J Am Coll Nutr.* 2006;25(6):514-522.

73. Yang CM, Li YQ. The therapeutic effects of eliminating allergic foods according to food-specific IgG antibodies in irritable bowel syndrome. *Zhonghua Nei Ke Za Zhi.* 2007;46(8):641-643.

74. Stefanini GF, Saggioro A, Alvisi V, et al. Oral cromolyn sodium in comparison with elimination diet in the irritable bowel syndrome, diarrheic type. Multicenter study of 428 patients. *Scand J Gastroenterol.* 1995;30(6):535-541.

75. Ducrotte P, Dapoigny M, Bonaz B, Siproudhis L. Symptomatic efficacy of beidellitic montmorillonite in irritable bowel syndrome: a randomized, controlled trial. *Aliment Pharmacol Ther.* 2005;21(4):435-444.

76. Chang FY, Lu CL, Chen CY, Luo JC. Efficacy of dioctahedral smectite in treating patients of diarrhea-predominant irritable bowel syndrome. *J Gastroenterol Hepatol.* 2007;22(12):2266-2272.

77. Taneja I, Deepak KK, Poojary G, et al. Yogic versus conventional treatment in diarrhea-predominant irritable bowel syndrome: a randomized control study. *Appl Psychophysiol Biofeedback.* 2004;29(1):19-33.

78. Kuttner L, Chambers CT, Hardial J, et al. A randomized trial of yoga for adolescents with irritable bowel syndrome. *Pain Res Manag.* 2006;11(4):217-223.

79. Browning JE. Chiropractic distractive decompression in treating pelvic pain and multiple system pelvic organic dysfunction. *J Manipulative Physiol Ther.* 1989;12(4):265-274.

80. Wiberg JM, Nordsteen J, Nilsson N. The short-term effect of spinal manipulation in the treatment of infantile colic: a randomized controlled clinical trial with a blinded observer. *J Manipulative Physiol Ther.* 1999;22(8):517-522.

81. Olafsdottir E, Forshei S, Fluge G, Markestad T. Randomised controlled trial of infantile colic treated with chiropractic spinal manipulation. *Arch Dis Child.* 2001;84(2):138-141.

82. Riot FM, Goudet P, Mouraux JP, Cougard P. Levator ani syndrome, functional intestinal disorders and articular abnormalities of the pelvis, the place of osteopathic treatment. Presse Med. 2004;33(13):852-857.

Chapter

45 *Ulcerative Colitis*

KEY POINTS

○ Patients with inflammatory bowel disease (IBD) frequently have micronutrient deficiencies.

○ Probiotics are helpful in maintaining remission in ulcerative colitis (UC).

○ Turmeric is effective in maintaining remission in UC.

○ The role of omega-3 fatty acids appears to be modest at best.

Thirty percent to 60% of patients with IBD have been reported to use complementary and alternative medicine.[1] The relative prevalence of different therapies was as follows: homeopathy (55%), probiotics (43%), classical naturopathy (38%), *Boswellia serrata* extracts (36%), and acupuncture/traditional Chinese medicine (33%). Numerous other herbal remedies being used include slippery elm, fenugreek, devil's claw, Mexican yam, tormentil, and wei tong ning (a traditional Chinese medicine).

In this chapter we will focus primarily on UC, even though there is likely to be an overlap with Crohn's disease (CD). (CD is discussed in Chapter 46.)

PROBIOTICS

Alterations of intestinal flora, such as a reduction in the concentration of *bifidobacteria* and increase of *Bacteroides* species, are associated with the severity of UC. Infusions of human fecal flora in patients with IBD and IBS have shown promising results.

Probiotics in Adults

Multiple studies have documented beneficial effects of both oral and intrarectal probiotics for the management of UC, especially for maintaining remission.[2-12] Effective probiotics include *E coli Nissle 1917*,[2,3] *Bifidobacterium*,[7,8] and VSL#3.

Probiotics in Children

VSL#3 treatment of mild to moderate UC results in a remission rate of 56% and a combined remission/response rate of 61%, without any adverse events.[13] Children on VSL#3 achieve greater remission and suffer a lower relapse rate compared to placebo.[14]

The Sang et al meta-analysis concluded that probiotics are more effective than placebo in maintaining remission in UC.[15] Patients receiving *B bifidum* treatment have a lower recurrence rate of 0.25 (95% CI: 0.12 to 0.50) compared to those in the nonprobiotic group.

Probiotics in Acute Pouchitis

Studies on the use of probiotics in acute pouchitis have yielded mixed and largely disappointing results.[16,17]

Pouchitis Prophylaxis

Beneficial effects of probiotics for prophylaxis has been documented by multiple studies.[18-22] Effective probiotics include Cultura (TINE Dairies BA, Oslo, Norway), containing live *lactobacilli (La-5)* and *bifidobacteria (Bb-12)*,[18] *L rhamnosus GG*,[19] and VSL#3.[20-22]

Experts have concluded that there is level I evidence for use of the VSL#3 in preventing pouchitis, and level II evidence for this agent in preventing relapse in patients with UC.[23,24]

An expert panel led by Floch et al gave an "A" recommendation for use of probiotics for preventing and maintaining remission in pouchitis.[25] The authors maintained "B" recommendations in several other areas of treating IBD.

PREBIOTICS

Germinated Barley Foodstuff

Germinated barley foodstuff (GBF) enhances luminal butyrate production, a preferred source of nutrition by colonocytes. The efficacy of GBF in the treatment of UC was examined in a randomized, multicenter, open-controlled trial. The control group was given baseline anti-inflammatory therapy for 4 weeks. In the GBF-treated group, patients received 20 to 30 g GBF daily, in addition to the baseline treatment. The GBF-treated group showed a significant decrease in clinical activity index scores compared with the control group.[26] Similar positive results were seen in another study combining GBF with conventional treatment for UC.[27]

Soy and Bowman-Birk Inhibitor Concentrate

Bowman-Birk inhibitor concentrate, a soy extract with high protease inhibitor activity, is efficacious in the treatment of animal models of colitis in mice. Bowman-Birk inhibitor concentrate for 12 weeks in patients with active UC results in lower index scores compared to placebo.[28]

Psyllium

A 4-month placebo-controlled trial of ispaghula in patients with UC in remission demonstrated a significantly higher rate of improvement of GI symptoms (69%) compared to placebo (24%).

Plantago ovata *Seeds*

Dietary fiber supplementation with *P ovata* seeds ameliorates colonic damage in HLA-B27 transgenic rats. Oral treatment with *P ovata* seeds (10 g bid) plus mesalamine (500 mg tid) results in a treatment failure rate of 30%, compared to 40% in the *P ovata* seed alone group and 35% in the mesalamine alone group.[29]

Wheat Fiber

Wheat fiber decreases the concentration of bile acids in feces in patients with UC, suggesting that it may have beneficial effect in this condition.

Wheat Grass

A randomized, double-blind, placebo-controlled study examined the effect of wheat grass (*Triticum aestivum*) juice in active distal UC.[30] Treatment was associated with significant reductions in the overall disease activity index and in the severity of rectal bleeding.

Use of prebiotics is beneficial in maintaining remission in UC.

MIND-BODY THERAPIES[31-39]

Results of longitudinal studies indicate a significant stress-inflammation relationship when UC and CD are studied independently; however, the results are negative when subjects in both diseases are lumped together.[31]

Specialist nurse-delivered counseling packages result in higher mental health scores at 6 months compared to those undergoing routine follow-up visits.[32] Psychoeducational group intervention has beneficial effects on coping, feelings of competence, and health-related quality of life in adolescents with IBD.[33]

Relaxation training is successful in ameliorating pain in patients with UC.[34] A comprehensive lifestyle and psychological program improves the quality of life greater than the usual-care waiting control group.[35]

Other effective modalities to improve psychological well-being include CBT,[36] hypnosis,[37,38] and psychological counseling.[39]

PHYTOBOTANICAL THERAPIES

Aloe vera *Gel*

A vera gel, taken for 4 weeks, is safe and results in a clinical response more often than placebo; it also reduces the histological disease activity in UC.[40]

Ambrotose Complex and Advanced Ambrotose

Ambrotose Complex and Advanced Ambrotose (Mannatech, Fallbrook, CA) are plant-derived polysaccharide dietary supplements that include *A vera* gel, arabinogalactan, fucoidan, and rice starch. All of these have shown to inhibit inflammatory activity in animal models of colitis. These formulations reduce colitis scores in animal models of dextran sodium sulfate-induced colitis.

Betel Nut

A comparative study of Asians found that 13% of male UC patients regularly used betel nut compared to 20% among controls (p<0.05).[41]

Boswellia, *aka Frankincense*

Prophylactic administration of *Boswellia* and antifibrotic *Scutellaria* extracts improves the course of experimental colitis in some, but not all, models of experimental colitis.[42] *B serrata* extract is superior to placebo for the treatment of collagenous colitis.[43] *B serrata* (*Salai guggal*) gum resin preparation is as effective as conventional medical treatment in patients with UC.[44,45]

Preliminary clinical evidence suggests efficacy of *Boswellia* extracts in some autoimmune diseases, including rheumatoid arthritis, Crohn's disease, ulcerative colitis, and bronchial asthma.[46]

Chlorella

Dietary supplements derived from *Chlorella pyrenoidosa*, a unicellular fresh water green algae, are rich in proteins, vitamins, and minerals. Administration of *Chlorella* each day accelerates healing in UC patients.[47]

Cordia myxa

Cordia myxa fruit treatment protects against acetic acid-induced colitis in animals.

Curcumin

A randomized, double-blind, placebo-controlled, multicenter trial assessed the efficacy of curcumin as maintenance therapy in patients with UC.[48] Patients received 1 g curcumin (or placebo) after breakfast and 1 g after the evening meal, plus sulfasalazine or mesalamine for 6 months. The relapse rate in the curcumin group was 5% compared to 21% in the placebo group.

Dandelion

Dandelion (*T officinale*) has been used for heartburn and GI distress. One supplement containing *T officinale*, *Hipericum perforatum*, *M officinalis*, *Calendula officinalis*, and *F vulgare* has been studied for the treatment of colitis in humans.[49] Authors have found the treatment to be effective.

Evening Primrose Oil

An RCT found that evening primrose oil significantly improves stool consistency, compared to fish oil (MaxEPA) and placebo at 6 months, and this difference is maintained 3 months after treatment is discontinued.[50] There is no effect on stool frequency, rectal bleeding, or disease relapse, suggesting only a modest positive effect.

Ginkgo

G biloba extract protects against inflammatory damage in several models of experimental colitis in animals.[51]

Ginseng

American ginseng extract inhibits leukocyte activation and epithelial cell DNA damage in dextran sodium sulfate-induced colitis in mice.[52] It suppresses colitis via apoptosis of inflammatory cells.

Grape Seeds

Proanthocyanidins from grape seeds protect against trinitrobenzene sulfonic acid-induced colitis in animals.[53] Treatment enhances recovery as seen by increased body weight, as well as improved colonic damage scores.

Lemon Balm

Citrus fruits are rich in hesperidin, a flavanone-type flavonoid. Oral administration of hesperidin significantly decreases disease activity index in animal models of dextran sodium sulfate-induced colitis. Human studies of nutritional factors suggest a negative correlation of citrus fruits and IBD.[54,55] One report indicated that treatment using an herbal combination including *C aurantium* (*Carum carvi*) is effective in chronic colitis.[49]

Radix Scutellariae

Extracts from *R Scutellariae* (roots of *Scutellaria baicalensis Georgi*) form a part of many traditional Chinese prescriptions. It is effective in treating acute dextran sodium sulfate-induced colitis.

Tormentil

Tormentil extracts have antioxidant properties and are used as a complementary therapy for IBD. Tormentil extracts (1200 to 3000 mg/d for 3 weeks) reduces the clinical activity index in patients with active UC.[56]

Herbal Combinations

A polyherbal Ayurvedic formulation from an ancient Ayurvedic text contains 4 different drugs: Bilwa (*A marmelos*), Dhanyak (*Coriandrum sativum*), Musta (*Cyperus rotundus*), and Vala (*V zizanioides*). It suppresses inflammatory activity in experimental colitis in mice to the same degree as the controls receiving prednisolone. [57]

ACUPUNCTURE[58-61]

Lee et al conducted a review of systematic reviews on the clinical efficacy of moxibustion in UC.[59] They found that there was a favorable effect of moxibustion on the response rate, compared to conventional drug therapy (RR = 1.24, 95% CI: 1.11 to 1.38, p<0.01). At the same time, the authors concluded that because of poor quality of trials, current evidence is insufficient. Mu et al performed a meta-analysis on the therapeutic effect of acupuncture and moxibustion on UC, and concluded that the treatment is superior to that of Western medicine with better safety and less adverse reactions.[61]

ENEMA THERAPY

Bovine Colostrum Enemas

A double-blind RCT studied 14 patients with mild to moderately severe distal colitis who received a colostrum enema (100 mL of 10% solution) or placebo (albumin solution) bid for 4 weeks.[62] Both groups also received mesalazine. The intervention group showed a significant reduction in symptom score, as well as histological score, compared to the placebo.

Butyrate Enema

Butyrate enemas (60 mL, containing 100 mM of sodium butyrate) result in only minor effects on markers of inflammation and oxidative stress.[63] Such enemas may offer benefit in refractory cases, however.[64]

Chinese Enema Therapy

Retention enema and per-colonoscopic spraying of Zhikang Compound Liquid (ZKCL) in patients with UC results in total effective rate of 90.38%, compared to 64.71% in controls.[65] Likewise, retention enema with quick-acting Kuijie powder (QAKJP) is effective in 99% of cases, compared to 71% in sulfasalazine group; the recurrence rate being 5.3% and 20.0%, respectively.[66]

The effect of a combined retention enema using Chinese and Western drugs for treating UC was examined in an RCT.[67] The total effective rate in the intervention group was 96.7% compared to 73.3% in the controls.

Vitamin E

An open-label study in 15 patients with UC found that rectal administration of d-alpha tocopherol (800 U/d) results in a positive response in 12 of the 15 patients. It may represent a novel therapy for mild to moderately active UC.[68]

SUPPLEMENTS

Dehydroepiandrosterone

A case of the beneficial effect of dehydroepiandrosterone 200 mg/d for 8 weeks in chronic active pouchitis in a 35-year-old female patient has been reported.[69] A pilot study demonstrated that dehydroepiandrosterone (200 mg/d) is effective and safe in patients with refractory UC.[70]

Fish Oil and Omega-3 Fatty Acids[71-78]

Patients with IBD frequently suffer from polyunsaturated fatty acid deficiency. De Ley et al[75] conducted a Cochrane database review and included 6 studies in analysis. While one study showed benefit for inducing remission, some other studies demonstrated positive impact on secondary outcomes. The authors concluded that the evidence does not allow for a definitive conclusion regarding the efficacy of fish oil. Turner et al's[78] meta-analysis, however, concluded that while it is effective in acute colitis, there is no difference in relapse rate when fish oil is used in patients with UC in remission.

A dose of fish oil (0.18 g EPA/capsule) is 15 to 18 capsules per day. Compliance is a problem because of fishy odor in the breath.

Glucosamine

Salvatore et al[79] conducted a study of N-acetylglucosamine, a nutritional substrate for glycosaminoglycan synthesis in children (n = 12). Subjects received N-acetylglucosamine as adjunct therapy for severe treatment-resistant IBD. Eight of the children given treatment showed significant improvement while 4 required resection.

Melatonin

Melatonin reduces colonic lesions and improves colitis symptoms in multiple animal models of colitis and carcinogenesis.[80-82] Use of melatonin in UC has been reported.[83-85] In contrast, melatonin administration may trigger CD symptoms.[86]

Short-Chain Fatty Acids

Colonic mucin is increased by sodium butyrate, and this may contribute to enhanced colonic repair mechanisms. Controlled trials on the use of SCFA enemas in distal UC have shown mixed results. Butyrate enema treatment is limited by its unpleasant smell. Other SCFAs, especially in large amounts, may disrupt the intestinal barrier and have the potential to worsen. (Also see Butyrate Enema section on page 224.)

Muscovite

Muscovite is a common rock-forming mineral also known as *common mica*, *isinglass*, or *potash mica*. It is made up of aluminum and potassium. Rectal administration of muscovite improves macroscopic and microscopic histological scores of trinitrobenzene sulfonic acid-induced colitis.

VITAMINS AND MINERALS

Special attention should be paid to the nutritional status of patients with IBD.[87] Abnormalities of trace elements can be demonstrated in children with IBD, probably as a result of inadequate intake, reduced absorption, as well as increased intestinal losses. Patients with UC have higher levels of copper and zinc than do controls. Men with pancolitis have significantly lower selenium and higher copper levels than men with proctitis.

Zinc

Zinc supplementation ameliorates colonic damage in the dextran sodium sulfate-induced model of colitis. Oral zinc supplementation (300 mg zinc aspartate, equal to 60 mg elemental zinc per day) in patients with inactive to moderately active IBD has no effect on the histology score, plasma albumin levels, or the disease activity index of the patients.[88]

Caution About Iron Supplements

Patients with IBD frequently develop iron deficiency and are prescribed oral iron therapy. Oral iron can, in some cases, potentiate the severity of colitis. In cases of intolerance and during acute exacerbations, consider intravenous iron.

REFERENCES

1.   Joos S, Rosemann T, Szecsenyi J, et al. Use of complementary and alternative medicine in Germany—a survey of patients with IBD. *BMC Complement Altern Med.* 2006;6:19.

2.   Rembacken BJ, Snelling AM, Hawkey PM, Chalmers DM, Axon AT. Non-pathogenic *Escherichia coli* versus mesalazine for the treatment of UC: a randomised trial. *Lancet*. 1999;354(9179):635-639.

3.   Kruis W, Fric P, Pokrotnieks J, et al. Maintaining remission of ulcerative colitis with the probiotic *Escherichia coli Nissle 1917* is as effective as with standard mesalazine. *Gut*. 2004;53(11):1617-1623.

4.   Tursi A, Brandimarte G, Giorgetti GM, et al. Low-dose balsalazide plus a high-potency probiotic preparation is more effective than balsalazide alone or mesalazine in the treatment of acute mild-to-moderate ulcerative colitis. *Med Sci Monit*. 2004;10(11):PI126-131.

5.   Furrie E, Macfarlane S, Kennedy A, et al. Synbiotic therapy (*Bifidobacterium longum*/Synergy 1) initiates resolution of inflammation in patients with active ulcerative colitis: a randomised controlled pilot trial. *Gut*. 2005;54(2):242-249.

6.   Zocco MA, dal Verme LZ, Cremonini F, et al. Efficacy of *Lactobacillus GG* in maintaining remission of ulcerative colitis. *Aliment Pharmacol Ther*. 2006;23(11):1567-1574.

7.   Ishikawa H, Akedo I, Umesaki Y, et al. Randomized controlled trial of the effect of *bifidobacteria*-fermented milk on ulcerative colitis. *J Am Coll Nutr*. 2003;22(1):56-63.

8.   Kato K, Mizuno S, Umesaki Y, et al. Randomized placebo-controlled trial assessing the effect of *bifidobacteria*-fermented milk on active ulcerative colitis. *Aliment Pharmacol Ther*. 2004;20(10):1133-1141.

9.   Sood A, Midha V, Makharia GK, et al. The probiotic preparation, VSL#3 induces remission in patients with mild-to-moderately active ulcerative colitis. *Clin Gastroenterol Hepatol*. 2009;7(11):1202-1209.

10.   Fujimori S, Gudis K, Mitsui K, et al. A randomized controlled trial on the efficacy of synbiotic versus probiotic or prebiotic treatment to improve the quality of life in patients with ulcerative colitis. *Nutrition*. 2009;25(5):520-525.

11.   Matthes H, Krummenerl T, Giensch M, Wolff C, Schulze J. Clinical trial: probiotic treatment of acute distal ulcerative colitis with rectally administered *Escherichia coli Nissle 1917* (EcN). *BMC Complement Altern* Med. 2010;10:13.

12.   Tursi A, Brandimarte G, Papa A, et al. Treatment of relapsing mild-to-moderate ulcerative colitis with the probiotic VSL#3 as adjunctive to a standard pharmaceutical treatment: a double-blind, randomized, placebo-controlled study. *Am J Gastroenterol*. 2010;105(10):2218-2227.

13.   Huynh HQ, deBruyn J, Guan L, et al. Probiotic preparation VSL#3 induces remission in children with mild to moderate acute ulcerative colitis: a pilot study. *Inflamm Bowel Dis*. 2009;15(5):760-768.

14.   Miele E, Pascarella F, Giannetti E, Quaglietta L, Baldassano RN, Staiano A. Effect of a probiotic preparation (VSL#3) on induction and maintenance of remission in children with ulcerative colitis. *Am J Gastroenterol*. 2009;104(2):437-443.

15. Sang LX, Chang B, Zhang WL, Wu XM, Li XH, Jiang M. Remission induction and maintenance effect of probiotics on ulcerative colitis: a meta-analysis. *World J Gastroenterol.* 2010;16(15):1908-1915.

16. Kuisma J, Mentula S, Jarvinen H, Kahri A, Saxelin M, Farkkila M. Effect of *Lactobacillus rhamnosus* GG on ileal pouch inflammation and microbial flora. *Aliment Pharmacol Ther.* 2003;17(4):509-515.

17. Gionchetti P, Rizzello F, Morselli C, et al. High-dose probiotics for the treatment of active pouchitis. *Dis Colon Rectum.* 2007;50(12):2075-2082.

18. Laake KO, Bjørneklett A, Aamodt G, et al. Outcome of four weeks' intervention with probiotics on symptoms and endoscopic appearance after surgical reconstruction with a J-configurated ileal-pouch-anal-anastomosis in ulcerative colitis. *Scand J Gastroenterol.* 2005;40(1):43-51.

19. Gosselink MP, Schouten WR, van Lieshout LM, et al. Delay of the first onset of pouchitis by oral intake of the probiotic strain *Lactobacillus rhamnosus* GG. *Dis Colon Rectum.* 2004;47(6):876-884.

20. Mimura T, Rizzello F, Helwig U, et al. Once daily high dose probiotic therapy (VSL#3) for maintaining remission in recurrent or refractory pouchitis. *Gut.* 2004;53(1):108-114.

21. Gionchetti P, Rizzello F, Venturi A, et al. Oral bacteriotherapy as maintenance treatment in patients with chronic pouchitis: a double-blind, placebo-controlled trial. *Gastroenterology.* 2000;119(2):305-309.

22. Gionchetti P, Rizzello F, Helwig U, et al. Prophylaxis of pouchitis onset with probiotic therapy: a double-blind, placebo-controlled trial. *Gastroenterology.* 2003;124(5):1202-1209.

23. Elahi B, Nikfar S, Derakhshani S, Vafaie M, Abdollahi M. On the benefit of probiotics in the management of pouchitis in patients underwent ileal pouch anal anastomosis: a meta-analysis of controlled clinical trials. *Dig Dis Sci.* 2008;53(5):1278-1284.

24. Pham M, Lemberg DA, Day AS. Probiotics: sorting the evidence from the myths. *Med J Aust.* 2008;188(5):304-308.

25. Floch MH, Walker WA, Guandalini S, et al. Recommendations for probiotic use—2008. *J Clin Gastroenterol.* 2008;42(Suppl 2):S104-108.

26. Kanauchi O, Mitsuyama K, Homma T, et al. Treatment of ulcerative colitis patients by long-term administration of germinated barley foodstuff: multi-center open trial. *Int J Mol Med.* 2003;12(5):701-704.

27. Hanai H, Kanauchi O, Mitsuyama K, et al. Germinated barley foodstuff prolongs remission in patients with ulcerative colitis. *Int J Mol Med.* 2004;13(5):643-647.

28. Lichtenstein GR, Deren JJ, Katz S, Lewis JD, Kennedy AR, Ware JH. Bowman-Birk inhibitor concentrate: a novel therapeutic agent for patients with active ulcerative colitis. *Dig Dis Sci.* 2008;53(1):175-180.

29. Fernández-Bañares F, Hinojosa J, Sánchez-Lombraña JL, et al. Randomized clinical trial of *Plantago ovata* seeds (dietary fiber) as compared with mesalamine in maintaining remission in ulcerative colitis. Spanish Group for the Study of Crohn's Disease and Ulcerative Colitis (GETECCU). *Am J Gastroenterol.* 1999;94(2):427-433.

30. Ben-Arye E, Goldin E, Wengrower D, Stamper A, Kohn R, Berry E. Wheat grass juice in the treatment of active distal ulcerative colitis: a randomized double-blind placebo-controlled trial. *Scand J Gastroenterol.* 2002;37(4):444-449.

31. Maunder RG, Levenstein S. The role of stress in the development and clinical course of inflammatory bowel disease: epidemiological evidence. *Curr Mol Med.* 2008;8(4):247-252.

32. Belling R, McLaren S, Woods L. Specialist nursing interventions for inflammatory bowel disease. *Cochrane Database Syst Rev.* 2009;(4):CD006597.

33. Díaz Sibaja MA, Comeche Moreno MI, Mas Hesse B. Protocolized cognitive-behavioural group therapy for inflammatory bowel disease. *Rev Esp Enferm Dig.* 2007;99(10):593-598.

34. Shaw L, Ehrlich A. Relaxation training as a treatment for chronic pain caused by ulcerative colitis. *Pain.* 1987;29(3):287-293.

35. Elsenbruch S, Langhorst J, Popkirowa K, et al. Effects of mind-body therapy on quality of life and neuroendocrine and cellular immune functions in patients with ulcerative colitis. *Psychother Psychosom.* 2005;74(5):277-287.

36. Mussell M, Böcker U, Nagel N, Olbrich R, Singer MV. Reducing psychological distress in patients with inflammatory bowel disease by cognitive-behavioural treatment: exploratory study of effectiveness. *Scand J Gastroenterol.* 2003;38(7):755-762.

37. Mawdsley JE, Jenkins DG, Macey MG, Langmead L, Rampton DS. The effect of hypnosis on systemic and rectal mucosal measures of inflammation in ulcerative colitis. *Am J Gastroenterol.* 2008;103(6):1460-1469.

38. Miller V, Whorwell PJ. Treatment of inflammatory bowel disease: a role for hypnotherapy? *Int J Clin Exp Hypn.* 2008;56(3):306-317.

39. Wahed M, Corser M, Goodhand JR, Rampton DS. Does psychological counseling alter the natural history of inflammatory bowel disease? *Inflamm Bowel Dis.* 2010;16(4):664-669.

40. Langmead L, Feakins RM, Goldthorpe S, et al. Randomized, double-blind, placebo-controlled trial of oral *Aloe vera* gel for active ulcerative colitis. *Aliment Pharmacol Ther.* 2004;19(7):739-747.

41. Lee CN, Jayanthi V, McDonald B, Probert CS, Mayberry JF. Betel nut and smoking. Are they both protective in ulcerative colitis? A pilot study. *Arq Gastroenterol.* 1996;33(1):3-5.

42. Kiela PR, Midura AJ, Kuscuoglu N, et al. Effects of *Boswellia serrata* in mouse models of chemically induced colitis. *Am J Physiol Gastrointest Liver Physiol.* 2005;288(4):G798-808.

43. Madisch A, Miehlke S, Eichele O, et al. *Boswellia serrata* extract for the treatment of collagenous colitis. A double-blind, randomized, placebo-controlled, multicenter trial. *Int J Colorectal Dis.* 2007;22(12):1445-1451.

44. Gupta I, Parihar A, Malhotra P, et al. Effects of *Boswellia serrata* gum resin in patients with ulcerative colitis. *Eur J Med Res.* 1997;2(1):37-43.

45. Gupta I, Parihar A, Malhotra P, et al. Effects of gum resin of *Boswellia serrata* in patients with chronic colitis. *Planta Med.* 2001;67(5):391-395.

46. Ammon HP. Boswellic acids in chronic inflammatory diseases. *Planta Med.* 2006;72(12):1100-1116.

47. Merchant RE, Andre CA. A review of recent clinical trials of the nutritional supplement *Chlorella pyrenoidosa* in the treatment of fibromyalgia, hypertension, and ulcerative colitis. *Altern Ther Health Med.* 2001;7(3):79-91.

48. Hanai H, Iida T, Takeuchi K, et al. Curcumin maintenance therapy for ulcerative colitis: randomized, multicenter, double-blind, placebo-controlled trial. *Clin Gastroenterol Hepatol.* 2006;4(12):1502-1506.

49. Chakurski I, Matev M, Koichev A, Angelova I, Stefanov G. Treatment of chronic colitis with an herbal combination of *Taraxacum officinale, Hipericum perforatum, Melissa officinaliss, Calendula officinalis* and *Foeniculum vulgare. Vutr Boles.* 1981;20(6):51-54.

50. Greenfield SM, Green AT, Teare JP, et al. A randomized controlled study of evening primrose oil and fish oil in ulcerative colitis. *Aliment Pharmacol Ther.* 1993;7(2):159-166.

51. Zhou YH, Yu JP, Liu YF, et al. Effects of *Ginkgo biloba* extract on inflammatory mediators (SOD, MDA, TNF-alpha, NF-kappaBp65, IL-6) in TNBS-induced colitis in rats. *Mediators Inflamm.* 2006;2006(5):92642.

52. Jin Y, Kotakadi VS, Ying L, et al. American ginseng suppresses inflammation and DNA damage associated with mouse colitis. *Carcinogenesis.* 2008;29(12):2351-2359.

53. Wang YH, Yang XL, Wang L, et al. Effects of proanthocyanidins from grape seed on treatment of recurrent ulcerative colitis in rats. *Can J Physiol Pharmacol.* 2010;88(9):888-898.

54. Magee EA, Edmond LM, Tasker SM, Kong SC, Curno R, Cummings JH. Associations between diet and disease activity in ulcerative colitis patients using a novel method of data analysis. *Nutr J.* 2005;4:7.

55. Russel MG, Engels LG, Muris JW, et al. Modern life' in the epidemiology of inflammatory bowel disease: a case-control study with special emphasis on nutritional factors. *Eur J Gastroenterol Hepatol.* 1998;10(3):243-249.

56. Huber R, Ditfurth AV, Amann F, et al. Tormentil for active ulcerative colitis: an open-label, dose-escalating study. *J Clin Gastroenterol.* 2007;41(9):834-838.

57. Jagtap AG, Shirke SS, Phadke AS. Effect of polyherbal formulation on experimental models of inflammatory bowel diseases. *J Ethnopharmacol.* 2004;90(2-3):195-204.

58. Wang SM, Li XG, Zhang LQ, Xu YC, Li Q. Clinical study on drug-separated moxibustion at Shenque (CV 8) for treatment of ulcerative colitis. *Zhongguo Zhen Jiu.* 2006;26(2):97-99.

59. Lee MS, Kang JW, Ernst E. Does moxibustion work? An overview of systematic reviews. *BMC Res Notes.* 2010;3:284.

60. Joos S, Wildau N, Kohnen R, et al. Acupuncture and moxibustion in the treatment of ulcerative colitis: a randomized controlled study. *Scand J Gastroenterol.* 2006;41(9):1056-1063.

61. Mu JP, Wu HG, Zhang ZQ, et al. Meta-analysis on acupuncture and moxibustion for treatment of ulcerative colitis. *Zhongguo Zhen Jiu.* 2007;27(9):687-690.

62. Khan Z, Macdonald C, Wicks AC, et al. Use of the 'nutriceutical', bovine colostrum, for the treatment of distal colitis: results from an initial study. *Aliment Pharmacol Ther.* 2002;16(11):1917-1922.

63. Hamer HM, Jonkers DM, Vanhoutvin SA, et al. Effect of butyrate enemas on inflammation and antioxidant status in the colonic mucosa of patients with ulcerative colitis in remission. *Clin Nutr.* 2010;29(6):738-744.

64. Steinhart AH, Brzezinski A, Baker JP. Treatment of refractory ulcerative proctosigmoiditis with butyrate enemas. *Am J Gastroenterol.* 1994;89(2):179-183.

65. Zhang J, Zeng YF, Xiao BQ, Wang J, Zhao A. Treatment of ulcerative colitis by combined therapy of retention enema and per-colonoscopic spraying with zhikang capsule compound liquid. *Zhongguo Zhong Xi Yi Jie He Za Zhi.* 2005;25(9):839-842.

66. Zhou Q, Yu J, Gu S. Clinical and experimental study on treatment of retention enema for chronic non-specific ulcerative colitis with quick-acting kuijie powder. *Zhongguo Zhong Xi Yi Jie He Za Zhi.* 1999;19(7):395-398.

67. Wang XY, Wu Y, Jiang XM. Observation on curative effect of chronic ulcerative colitis treated by retention enema with combination of Chinese and Western drugs. *Zhongguo Zhong Xi Yi Jie He Za Zhi.* 2007;27(12):1123-115.

68. Mirbagheri SA, Nezami BG, Assa S, Hajimahmoodi M. Rectal administration of d-alpha tocopherol for active ulcerative colitis: a preliminary report. *World J Gastroenterol.* 2008;14(39):5990-5995.

69. Klebl FH, Bregenzer N, Rogler G, Straub RH, Schölmerich J, Andus T. Treatment of pouchitis with dehydroepiandrosterone (DHEA)—a case report. *Z Gastroenterol.* 2003;41(11):1087-1090.

70. Andus T, Klebl F, Rogler G, Bregenzer N, Schölmerich J, Straub RH. Patients with refractory Crohn's disease or ulcerative colitis respond to dehydroepiandrosterone: a pilot study. *Aliment Pharmacol Ther.* 2003;17(3):409-414.

71. Salomon P, Kornbluth AA, Janowitz HD. Treatment of ulcerative colitis with fish oil n-3-omega-fatty acid: an open trial. *J Clin Gastroenterol.* 1990;12(2):157-161.

72. Aslan A, Triadafilopoulos G. Fish oil fatty acid supplementation in active ulcerative colitis: a double-blind, placebo-controlled, crossover study. *Am J Gastroenterol.* 1992;87(4):432-437.

73. Stenson WF, Cort D, Rodgers J, et al. Dietary supplementation with fish oil in ulcerative colitis. *Ann Intern Med.* 1992;116(8):609-614.

74. Dichi I, Frenhane P, Dichi JB, et al. Comparison of omega-3 fatty acids and sulfasalazine in ulcerative colitis. *Nutrition*. 2000;16(2):87-90.

75. De Ley M, de Vos R, Hommes DW, Stokkers P. Fish oil for induction of remission in ulcerative colitis. *Cochrane Database Syst Rev*. 2007;(4):CD005986.

76. Middleton SJ, Naylor S, Woolner J, Hunter JO. A double-blind, random-ized, placebo-controlled trial of essential fatty acid supplementation in the maintenance of remission of ulcerative colitis. *Aliment Pharmacol Ther*. 2002;16(6):1131-1135.

77. Loeschke K, Ueberschaer B, Pietsch A, et al. N-3 fatty acids only delay early relapse of ulcerative colitis in remission. *Dig Dis Sci*. 1996;41(10):2087-2094.

78. Turner D, Shah PS, Steinhart AH, Zlotkin S, Griffiths AM. Maintenance of remission in inflammatory bowel disease using omega-3 fatty acids (fish oil): a systematic review and meta-analyses. *Inflamm Bowel Dis*. 2011;17(1):336-345.

79. Salvatore S, Heuschkel R, Tomlin S, et al. A pilot study of N-acetyl glu-cosamine, a nutritional substrate for glycosaminoglycan synthesis, in paediatric chronic inflammatory bowel disease. *Aliment Pharmacol Ther*. 2000;14(12):1567-1579.

80. Tahan G, Gramignoli R, Marongiu F, et al. Melatonin expresses power-ful anti-inflammatory and antioxidant activities resulting in complete improvement of acetic-acid-induced colitis in rats. *Dig Dis Sci*. 2011;56(3):715-720.

81. Pentney PT, Bubenik GA. Melatonin reduces the severity of dextran-induced colitis in mice. *J Pineal Res*. 1995;19(1):31-39.

82. Tanaka T, Yasui Y, Tanaka M, Tanaka T, Oyama T, Rahman KM. Melatonin suppresses AOM/DSS-induced large bowel oncogenesis in rats. *Chem Biol Interact*. 2009;177(2):128-136.

83. Maldonado MD, Calvo JR. Melatonin usage in ulcerative colitis: a case report. *J Pineal Res*. 2008;45(3):339-340.

84. Boznanska P, Wichan P, Stepien A, et al. 24-hour urinary 6-hydrox-ymelatonin sulfate excretion in patients with ulcerative colitis. *Pol Merkur Lekarski*. 2007;22(131):369-372.

85. Terry PD, Villinger F, Bubenik GA, Sitaraman SV. Melatonin and ulcer-ative colitis: evidence, biological mechanisms, and future research. *Inflamm Bowel Dis*. 2009;15(1):134-140.

86. Calvo JR, Guerrero JM, Osuna C, Molinero P, Carrillo-Vico A. Melatonin triggers Crohn's disease symptoms. *J Pineal Res*. 2002;32(4):277-278.

87. Goh J, O'Morain CA. Review article: nutrition and adult inflammatory bowel disease. *Aliment Pharmacol Ther*. 2003;17(3):307-320.

88. Mulder TP, van der Sluys Veer A, Verspaget HW, et al. Effect of oral zinc supplementation on metallothionein and superoxide dismutase con-centrations in patients with inflammatory bowel disease. *J Gastroenterol Hepatol*. 1994;9(5):472-477.

Chapter

46 *Crohn's Disease*

KEY POINTS

- ○ Clinical studies using probiotics have been disappointing.
- ○ Acupuncture may be of benefit.
- ○ Patients with Crohn's disease (CD) should be screened for micronutrient deficiencies.
- ○ Data supporting the use of complementary and alternative medicine in CD are scanty.

PROBIOTICS[1]

A dysfunctional mucosal barrier[2] with or without an alteration of bacterial composition has the potential to allow luminal bacterial antigens to initiate the chronic inflammatory cascade in CD.

Studies using probiotics in CD have largely been disappointing.[3-9] Probiotics studied include *Lactobacillus johnsonii, L GG,* and *S boulardii.* Butterworth et al used a Cochrane database review[9] and concluded that there is insufficient evidence to make any conclusions about the efficacy of probiotics for induction of remission in CD. A recent meta-analysis of studies concluded that the probiotics do not reduce the risk of postoperative recurrence, compared to placebo.[10]

MIND-BODY MEDICINE

Psychotherapy

Psychotherapy does not have an impact on the course of CD, although patients with psychological issues may benefit from it.[11-14]

ACUPUNCTURE

Limited evidence supports the use of acupuncture in CD.[15,16] Schneider et al, in a systematic review, concluded that real acupuncture is superior to sham acupuncture in improving disease activity.[16]

SUPPLEMENTS

Dehydroepiandrosterone

Dehydroepiandrosterone sulfate concentrations are decreased in patients with IBD. A pilot study reported that dehydroepiandrosterone is effective and safe in patients with refractory CD or UC.[17]

Melatonin

Melatonin has been reported to trigger CD symptoms. Preliminary data regarding the utility of melatonin in the treatment of CD are ambiguous or negative.

Omega-3 Fatty Acids[18-23]

Turner et al's meta-analysis concluded that there was a statistically significant advantage for omega-3 fatty acids in CD.[21] However, the studies were heterogeneous and, therefore, there are insufficient data to make a firm recommendation about its use.

Glucosamine

Abnormalities in colonic glycoprotein synthesis have been implicated in the pathogenesis of IBD. N-acetylglucosamine is incorporated into glycosaminoglycans and glycoproteins and may lead to enhanced tissue repair mechanisms. A pilot study reported that children with IBD, when given N-acetylglucosamine, show clinical as well as histological improvement.[24]

Glutamine

Glutamine-enriched enteral diets decrease intestinal damage and disease activity while improving nitrogen balance in animal models of IBD. However, clinical data in humans have been disappointing.[25,26]

Short-Chain Fatty Acids

Intestinal biopsies from CD patients were examined with and without exposure to butyric acid. Treatment resulted in decreased TNF-alpha, providing a plausible mechanism for its potential use in CD. An open-label study found that the use of enteric-coated butyrate (4 g/d for 8 weeks) results in improvement in 69% of the patients, including 53% who achieved remission.[27]

Colostrum

Administration of multiple nutraceuticals, consisting of fish peptides, bovine colostrum, boswellia serrata, curcumin, and a multivitamin, probiotics and recombinant human GH (rhGH) along with exclusion of dairy products, certain grains, and carrageenan-containing foods, results in prolonged remission and restoration of weight in subjects with CD.[28] There is a lack of data for its use alone in CD.

Insulin-Like Growth Factor-1

Low serum levels of insulin-like growth factor-1 have been implicated in growth stunting in pediatric CD. There is a lack of evidence documenting its beneficial role in patients.

Vitamins and Minerals[29-31]

A majority of patients with CD demonstrate low plasma concentrations of vitamin C (84%), copper (84%), niacin (77%), and zinc (65%). Although most patients with IBD (74%) are well nourished, there is a decrease in body cell mass as well as handgrip strength in patients with CD and UC, compared to controls.[29] Serum selenium and zinc levels are lower, and serum copper levels are higher in patients with CD.[31] In contrast, men and women with UC have higher levels of copper and zinc than did controls. Zinc supplementation tightens "leaky gut" in CD, as measured by lactulose/mannitol ratio, and potentially can reduce relapse.[32]

HERBAL THERAPIES

There is a huge overlap between UC and CD, especially in experimental evidence related to herbal therapies.

Cat's Claw

Uncaria tomentosa, also known as cat's claw, has been used to treat chronic disorders including IBD and arthritis since ancient times. There is a lack of data for its use in CD.

Curcumin (Turmeric)

Human studies for its use in CD are lacking.[33]

Berberine

Berberine is an active constituent of several botanicals. It protects against experimental colonic tissue damage in animal models of colitis. There is a lack of human studies.

Boswellia

Results of studies in animals[34] as well as human CD have been mixed.[35,36]

Lemon Balm

A case-controlled study of nutritional factors found a negative correlation of citrus fruits and CD.[37]

ELIMINATION DIETS

Food sensitivities have been implicated in the pathogenesis of CD. Similarly, high FODMAP diets have been implicated in the rise of CD and celiac disease in recent times. Results using elimination diets in CD have been mixed.[38-40]

Patients may identify potential symptom-provoking foods using a food-symptom diary, and then try elimination diets for 2 to 4 weeks at a time to see if any part of the elimination diet is helpful. On the other hand, adopting a Six Food Elimination Diet or the FODMAP diet (see Chapter 10) globally might be an easier strategy, with a greater chance for success and compliance, and may be undertaken as the first step.

REFERENCES

1. Reiff C, Kelly D. Inflammatory bowel disease, gut bacteria and probiotic therapy. *Int J Med Microbiol.* 2010;300(1):25-33.

2. Hering NA, Schulzke JD. Therapeutic options to modulate barrier defects in inflammatory bowel disease. *Dig Dis.* 2009;27(4):450-454.

3. Van Gossum A, Dewit O, Louis E, et al. Multicenter randomized-controlled clinical trial of probiotics (*Lactobacillus johnsonii*, LA1) on early endoscopic recurrence of Crohn's disease after ileo-caecal resection. *Inflamm Bowel Dis.* 2007;13(2):135-142.

4. Prantera C, Scribano ML, Falasco G, Andreoli A, Luzi C. Ineffectiveness of probiotics in preventing recurrence after curative resection for Crohn's disease: a randomised controlled trial with Lactobacillus GG. *Gut.* 2002;51(3):405-409.

5. Garcia Vilela E, De Lourdes De Abreu Ferrari M, Oswaldo Da Gama Torres H, et al. Influence of *Saccharomyces boulardii* on the intestinal permeability of patients with Crohn's disease in remission. *Scand J Gastroenterol.* 2008;43(7):842-848.

6. Guslandi M, Mezzi G, Sorghi M, Testoni PA. *Saccharomyces boulardii* in maintenance treatment of Crohn's disease. *Dig Dis Sci.* 2000;45(7):1462-1464.

7. Plein K, Hotz J. Therapeutic effects of *Saccharomyces boulardii* on mild residual symptoms in a stable phase of Crohn's disease with special respect to chronic diarrhea—a pilot study. *Z Gastroenterol.* 1993;31:129-134.

8. Malin M, Suomalainen H, Saxelin M, Isolauri E. Promotion of IgA immune response in patients with Crohn's disease by oral bacteriotherapy with *Lactobacillus GG. Ann Nutr Metab.* 1996;40(3):137-145.

9. Butterworth AD, Thomas AG, Akobeng AK. Probiotics for induction of remission in Crohn's disease. *Cochrane Database Syst Rev.* 2008;(3):CD006634.

10. Doherty GA, Bennett GC, Cheifetz AS, Moss AC. Meta-analysis: targeting the intestinal microbiota in prophylaxis for post-operative Crohn's disease. *Aliment Pharmacol Ther.* 2010;31(8):802-809.

11. Wahed M, Corser M, Goodhand JR, Rampton DS. Does psychological counseling alter the natural history of inflammatory bowel disease? *Inflamm Bowel Dis.* 2010;16(4):664-669.

12. Deter HC, Keller W, von Wietersheim J, et al; German Study Group on Psychosocial Intervention in Crohn's Disease. Psychological treatment may reduce the need for healthcare in patients with Crohn's disease. *Inflamm Bowel Dis.* 2007;13(6):745-752.

13. von Wietersheim J, Scheib P, Keller W, et al. The effects of psychotherapy on Crohn's disease patients—results of a randomized multicenter study. *Psychother Psychosom Med Psychol.* 2001;51(1):2-9.

14. Keller W, Pritsch M, Von Wietersheim J, et al; German Study Group on Psychosocial Intervention in Crohn's Disease. Effect of psychotherapy and relaxation on the psychosocial and somatic course of Crohn's disease: main results of the German Prospective Multicenter Psychotherapy Treatment study on Crohn's disease. *J Psychosom Res.* 2004;56(6):687-696.

15. Joos S, Brinkhaus B, Maluche C, et al. Acupuncture and moxibustion in the treatment of active Crohn's disease: a randomized controlled study. *Digestion.* 2004;69(3):131-139.

16. Schneider A, Streitberger K, Joos S. Acupuncture treatment in gastrointestinal diseases: a systematic review. *World J Gastroenterol.* 2007;13:3417-3424.

17. Andus T, Klebl F, Rogler G, Bregenzer N, Schölmerich J, Straub RH. Patients with refractory Crohn's disease or ulcerative colitis respond to dehydroepiandrosterone: a pilot study. *Aliment Pharmacol Ther.* 2003;17(3):409-414.

18. Romano C, Cucchiara S, Barabino A, Annese V, Sferlazzas C. Usefulness of omega-3 fatty acid supplementation in addition to mesalazine in maintaining remission in pediatric Crohn's disease: a double-blind, randomized, placebo-controlled study. *World J Gastroenterol.* 2005;11:7118-7121.

19. Lorenz-Meyer H, Bauer P, Nicolay C, et al. Omega-3 fatty acids and low carbohydrate diet for maintenance of remission in Crohn's disease. A randomized controlled multicenter trial. Study Group Members (German Crohn's Disease Study Group. *Scand J Gastroenterol.* 1996;31(8):778-785.

20. Feagan BG, Sandborn WJ, Mittmann U, et al. Omega-3 free fatty acids for the maintenance of remission in Crohn disease: the EPIC Randomized Controlled Trials. *JAMA.* 2008;299(14):1690-1697.

21. Turner D, Shah PS, Steinhart AH, Zlotkin S, Griffiths AM. Maintenance of remission in inflammatory bowel disease using omega-3 fatty acids (fish oil): a systematic review and meta-analyses. *Inflamm Bowel Dis.* 2011;17(1):336-345.

22. Bjørkkjaer T, Brunborg LA, Arslan G, et al. Reduced joint pain after short-term duodenal administration of seal oil in patients with inflammatory bowel disease: comparison with soy oil. *Scand J Gastroenterol.* 2004;39(11):1088-1094.

23. Brunborg LA, Madland TM, Lind RA, et al. Effects of short-term oral administration of dietary marine oils in patients with inflammatory bowel disease and joint pain: a pilot study comparing seal oil and cod liver oil. *Clin Nutr.* 2008;27(4):614-622.

24. Salvatore S, Heuschkel R, Tomlin S, et al. A pilot study of N-acetyl glucosamine, a nutritional substrate for glycosaminoglycan synthesis, in paediatric chronic inflammatory bowel disease. *Aliment Pharmacol Ther.* 2000;14(12):1567-1579.

25. Akobeng AK, Miller V, Thomas AG, Richmond K. Glutamine supplementation and intestinal permeability in Crohn's disease. *J Parenter Enteral Nutr.* 2000;24(3):196.

26. Akobeng AK, Miller V, Stanton J, Elbadri AM, Thomas AG. Double-blind randomized controlled trial of glutamine-enriched polymeric diet in the treatment of active Crohn's disease. *J Pediatr Gastroenterol Nutr.* 2000;30(1):78-84.

27. Di Sabatino A, Morera R, Ciccocioppo R, et al. Oral butyrate for mildly to moderately active Crohn's disease. *Aliment Pharmacol Ther.* 2005;22(9):789-794.

28. AE, Grovit M, Bulone L. Effect of exclusion diet with nutraceutical therapy in juvenile Crohn's disease. *J Am Coll Nutr.* 2009;28(3):277-285.

29. Valentini L, Schaper L, Buning C, et al. Malnutrition and impaired muscle strength in patients with Crohn's disease and ulcerative colitis in remission. *Nutrition.* 2008;24(7-8):694-702.

30. Younes-Mhenni S, Derex L, Berruyer M, et al. Large-artery stroke in a young patient with Crohn's disease. Role of vitamin B_6 deficiency-induced hyperhomocysteinemia. *J Neurol Sci.* 2004;221(1-2):113-115.

31. Ringstad J, Kildebo S, Thomassen Y. Serum selenium, copper, and zinc concentrations in Crohn's disease and ulcerative colitis. *Scand J Gastroenterol.* 1993;28(7):605-608.

32. Sturniolo GC, Di Leo V, Ferronato A, D'Odorico A, D'Incà R. Zinc supplementation tightens "leaky gut" in Crohn's disease. *Inflamm Bowel Dis.* 2001;7(2):94-98.

33. Sugimoto K, Hanai H, Tozawa K, et al. Curcumin prevents and ameliorates trinitrobenzene sulfonic acid-induced colitis in mice. *Gastroenterology.* 2002;123(6):1912-1922.

34. Kiela PR, Midura AJ, Kuscuoglu N, et al. Effects of *Boswellia serrata* in mouse models of chemically induced colitis. *Am J Physiol Gastrointest Liver Physiol.* 2005;288(4):G798-808.

35. Gerhardt H, Seifert F, Buvari P, Vogelsang H, Repges R. Therapy of active Crohn disease with *Boswellia serrata* extract H 15. *Z Gastroenterol.* 2001;39(1):11-17.

36. Holtmeier W, Zeuzem S, Preiss J, et al. Randomized, placebo-controlled, double-blind trial of *Boswellia serrata* in maintaining remission of Crohn's disease: good safety profile but lack of efficacy. *Inflamm Bowel Dis.* 2011;17(2):573-582.

37. Russel MG, Engels LG, Muris JW, et al. Modern life' in the epidemiology of inflammatory bowel disease: a case-control study with special emphasis on nutritional factors. *Eur J Gastroenterol Hepatol.* 1998;10(3):243-249.

38. Heaton KW, Thornton JR, Emmett PM. Treatment of Crohn's disease with an unrefined-carbohydrate, fibre-rich diet. *BMJ.* 1979;2(6193):764-766.

39. Jones VA, Dickinson RJ, Workman E, et al. Crohn's disease: maintenance of remission by diet. *Lancet.* 1985;2(8448):177-180.

40. Ritchie JK, Wadsworth J, Lennard-Jones JE, Rogers E. Controlled multicentre therapeutic trial of an unrefined carbohydrate, fibre rich diet in Crohn's disease. *BMJ (Clin Res Ed).* 1987;295(6597):517-520.

Chapter 47 *Role of Probiotics in Diarrhea*

KEY POINTS

○ Probiotics are effective for the primary and secondary prevention of acute gastroenteritis in children.

○ Taken along with hydration therapy, probiotics reduce stool frequency and the duration of diarrhea in children.

○ Probiotics reduce the risk of traveler's diarrhea, as well as chemoradiation-induced diarrhea.

PREVENTING ACUTE DIARRHEA

Preventing Necrotizing Enterocolitis

A Cochrane database review concluded that enteral supplementation of probiotics reduces the risk of severe necrotizing enterocolitis and mortality in preterm infants.[1]

Preventing Infections in Day Care Facilities

Multiple studies have documented the beneficial effects of probiotics[2,3] in preventing infections in day care. Probiotics studied include formula supplemented with *B lactis (BB-12), L reuteri,* as well as milk products containing probiotics and prebiotics (Curtin University Probiotics in Daycare [CUPDAY] Milk).[3]

PREVENTING TRAVELER'S DIARRHEA

McFarland's meta-analysis concluded that probiotics result in significant reduction of relative risk of traveler's diarrhea, and that several probiotics *(S boulardii* and a mixture of *L acidophilus* and *B bifidum)* are effective for this indication.[4]

PREVENTING RADIATION-INDUCED DIARRHEA[5-7]

Most management strategies are based on anecdotal evidence or case series.

Delia et al conducted a double-blind, placebo-controlled trial to investigate the efficacy of VSL#3 on the prevention of radiation-induced diarrhea in cancer patients.[5] There was higher incidence of radiation-induced diarrhea in the placebo group compared to VSL#3 patients (51.8% versus 31.6%). Other studies using *L casei DN-114 001* or *L acidophilus* plus *B bifidum* have reported similar positive results.[6,7]

PREVENTING FEEDING TUBE DIARRHEA[8-10]

Several experts have recommended the use of pre- and/or probiotics in feeding formula.[8] Bleichner et al studied 128 patients on enteral tube feeding in a prospective, randomized, placebo-controlled fashion.[9] Treatment with *S boulardii* reduced the mean percentage of days with diarrhea per feeding days from 18.9% to 14.2% (p<0.01). Beneficial results have also been documented using VSL#3.[10]

PREVENTING CHEMOTHERAPY-INDUCED DIARRHEA

VSL#3 is effective in reducing chemotherapy-induced diarrhea in rats.[11] Compared to controls, patients consuming *L rhamnosus GG* and fiber during chemotherapy have lesser grade (3 or 4) diarrhea, less abdominal discomfort, and fewer chemotherapy dose reductions due to bowel toxicity.[12]

Evidence indicates that probiotics reduce the risk, as well as severity, of diarrhea associated with tube feeding, radiation therapy, and/or chemotherapy.

PREVENTING DIARRHEA IN NURSING HOMES

A randomized, double-blind, placebo-controlled trial conducted in 2 nursing homes in Finland assessed the impact of fermented oat drink containing *B longum* on bowel movements among elderly nursing home residents.[13] Probiotic use helped normalize bowel movements in frail nursing home patients.

Evidence on the beneficial effect of probiotics in preventing diarrhea is accumulating. Trials of probiotics, singly or as part of various combinations including *S boulardii*, *L rhamnosus GG*, and *L acidophilus*, may be worth the cost in many cases (depending upon the indication and the product used).

REFERENCES

1. Alfaleh K, Anabrees J, Bassler D, Al-Kharfi T. Probiotics for prevention of necrotizing enterocolitis in preterm infants. *Cochrane Database Syst* Rev. 2011;3:CD005496.

2. Weizman Z, Asli G, Alsheikh A. Effect of a probiotic infant formula on infections in child care centers: comparison of two probiotic agents. *Pediatrics.* 2005;115(1):5-9.

3. Binns CW, Lee AH, Harding H, Gracey M, Barclay DV. The CUPDAY Study: prebiotic-probiotic milk product in 1-3-year-old children attending childcare centres. *Acta Paediatr.* 2007;96(11):1646-1650.

4. McFarland LV. Meta-analysis of probiotics for the prevention of traveler's diarrhea. *Travel Med Infect Dis.* 2007;5(2):97-105.

5. Delia P, Sansotta G, Donato V, et al. Use of probiotics for prevention of radiation-induced diarrhea. *World J Gastroenterol.* 2007;13(6):912-915.

6. Giralt J, Regadera JP, Verges R, et al. Effects of probiotic *Lactobacillus casei DN-114 001* in prevention of radiation-induced diarrhea: results from multicenter, randomized, placebo-controlled nutritional trial. *Int J Radiat Oncol Biol Phys.* 2008;71(4):1213-1219.

7. Chitapanarux I, Chitapanarux T, Traisathit P, et al. Randomized controlled trial of live *Lactobacillus acidophilus* plus *Bifidobacterium bifidum* in prophylaxis of diarrhea during radiotherapy in cervical cancer patients. *Radiat Oncol.* 2010;5:31.

8. Dobb GJ. Diarrhoea in the critically ill. *Intensive Care Med.* 1986;12(3):113-115.

9. Bleichner G, Bléhaut H, Mentec H, Moyse D. *Saccharomyces boulardii* prevents diarrhea in critically ill tube-fed patients. A multicenter, randomized, double-blind placebo-controlled trial. *Intensive Care Med.* 1997;23(5):517-523.

10. Frohmader TJ, Chaboyer WP, Robertson IK, Gowardman J. Decrease in frequency of liquid stool in enterally fed critically ill patients given the multispecies probiotic VSL#3: a pilot trial. *Am J Crit Care.* 2010;19(3):e1-11.

11. Bowen JM, Stringer AM, Gibson RJ, Yeoh AS, Hannam S, Keefe DM. VSL#3 probiotic treatment reduces chemotherapy-induced diarrhea and weight loss. *Cancer Biol Ther.* 2007;6(9):1449-1454.

12. Osterlund P, Ruotsalainen T, Korpela R, et al. *Lactobacillus* supplementation for diarrhoea related to chemotherapy of colorectal cancer: a randomised study. *Br J Cancer.* 2007;97(8):1028-1034.

13. Pitkala KH, Strandberg TE, Finne Soveri UH, et al. Fermented cereal with specific *bifidobacteria* normalizes bowel movements in elderly nursing home residents. A randomized, controlled trial. *J Nutr Health Aging.* 2007;11(4):305-311.

Chapter

48 Nonprobiotic Management of Diarrhea

KEY POINTS

- ◯ In vitro and in vivo data lend support to the use of many phytobotanicals in the treatment of diarrhea.
- ◯ Bovine colostrum is effective for the treatment of diarrhea.
- ◯ Zinc supplementation helps in the treatment and prevention of diarrhea in children.

BOVINE COLOSTRUM

The biological value of bovine colostrum has been well documented in clinical trials involving bacteria and viruses including diarrhea in HIV-infected patients. Evidence indicates that it has synergistic effects with antibiotics used for infections.

Diarrhea in Children

Most, but not all, studies have shown bovine colostrum to be effective against diarrhea in children.[1-5] It is effective in infants with hemorrhagic diarrhea caused by infections with enterohemorrhagic *E coli*. It reduces the likelihood of infantile hemorrhagic diarrhea disease progressing to hemolytic uremic syndrome.

Bovine colostrum is effective for the treatment of diarrhea, although the efficacy may be less in immunocompromised patients.[6]

HIV Diarrhea[7-9]

AIDS patients with *Cryptosporidium parvum* diarrhea taking colostrum-derived bovine immunoglobulin concentrate for 21 days achieved a significant decrease in stool weight, as well as frequency.[8]

HEN-BASED HYPERIMMUNE EGG YOLK

A randomized, double-blind, placebo-controlled study examined the effect of 10 g/d hyperimmune egg yolk in 79 children with known rotavirus diarrhea.[10] The hyperimmune egg yolk group had a significant reduction in both stool output and need for hydration solution.

PHYTOBOTANICALS

Aegle marmelos

Pretreatment of mice with unripe fruit extract results in the inhibition of both the intestinal transit, as well as the accumulation of intestinal fluids induced by castor oil in mice.

Albizia lebbeck

The seed extract of *A lebbeck* possesses antidiarrheal activity and potentiates the antidiarrheal activity of loperamide in experimental models.

Alchornea cordifolia

Leaf extract of *A cordifolia* delays mouse intestinal transit accelerated by castor oil and decreases loose stools. There is lack of human studies.

Artemisia ludoviciana

In vitro experiments reveal that leaf extracts from mature plants are active antiparasitic agents. Human studies are needed.

Asparagus

A racemosus wild root extract inhibits castor oil-induced diarrhea, along with reduction in GI motility, in a charcoal meal test in rats.[11] *Asparagus pubescens* root inhibits intestinal propulsion, castor oil-induced diarrhea, and intestinal fluid accumulation.[12]

Baicalin

Kampo medicines TJ-14 and TJ-114 contain baicalin. Treatment with either baicalin or Kampo medicines TJ-14 and TJ-114 improves chemotherapy-induced anorexia and delays onset of diarrheal symptoms in animal models.[13]

Berberine

Berberine has antimicrobial activity against a variety of bacteria, viruses, fungi, protozoans, helminths, and chlamydia. It reduces castor oil-induced diarrhea.

Boswellia serrata

B serrata prevents diarrhea and normalizes intestinal motility in animal models of diarrhea, without slowing the rate of transit in control animals.[14]

Butea monosperma

The extracts from the stem bark of *B monosperma* inhibit castor oil-induced diarrhea in rats, in addition to reducing GI motility.

Byrsocarpus coccineus

B coccineus is used as an antidiarrheal in Africa and its effects are mediated via actions at multiple levels.[15] Aqueous leaf extract of *B coccineus* causes a decrease in propulsion in the castor oil-induced intestinal transit in mice. It slows normal intestinal transit.

Calendula officinalis

Extract of *C officinalis* flowers contains both spasmolytic and spasmogenic constituents, supporting its use in abdominal cramps, diarrhea, and constipation.

Calotropis

It reduces fecal output, frequency, and severity of diarrhea in rats treated with castor oil.[16]

Camellia sinensis

The hot water extract of black tea (*C sinensis*) exerts antidiarrheal activity in animal models of diarrhea.[17]

Carpolobia lutea

The ethanol extract of *C lutea* leaves reduces castor oil-induced diarrhea and fluid accumulation in rodents.[18]

Casimiroa tetrameria

The leaves of *C tetrameria* are used by the Mayans of the Yucatán peninsula for treating GI disorders, such as diarrhea and GI cramps. The mechanisms of action include inhibition of peristalsis.[19]

Cassia nigricans

Methanol extract of *C nigricans* leaves cause a dose-dependent decline in both the small intestinal propulsive movement, as well as castor oil-induced fluid accumulation.

Chaenomeles speciosa

Fruit of *Chaenomeles* inhibits the heat-labile enterotoxin-induced diarrhea in mice by blocking the binding of the toxin to the surface of intestinal epithelial cells.[20]

Cleome viscosa

C viscosa extract inhibits castor oil-induced diarrhea and PGE2-induced enteropooling in rats.[21] There is also a decrease in GI motility in the charcoal meal test.

Clerodendrum phlomidis

It is effective in experimentally induced diarrhea in animals. Human studies are lacking.

Cortex magnoliae officinalis

Ethanol extract of *C magnoliae officinalis* inhibits experimental diarrhea in mice.

Croton lechleri

A proanthocyanidin extract of the bark latex of *C lechleri* inhibits cholera toxin-induced fluid accumulation and chloride secretion.[22] These extracts are present in several commercial formulations.

Curcumin (Turmeric)

An open-label study examined the effect of curcumin for 41 weeks in patients with HIV-associated diarrhea.[23] Diarrhea resolved in all patients in 13 days. The average number of bowel movements declined from 7 to 1.7 per day, and this was accompanied by significant weight gain.

Egletes viscosa

This plant flavonoid has antidiarrheal actions, including inhibition of intestinal transit in vitro and vivo.[24]

Epilobium

In vitro and in vivo data support the use of extracts of various *Epilobium* species as antidiarrheal agents.[25]

Evodiae fructus

Dried, unripe fruit of the *Evodia rutaecarpa* inhibits intestinal transit in mice, as assessed by the charcoal meal test.[26]

Ferula gummosa Boiss

F gummosa Boiss is used as herbal therapy for the treatment of GI disorders in the Middle East. *F gummosa* oil relaxes isolated rat ileum.[27]

Ficus hispida

Experimental data support the use of extract of *F hispida* as an antidiarrheal agent.[28]

Galla chinensis

G chinensis extract inhibits heat-labile toxin-induced diarrhea by inhibiting it's binding to intestinal epithelium.

Ginger (Zingiber officinale)

Zingerone (vanillylacetone) is the bioactive component responsible for its antidiarrheal properties. It demonstrates both pre- and postjunctional inhibitory effects on ileal contractility.[29]

Guava (Psidium guajava)

Although mostly used as an antispasmodic, antibacterial, and antidiarrheal, its actions include cytoprotection, antimicrobial, anti-inflammatory, and antinociceptive properties—allowing its use in diverse illnesses.[30] Its antibacterial properties can potentially be useful to control foodborne pathogens and spoilage organisms.[31] An RCT examined the effect of *P guajava* for the treatment of rotaviral enteritis in infants.[32] Treatment resulted in recovery in 87.1% of patients at 3 days compared to 58% in controls.

Guiera senegalensis

G senegalensis is a popular and potent antidiarrheal herbal remedy used in Nigeria. It inhibits intestinal motility.

Hemidesmus indicus *(Indian Sarsaparilla)*

It inhibits GI motility, and its antidiarrheal effect may be superior to lomotil.[33]

Herba pogostemonis

H pogostemonis inhibits acetyl choline, as well as barium chloride-induced spasmodic contractions of isolated rabbit intestine,[34] along with an inhibition of intestinal propulsion.

Hibiscus rosa-sinensis

H rosa-sinensis is used for a variety of GI disorders, including constipation and diarrhea.[35]

Irvingia gabonensis

The aqueous leaf extract of *I gabonensis* is an effective antidiarrheal remedy. It inhibits histamine-induced contractions of guinea pig ileum[36] and decreases GI motility in mice. It ameliorates castor oil-induced diarrhea.

Jussiaea suffruticosa

Extracts from aerial parts of *J suffruticosa* inhibit castor oil-induced diarrhea and enteropooling in rats.

Kakkonto

It is beneficial in mouse models of food allergy with GI symptoms.[37]

Lantana camara

L camara inhibits neostigmine-induced motility, suggesting an anticholinergic effect.[38]

Litsea polyantha

Methanol extract of *L polyantha* inhibits GI motility and reduces fecal excretion in mice.[39]

Mebarid[40]

Mebarid retards intestinal motility on charcoal meal test in mice (Table 48-1).

Mezoneuron benthamianum[41]

The extract of *M benthamianum* inhibits diarrhea via the alpha-2 adrenergic system. It decreases gut propulsion and delays the onset and severity of diarrhea.

Neem (Azadirachta indica)

A indica is known as neem in India. It exerts antibacterial activity against the multidrug-resistant *Vibrio cholerae*, as well as several food-borne pathogens.[31,42]

Nigella sativa

The seeds of *Nigella sativa* are also known as "Kalonji." It has antioxidant, antihypertensive, analgesic, antipyretic, antimicrobial, and antineoplastic properties.[43] It relaxes spontaneous contractions in isolated rabbit jejunum.[44]

Table 48-1. Some Antidiarrheal Agents Used in Mexico[45]

Chiranthodendron pentadactylon	Inhibits cholera toxin-induced intestinal secretion in a rat model; active against *Entamoeba histolytica*
Hippocratea excelsa	Inhibits cholera toxin-induced intestinal secretion in a rat model
Ocimum basilicum	Inhibits cholera toxin-induced intestinal secretion in a rat model
Geranium mexicanum	Inhibits cholera toxin-induced intestinal secretion in a rat model
Bocconia frutescens	Inhibit cholera toxin-induced intestinal secretion in a rat model
Caesalpinia pulcherrima[46]	Antibacterial activity against *E coli*, *Shigella*, and *Salmonella*
C pentadactylon	Antibacterial activity against *E coli*, *Shigella*, and *Salmonella*
Cocos nucifera	Antibacterial activity against *E coli*, *Shigella*, and *Salmonella*
G mexicanum	Antibacterial activity against *E coli*, *Shigella*, and *Salmonella*
Helianthemum glomeratum: Bioactive flavonol glycosides isolated from the plant include tiliroside, and quercitrin[47]	Antiamoebic and antigiardial activity, but less active than metronidazole and emetine
H excelsa	Antibacterial activity against *E coli*, *Shigella*, and *Salmonella*
Punica granatum	Antibacterial activity against *E coli*, *Shigella*, and *Salmonella*; active against *E histolytica*
Annona cherimola[48]	Active against *E histolytica*
Dorstenia contrajerva	Active against *Giardia lamblia* in vitro

(continued)

Table 48-1 (continued). Some Antidiarrheal Agents Used in Mexico[45]

Senna villosa[48]	Active against *G lamblia* in vitro
Ruta chalepensis	Active against *G lamblia* in vitro
Rubus coriifolius: Active compounds include epicatechin, catechin, hyperin, gallic acid, and ellagic acid[49]	Antiprotozoal action against *E histolytica* and *G lamblia*, with epicatechin being the most active
Teloxys graveolens: Bioactive compounds include 1 coumarinic acid derivative, melilotoside, and 5 flavonoids	Active against *E histolytica* and *G lamblia*
Loeselia mexicana[50]	Reduces chemically induced diarrhea and slows intestinal transit
Zanthoxylum liebmannianum[51]: Bioactive component is asarinin isolated from its extract	Leaves inhibit reproduction of trophozoites of *E histolytica* and *G lamblia*

Nutmeg

Nutmeg is one of the Ayurvedic medicines used to treat diarrhea. It inhibits chemically induced contractions in guinea pig ileum and reduces diarrhea.[52]

Papaya (Carica papaya)

Papaya latex (*C papaya*) is used for worm infections. Administration of papaya latex to naturally infected pigs results in significant reduction in worm counts.[53]

Pentaclethra macrophylla

Leaf extracts are used for diarrhea. It reduces fecal output in chemically induced diarrhea.

Piper betle *Leaves*

It inhibits spontaneous, as well as chemically induced, intestinal contractions.[54]

Plantain

A controlled study compared the efficacy of a precooked plantain flour-based solution and standard rehydration electrolytes for treating dehydration and diarrhea.[55] Children received either the oral rehydration salt/World Health Organization standard treatment, or a solution with electrolytes similar to oral rehydration salts/World Health Organization and 50 g of precooked plantain flour instead of glucose (oral rehydration salts/plantain). Both solutions were equally effective.

Salicairine

It inhibits bisacodyl-induced increase in colonic transit in rats,[56] and increases net fluid absorption.

Sangre de Grado

Sangre de grado is an herbal medicine used in the Amazon region. It inhibits the secretory response to capsaicin in guinea pig ileum.

Seirogan (Wood Creosote)

Seirogan, an herbal medication containing wood creosote, is used as an antidiarrheal and antispasmodic remedy. A multicenter, randomized, double-blind study compared the effect of wood creosote to loperamide in patients with acute, nonspecific diarrhea.[57] Wood creosote and loperamide were equally effective.

Senna racemosa

Extracts from leaves, roots, and bark of *S racemosa* show good antiprotozoal activity against *Giardia intestinalis* and *Entamoeba histolytica* in vitro.

Shakhotaka or Siora (Streblus asper Lour)

S asper Lour is a small tree that has been a part of Ayurvedic medicine for a variety of diverse illnesses like diarrhea, dysentery, etc.[58] It is also reputed for oral health.[59]

Sphaeranthus senegalensis

It is effective in castor oil-induced diarrhea, and slows transit on GI charcoal meal test in animals.[60]

St. John's Wort (Hypericum perforatum)

Its spasmolytic effects are mediated through inhibition of calcium influx and phosphodiesterase-like mechanisms, supporting its use in GI disorders.[61]

Sumac (Rhus)

Rhus coriaria (sumac) demonstrates antibacterial activity against a variety of foodborne pathogens, including *Bacillus cereus*.[62] Mice treated with *Rhus javanica* fruit extract demonstrated a significant reduction in fecal output.[63]

Terminalia avicennioides

It inhibits spontaneous movements, as well as acetylcholine-induced contractions.[64]

Tormentil Root Extract (Potentilla tormentilla)

A randomized, double-blinded, placebo-controlled trial studied the effect of tormentil root extract in 40 children with rotavirus diarrhea.[65] Complete resolution of diarrhea within 48 hours in the treatment group was significantly superior to the response in the placebo group.

Trichodesma indicum *Root Extract*

T indicum root extract has been used for diarrhea, dysentery, and fever in Indian folk medicine. It slows the transit time of charcoal meal in animal models.[66]

Tulsi (Ocimum sanctum)

Different parts of tulsi are used for a variety of disorders in Ayurvedic medicine, including infections. Other suggested actions promoting its use include hepatoprotective, cardioprotective, anti-emetic, antineoplastic, antispasmodic, analgesic, adaptogenic, and diaphoretic actions.[67] The aqueous extract of the leaves of *Ocimum gratissimum* inhibits castor oil-induced diarrhea in rats.[68]

Xylocarpus

It has antidiarrheal activity in castor oil- and magnesium sulfate-induced models of diarrhea in mice.[69] It inhibits multiple foodborne pathogens.[70]

Zuccagnia punctata

Extracts of *Z punctata* slow the intestinal transit in rats and mice.

Herbal Combinations

APPLE PECTIN-CHAMOMILE EXTRACT[71,72]

A commercial preparation containing apple pectin and chamomile extract in addition to the usual rehydration and realimentation diet results in a significant decrease in the duration of diarrhea.[71]

DA-CHENG-QI DECOCTION (DCQ)

In vitro experiments on spontaneous cellular electrical activities of guinea-pig's taenia coli support antidiarrheal potential of this concoction. It accelerates the burst of slow wave potential.[713]

FUKEAN TABLET

In vitro and in vivo data support the use of FuKean Tablet (Guangdong Zaitian Pharmaceutical Co, Guangdong, China), a traditional Chinese medicine, for diarrhea.[74]

GRANULE OF CHILDREN-DIARRHEA FAST-STOPPING

It is composed of 7 medical herbs including *Poria cocos*, haw charcoal, *Euphorbia humifusa*, etc. A case series of 419 cases reported it to have a total effective rate of 96%.[75]

HANGE-SHASHIN-TO (TJ-14)[76-79]

Hange-shashin-to (TJ-14) is a Kampo medicine widely used as an antidiarrheal agent. It reduces the diarrhea induced by CPT-11or irinotecan in humans.[78,79]

HUANG QIN DECOCTION

The antispasmodic effect of the compound prescription occurs via the synergistic interaction between *Radix Paeoniae alba* and *R Glycyrrhiza*, whereas the antidiarrheal effects are mediated via *R Scutellariae*.[80] A Cochrane database review on Chinese medicinal herbs for chemotherapy side effects in colorectal cancer patients concluded that decoctions of Huang Qin compounds may stimulate immunocompetent cells and decrease side effects in patients treated with chemotherapy.[81]

HUOXIANG ZHENGQI LIQUID

Huoxiang Zhengqi Liquid is a traditional Chinese herbal combination, including *Rhizoma atractylodis*, *C magnoliae officinalis*, and *Pericarpium citri reticulatae*. The antidiarrheal effects are mediated via immunomodulation.[82]

HYUNGBANGJIHWANGTANG

Hyungbangjihwangtang is a multiherbal decoction used as an antidiarrheal agent, especially in Korea. The drug inhibits lipopolysaccharide-induced inflammatory cytokine production, suggesting a potential role as an anti-inflammatory agent.[83]

JIANPI WENSHEN DECOCTION

This Chinese decoction is useful for diabetic diarrhea, mediated likely via restoration of serum gastrin and somatostatin toward the normal range.[84]

JIAWEI SIJUNZI DECOCTION

Treatment with Jiawei Sijunzi decoction after radiation normalizes the migrating motor complexes or migrating myoelectric complexes.[85] This lends support for its use in radiation-induced diarrhea.

KO-KEN-HUANG-LIEN-HUANG-CHIN-TANG

It is a combination of *Pueraria,* coptis, scute, and licorice. Administration to piglets reduces diarrhea and enhances weight gain.[86]

PAEONIA-GLYCYRRHIZA DECOCTION

Oral administration of *Paeonia-Glycyrrhiza* decoction (PGD) results in attenuating alterations in migrating motor complexes and may be one mechanism for relieving diarrhea.[87]

PORIA-POLYPORUS ANTIDIARRHEA MIXTURE

A controlled study compared the efficacy of the Chinese remedy Poria-Polyporus Antidiarrhea Mixture with Smecta (Beaufour Ipsen Industrie, Dreux, France) in infants with rotavirus diarrhea.[88] The effective rate in the Poria-Polyporus Antidiarrhea Mixture group and Smecta groups were 83% and 90%, respectively.

QILIAN LIQUID

A controlled study examined the effect of retention enema with Qilian Liquid for infantile autumn diarrhea. The treatment provided symptomatic improvement.[89]

QIWEI BAIZHU POWDER

A controlled trial of patients with rotaviral enteritis treated with Qiwei Baizhu powder[89] demonstrated Qiwei Baizhu powder to be superior to the controls.

SOONKIJANGQUEBO

Soonkijangquebo[90] is a Korean herbal formulation. It inhibits castor oil-induced diarrhea in mice.

SOURCE QI

An open-label study examined the effect of Source Qi, a Chinese herbal formulation for HIV-associated, pathogen-negative, chronic diarrhea. Treatment resulted in a modest, but sustained, decrease in the number of stools per day.[91]

TAO HUA ZHI XIE GRANULE

Tao Hua Zhi Xie granule reduces the incidence and frequency of diarrhea induced by *Sennae folium* and castor oil.[92]

TJ-60 (Keishi-Ka-Shakuyaku-To, Gui-Zhi-Jia-Shao-Yao-Tang)

TJ-60 inhibits diarrhea induced by pilocarpine, barium chloride, or castor oil.[93]

TJ-14 and TJ-114

Kampo medicines TJ-14 and TJ-114 are useful for chemotherapy-induced diarrhea. The bioactive component is baicalin. It protects against chemotherapy-induced diarrheal weight loss.[94]

Triphala

It has 3 active constituents, including Amalaki (*E officinalis*), Haritaki (*Chebulic myrobalan*), and Bibhitaki (*Beleric myrobalan*). It has anti-inflammatory and antidiarrheal properties against castor oil-induced diarrhea in animals.[95] It ameliorates radiation-induced GI damage via its free radical scavenging activity.[96]

Wenchangning Oral Liquor

Treatment of infantile autumn diarrhea with Wenchangning Oral Liquor shows a cure rate of 82% and is superior to gentamicin.[97]

Xiang Cheng San

An RCT of children suffering from chronic, protracted diarrhea examined the effect of Xiang Cheng San application externally applied to the umbilicus.[98] Xiang Cheng San-treated patients demonstrated superior results, compared to Western medicine.

Xi Xie Ting

Treatment of diarrhea in children by bathing their legs and feet with Xi Xie Ting results in decreased frequency, amount, and improved consistency of stool.[99]

Yunpi Zhixie Granule

An RCT examined the effect of Yunpi Zhixie granule in 300 children with diarrhea.[100] Yunpi Zhixie granule was significantly more effective, especially for chronic diarrhea.

Zhixie Buye Mixture

The Zhixie Buye mixture[101] is effective for the treatment of infantile diarrhea. It is significantly more effective in eliminating vomiting and abdominal distension, compared to controls.

Miscellaneous Herbal Combinations

Berberine and *Geranii Herba*

Berberine and *Geranii Herba* inhibits experimentally induced contractions of the ileum and colon.[102] Berberine and *Geranii Herba* inhibits diarrhea induced by castor oil or barium chloride, but not the diarrhea induced by pilocarpine or serotonin.

CIMICIFUGA RHIZOMA, MELIAE CORTEX, RHIZOMA COPTIDIS, PHELLODENDRON CORTEX, AND SOPHORA SUBPROSTRATA RADIX

The combined extracts of these herbs significantly decrease porcine epidemic diarrhea.[103]

ACUPUNCTURE[104-107]

Acupuncture at acupoint GV1 (Jiaochao) for the treatment of a piglet model of enteropathogenic *E coli* diarrhea is just as effective as antibiotics.[104] Application of shallow needling at acupoints Qihai (Ren 6), Shuifen (Ren 9), bilateral Tianshu (St 25), and bilateral Zusanli (St 36), along with adjuvant acupoints Taibai (Sp 3) and Gongsun (Sp 4), results in a significantly superior response in children with diarrhea, compared to those treated with conventional medicines (including antibiotics).[106]

MASSAGE THERAPY[108,109]

An RCT examined the effect of therapeutic massage on diarrhea in infants living in orphanages in Ecuador.[108] The subjects receiving daily infant massage suffered a 50% less risk of diarrhea than controls (RR = 1.54, $p<0.001$).

ACUPUNCTURE PLUS MASSAGE

Acupuncture plus massage therapy results in a 55% response rate, compared to 35% for Western medicine, for the control of infantile diarrhea.[110]

HOMEOPATHY

A systematic review found 3 RCTs examining the effect of home-opathy in acute childhood diarrhea.[111] Two of these trials found that homeopathy was effective in improving the duration of diarrhea and the number of unformed stools.

DIETARY MEASURES

Lactose-Free Formula

Lactose-free formula is more effective in reducing the duration of diarrhea and stool frequency in subjects with acute diarrhea, compared to controls.[112]

Vitamins and Minerals

Zinc

A systematic review concluded that zinc supplementation is an effective treatment for acute diarrhea and is likely to reduce related morbidity and mortality.[113] Similarly, preventive zinc supplementation improves mortality and morbidity due to diarrhea in developing countries.[114]

Vitamin A

A double-blind, randomized, placebo-controlled study of 900 children aged 12 to 60 months with acute diarrhea found a 36% reduction in the mean daily prevalence of diarrhea associated with fever in vitamin A-supplemented children.[115] A Cochrane database meta-analysis review concluded that vitamin A reduces mortality in HIV-infected children.[116] The effect on diarrhea-specific mortality, however, did not reach statistical significance.

References

1. Tawfeek HI, Najim NH, Al-Mashikhi S. Efficacy of an infant formula containing anti-*Escherichia coli* colostral antibodies from hyperimmunized cows in preventing diarrhea in infants and children: a field trial. *Int J Infect Dis.* 2003;7(2):120-128.

2. Huppertz HI, Rutkowski S, Busch DH, et al. Bovine colostrum ameliorates diarrhea in infection with diarrheagenic *Escherichia coli,* shiga toxin-producing *E. coli*, and *E. coli* expressing intimin and hemolysin. *J Pediatr Gastroenterol Nutr.* 1999;29(4):452-456.

3. Sarker SA, Casswall TH, Mahalanabis D, et al. Successful treatment of rotavirus diarrhea in children with immunoglobulin from immunized bovine colostrum. *Pediatr Infect Dis J.* 1998;17(12):1149-1154.

4. Ebina T. Prophylaxis of rotavirus gastroenteritis using immunoglobulin. *Arch Virol Suppl.* 1996;12:217-223.

5. Ashraf H, Mahalanabis D, Mitra AK, Tzipori S, Fuchs GJ. Hyperimmune bovine colostrum in the treatment of shigellosis in children: a double-blind, randomized, controlled trial. *Acta Paediatr.* 2001;90(12):1373-1378.

6. Struff WG, Sprotte G. Bovine colostrum as a biologic in clinical medicine: a review—part II: clinical studies. *Int J Clin Pharmacol Ther.* 2008;46(5):211-225.

7. Okhuysen PC, Chappell CL, Crabb J, Valdez LM, Douglass ET, DuPont HL. Prophylactic effect of bovine anti-*Cryptosporidium* hyperimmune colostrum immunoglobulin in healthy volunteers challenged with *Cryptosporidium parvum. Clin Infect Dis.* 1998;26(6):1324-1329.

8.   Greenberg PD, Cello JP. Treatment of severe diarrhea caused by *Cryptosporidium parvum* with oral bovine immunoglobulin concentrate in patients with AIDS. *J Acquir Immune Defic Syndr Hum Retrovirol.* 1996;13(4):348-354.

9.   Florén CH, Chinenye S, Elfstrand L, Hagman C, Ihse I. ColoPlus, a new product based on bovine colostrum, alleviates HIV-associated diarrhea. *Scand J Gastroenterol.* 2006;41(6):682-686.

10. Sarker SA, Casswall TH, Juneja LR, et al. Randomized, placebo-controlled, clinical trial of hyperimmunized chicken egg yolk immunoglobulin in children with rotavirus diarrhea. *Pediatr Gastroenterol Nutr.* 2001;32(1):19-25.

11. Venkatesan N, Thiyagarajan V, Narayanan S, et al. Anti-diarrhoeal potential of *Asparagus racemosus* wild root extracts in laboratory animals. *J Pharm Pharm Sci.* 2005;8(1):39-46.

12. Nwafor PA, Okwuasaba FK, Binda LG. Antidiarrhoeal and antiulcerogenic effects of methanolic extract of *Asparagus pubescens* root in rats. *J Ethnopharmacol.* 2000;72(3):421-427.

13. Takasuna K, Kasai Y, Kitano Y, et al. Protective effects of kampo medicines and baicalin against intestinal toxicity of a new anticancer camptothecin derivative, irinotecan hydrochloride (CPT-11), in rats. *Jpn J Cancer Res.* 1995;86(10):978-984.

14. Borrelli F, Capasso F, Capasso R, et al. Effect of *Boswellia serrata* on intestinal motility in rodents: inhibition of diarrhoea without constipation. *Br J Pharmacol.* 2006;148(4):553-560.

15. Akindele AJ, Adeyemi OO. Evaluation of the antidiarrhoeal activity of *Byrsocarpus coccineus. J Ethnopharmacol.* 2006;108(1):20-25.

16. Kumar S, Dewan S, Sangraula H, Kumar VL. Anti-diarrhoeal activity of the latex of *Calotropis procera. J Ethnopharmacol.* 2001;76(1):115-118.

17. Besra SE, Gomes A, Ganguly DK, Vedasiromoni JR. Antidiarrhoeal activity of hot water extract of black tea (*Camellia sinensis*). *Phytother Res.* 2003;17(4):380-384.

18. Nwafor PA, Bassey AI. Evaluation of anti-diarrhoeal and anti-ulcerogenic potential of ethanol extract of *Carpolobia lutea* leaves in rodents. *J Ethnopharmacol.* 2007;111(3):619-624.

19. Heinrich M, Heneka B, Ankli A, Rimpler H, Sticher O, Kostiza T. Spasmolytic and antidiarrhoeal properties of the Yucatec Mayan medicinal plant *Casimiroa tetrameria. J Pharm Pharmacol.* 2005;57(9):1081-1085.

20. Chen JC, Chang YS, Wu SL, et al. Inhibition of *Escherichia coli* heat-labile enterotoxin-induced diarrhea by *Chaenomeles speciosa. J Ethnopharmacol.* 2007;113(2):233-239.

21. Devi BP, Boominathan R, Mandal SC. Evaluation of anti-diarrheal activity of *Cleome viscosa L.* extract in rats. *Phytomedicine.* 2002;9(8):739-742.

22. Fischer H, Machen TE, Widdicombe JH, et al. A novel extract SB-300 from the stem bark latex of *Croton lechleri* inhibits CFTR-mediated chloride secretion in human colonic epithelial cells. *J Ethnopharmacol.* 2004;93(2-3):351-357.

23. Conteas CN, Panossian AM, Tran TT, Singh HM. Treatment of HIV-associated diarrhea with curcumin. *Dig Dis Sci.* 2009;54(10):2188-2191.

24. Rao VS, Santos FA, Sobreira TT, Souza MF, Melo CL, Silveira ER. Investigations on the gastroprotective and antidiarrhoeal properties of ternatin, a tetramethoxyflavone from *Egletes viscosa. Planta Med.* 1997;63(2):146-149.

25. Vitali F, Fonte G, Saija A, Tita B. Inhibition of intestinal motility and secretion by extracts of *Epilobium spp.* in mice. *J Ethnopharmacol.* 2006;107(3):342-348.

26. Yu LL, Liao JF, Chen CF. Effect of the crude extract of *Evodiae fructus* on the intestinal transit in mice. *Planta Med.* 1994;60(4):308-312.

27. Sadraei H, Asghari GR, Hajhashemi V, Kolagar A, Ebrahimi M. Spasmolytic activity of essential oil and various extracts of *Ferula gummosa Boiss* on ileum contractions. *Phytomedicine.* 2001;8(5):370-376.

28. Mandal SC, Ashok Kumar CK. Studies on anti-diarrhoeal activity of *Ficus hispida* leaf extract in rats. *Fitoterapia.* 2002;73(7-8):663-667.

29. Borrelli F, Capasso R, Pinto A, Izzo AA. Inhibitory effect of ginger (*Zingiber officinale*) on rat ileal motility in vitro. *Life Sci.* 2004;74(23):2889-2896.

30. Gutiérrez RM, Mitchell S, Solis RV. *Psidium guajava*: a review of its traditional uses, phytochemistry and pharmacology. *J Ethnopharmacol.* 2008;117(1):1-27.

31. Mahfuzul Hoque MD, Bari ML, Inatsu Y, Juneja VK, Kawamoto S. Antibacterial activity of guava (*Psidium guajava L.*) and neem (*Azadirachta indica A. Juss.*) extracts against foodborne pathogens and spoilage bacteria. *Foodborne Pathog Dis.* 2007;4(4):481-488.

32. Wei L, Li Z, Chen B. Clinical study on treatment of infantile rotaviral enteritis with *Psidium guajava L. Zhongguo Zhong Xi Yi Jie He Za Zhi.* 2000;20(12):893-895.

33. Das S, Prakash R, Devaraj SN. Antidiarrhoeal effects of methanolic root extract of *Hemidesmus indicus* (Indian sarsaparilla)—an in vitro and in vivo study. *Indian J Exp Biol.* 2003;41(4):363-366.

34. Chen X, He B, Li X, Luo J. Effects of *herba Pogostemonis* on gastrointestinal tract. *Zhong Yao Cai.* 1998;21(9):462-466.

35. Gilani AH, Bashir S, Janbaz KH, Shah AJ. Presence of cholinergic and calcium channel blocking activities explains the traditional use of *Hibiscus rosasinensis* in constipation and diarrhoea. *J Ethnopharmacol.* 2005;102(2):289-294.

36. Abdulrahman F, Inyang IS, Abbah J, Binda L, Amos S, Gamaniel K. Effect of aqueous leaf extract of *Irvingia gabonensis* on gastrointestinal tract in rodents. *Indian J Exp Biol.* 2004;42(8):787-791.

37. Yamamoto T, Fujiwara K, Yoshida M, et al. Therapeutic effect of kakkonto in a mouse model of food allergy with gastrointestinal symptoms. *Int Arch Allergy Immunol.* 2009;148(3):175-185.

38. Sagar L, Sehgal R, Ojha S. Evaluation of antimotility effect of *Lantana camara L. var. acuelata* constituents on neostigmine induced gastrointestinal transit in mice. *BMC Complement Altern Med.* 2005;5:18.

39. Poonia BS, Sasmal D, Mazumdar PM. Anti-diarrheal activity of methanol extract of *Litsea polyantha* bark in mice. *Fitoterapia*. 2007;78(3):171-174.

40. Bafna P, Bodhankar S. Gastrointestinal effects of Mebarid, an Ayurvedic formulation, in experimental animals. *J Ethnopharmacol*. 2003;86(2-3):173-176.

41. Mbagwu HO, Adeyemi OO. Anti-diarrhoeal activity of the aqueous extract of *Mezoneuron benthamianum Baill* (*Caesalpiniaceae*). *J Ethnopharmacol*. 2008;116(1):16-20.

42. Thakurta P, Bhowmik P, Mukherjee S, et al. Antibacterial, antisecretory and antihemorrhagic activity of *Azadirachta indica* used to treat cholera and diarrhea in India. *J Ethnopharmacol*. 2007;111(3):607-612.

43. Ali BH, Blunden G. Pharmacological and toxicological properties of *Nigella sativa*. *Phytother Res*. 2003;17(4):299-305.

44. Gilani AH, Aziz N, Khurram IM, Chaudhary KS, Iqbal A. Bronchodilator, spasmolytic and calcium antagonist activities of *Nigella sativa* seeds (Kalonji): a traditional herbal product with multiple medicinal uses. *J Pak Med Assoc*. 2001;51(3):115-120.

45. Velázquez C, Calzada F, Torres J, González F, Ceballos G. Antisecretory activity of plants used to treat gastrointestinal disorders in Mexico. *J Ethnopharmacol*. 2006;103(1):66-70.

46. Alanís AD, Calzada F, Cervantes JA, Torres J, Ceballos GM. Antibacterial properties of some plants used in Mexican traditional medicine for the treatment of gastrointestinal disorders. *J Ethnopharmacol*. 2005;100(1-2):153-157.

47. Calzada F, Alanís AD. Additional antiprotozoal flavonol glycosides of the aerial parts of *Helianthemum glomeratum*. *Phytother Res*. 2007;21(1):78-80.

48. Calzada F, Yépez-Mulia L, Aguilar A. In vitro susceptibility of *Entamoeba histolytica* and *Giardia lamblia* to plants used in Mexican traditional medicine for the treatment of gastrointestinal disorders. *J Ethnopharmacol*. 2006;108(3):367-370.

49. Alanís AD, Calzada F, Cedillo-Rivera R, Meckes M. Antiprotozoal activity of the constituents of *Rubus coriifolius*. *Phytother Res*. 2003;17(6):681-682.

50. Pérez GS, Pérez GC, Zavala MA. A study of the antidiarrheal properties of *Loeselia mexicana* on mice and rats. *Phytomedicine*. 2005;12(9):670-674.

51. Arrieta J, Reyes B, Calzada F, Cedillo-Rivera R, Navarrete A. Amoebicidal and giardicidal compounds from the leaves of *Zanthoxylum liebmannianun*. *Fitoterapia*. 2001;72(3):295-297.

52. Grover JK, Khandkar S, Vats V, Dhunnoo Y, Das D. Pharmacological studies on *Myristica fragrans*—antidiarrheal, hypnotic, analgesic and hemodynamic (blood pressure) parameters. *Methods Find Exp Clin Pharmacol*. 2002;24(10):675-680.

53. Satrija F, Nansen P, Bjørn H, Murtini S, He S. Effect of papaya latex against *Ascaris suum* in naturally infected pigs. *J Helminthol*. 1994;68(4):343-346.

54. Gilani AH, Aziz N, Khurram IM, Rao ZA, Ali NK. The presence of cholinomimetic and calcium channel antagonist constituents in *Piper betle* linn. *Phytother Res.* 2000;14(6):436-442.

55. Bernal C, Alcaraz GM, Botero JE. Oral rehydration with a plantain flour-based solution precooked with standardized electrolytes. *Biomedica.* 2005;25(1):11-21.

56. Brun Y, Wang XP, Willemot J, Sevenet T, Demenge P. Experimental study of antidiarrheal activity of Salicairine. *Fundam Clin Pharmacol.* 1998;12(1):30-36.

57. Kuge T, Shibata T, Willett MS. Multicenter, double-blind, randomized comparison of wood creosote, the principal active ingredient of Seirogan, an herbal antidiarrheal medication, and loperamide in adults with acute nonspecific diarrhea. *Clin Ther.* 2004;26(10):1644-1651.

58. Rastogi S, Kulshreshtha DK, Rawat AK. *Streblus asper Lour.* Shakhotaka: a review of its chemical, pharmacological and ethnomedicinal properties. *Evid Based Complement Alternat Med.* 2006;3(2):217-222.

59. Taweechaisupapong S, Intaranongpai K, Suwannarong W, et al. Clinical and microbiological effects of subgingival irrigation with *Streblus asper* leaf extract in chronic periodontitis. *J Clin Dent.* 2006;17(3):67-71.

60. Adzu B, Tarfa F, Amos S, Gamaniel KS. The efficacy of *Sphaeranthus senegalensis Vaill* extract against diarrhoea in rats. *J Ethnopharmacol.* 2004;95(2-3):173-176.

61. Gilani AH, Khan AU, Subhan F, Khan M. Antispasmodic and broncho-dilator activities of St John's wort are putatively mediated through dual inhibition of calcium influx and phosphodiesterase. *Fundam Clin Pharmacol.* 2005;19(6):695-705.

62. Nasar-Abbas SM, Halkman AK. Antimicrobial effect of water extract of sumac (*Rhus coriaria L.*) on the growth of some food borne bacteria including pathogens. *Int J Food Microbiol.* 2004;97(1):63-69.

63. Tangpu V, Yadav AK. Antidiarrhoeal activity of *Rhus javanica* ripen fruit extract in albino mice. *Fitoterapia.* 2004;75(1):39-44.

64. Ali A, Kaur G, Hamid H, et al. Terminoside A, a new triterpene glyco-side from the bark of *Terminalia arjuna* inhibits nitric oxide production in murine macrophages. *J Asian Nat Prod Res.* 2003;5(2):137-142.

65. Subbotina MD, Timchenko VN, Vorobyov MM, et al. Effect of oral administration of tormentil root extract (*Potentilla tormentilla*) on rotavi-rus diarrhea in children: a randomized, double blind, controlled trial. *Pediatr Infect Dis J.* 2003;22(8):706-711.

66. Perianayagam JB, Sharma SK, Pillai KK. Evaluation of antidiarrheal potential of *Trichodesma indicum* root extract in rats. *Methods Find Exp Clin Pharmacol.* 2005;27(8):533-537.

67. Prakash P, Gupta N. Therapeutic uses of *Ocimum sanctum Linn* (Tulsi) with a note on eugenol and its pharmacological actions: a short review. *Indian J Physiol Pharmacol.* 2005;49(2):125-131.

68. Offiah VN, Chikwendu UA. Antidiarrhoeal effects of *Ocimum gratissi-mum* leaf extract in experimental animals. *J Ethnopharmacol.* 1999;68(1-3):327-330.

69. Rouf R, Uddin SJ, Shilpi JA, Alamgir M. Assessment of antidiarrhoeal activity of the methanol extract of *Xylocarpus granatum* bark in mice model. *J Ethnopharmacol.* 2007;109(3):539-542.

70. Uddin SJ, Shilpi JA, Alam SM, Alamgir M, Rahman MT, Sarker SD. Antidiarrhoeal activity of the methanol extract of the barks of *Xylocarpus moluccensis* in castor oil- and magnesium sulphate-induced diarrhoea models in mice. *J Ethnopharmacol.* 2005;101(1-3):139-143.

71. de la Motte S, Böse-O'Reilly S, Heinisch M, Harrison F. Double-blind comparison of an apple pectin-chamomile extract preparation with placebo in children with diarrhea. *Arzneimittelforschung.* 1997;47(11): 1247-1249.

72. Becker B, Kuhn U, Hardewig-Budny B. Double-blind, randomized evaluation of clinical efficacy and tolerability of an apple pectin-chamomile extract in children with unspecific diarrhea. *Arzneimittelforschung.* 2006;56(6):387-393.

73. Yang WX, Jin ZG, Tian ZS. Effects of dachengqi decoction and rhubarb on cellular electrical activities in smooth muscle of the guinea-pig taenia coli. *Zhongguo Zhong Xi Yi Jie He Za Zhi.* 1993;13(1):33-36.

74. Zhou J, Li R, Ye M, Huang G, Liao H. Experimental study on pharmacological action of Fukean tablet on gastrointestinal tract. *Zhong Yao Cai.* 1999;22(9):465-467.

75. Li YL. Clinical and experimental study on the treatment of children diarrhea by granule of children-diarrhea fast-stopping. *Zhong Xi Yi Jie He Za Zhi.* 1991;11(2):79-82,67.

76. Kase Y, Saitoh K, Makino B, et al. Relationship between the antidiarrhoeal effects of Hange-Shashin-To and its active components. *Phytother Res.* 1999;13(6):468-473.

77. Kase Y, Hayakawa T, Aburada M, Komatsu Y, Kamataki T. Preventive effects of Hange-shashin-to on irinotecan hydrochloride-caused diarrhea and its relevance to the colonic prostaglandin E2 and water absorption in the rat. *Jpn J Pharmacol.* 1997;75(4):407-413.

78. Sakata Y, Suzuki H, Kamataki T. Preventive effect of TJ-14, a kampo (Chinese herb) medicine, on diarrhea induced by irinotecan hydrochloride (CPT-11). *Gan To Kagaku Ryoho.* 1994;21(8):1241-1244.

79. Mori K, Kondo T, Kamiyama Y, Kano Y, Tominaga K. Preventive effect of Kampo medicine (Hangeshashin-to) against irinotecan-induced diarrhea in advanced non-small-cell lung cancer. *Cancer Chemother Pharmacol.* 2003;51(5):403-406.

80. Huang L, Liu J, Li D, et al. A study on components and compound prescription of huangqin decoction. *Zhongguo Zhong Yao Za Zhi.* 1991;16(3):177-181, back cover.

81. Taixiang W, Munro AJ, Guanjian L. Chinese medical herbs for chemotherapy side effects in colorectal cancer patients. *Cochrane Database Syst Rev.* 2005;(1):CD004540.

82. He YH, Zhao HY, Liu ZL, et al. Effects of huoxiangzhengqi liquid on enteric mucosal immune responses in mice with *Bacillus dysenteriae* and *Salmonella typhimurium* induced diarrhea. *World J Gastroenterol.* 2006;12(45):7346-7349.

83. Moon PD, Jeong HJ, Um JY, Kim HM, Hong SH. LPS-induced inflammatory cytokine production was inhibited by HyungbangJihwangTang through blockade of NF-kappaB in peripheral blood mononuclear cells. *Int J Neurosci.* 2007;117(9):1315-1329. Erratum in: 2007;117(11):1639.

84. Xiao W, Liu J, Liu LY. Effect of jianpi wenshen decoction on serum gastrin, plasma motilin and somatostatin in patients of diabetic diarrhea. *Zhongguo Zhong Xi Yi Jie He Za Zhi.* 2002;22(8):587-589.

85. Chen GZ, Fu D. Effect of jiawei sijunzi decoction on migrating myoelectric complex in 8 Gy irradiated rats. *Zhongguo Zhong Xi Yi Jie He Za Zhi.* 1996;16(4):221-223.

86. Lin JH, Lo YY, Shu NS, et al. Control of preweaning diarrhea in piglets by acupuncture and Chinese medicine. *Am J Chin Med.* 1988;16(1-2):75-80.

87. Xu JD, Liu ZH, Chen SZ. Effects of *Paeonia-Glycyrrhiza* decoction on changes induced by cisplatin in rats. *Zhongguo Zhong Xi Yi Jie He Za Zhi.* 1994;14(11):673-674.

88. Wang SS, Yang S, Ma Y. Efficacy of poria-polyporus anti-diarrhea oral liquor in treating infantile rotavirus diarrhea: a controlled study with smicta. *Zhongguo Zhong Xi Yi Jie He Za Zhi.* 1995;15(5):284-286.

89. He ST, He FZ, Wu CR, et al. Treatment of rotaviral gastroenteritis with Qiwei Baizhu powder. *World J Gastroenterol.* 2001;7(5):735-740.

90. Ryu SD, Park CS, Baek HM, et al. Anti-diarrheal and spasmolytic activities and acute toxicity study of Soonkijangquebo, a herbal antidiarrheal formula. *J Ethnopharmacol.* 2004;91(1):75-80.

91. Cohen MR, Mitchell TF, Bacchetti P, et al. Use of a chinese herbal medicine for treatment of HIV-associated pathogen-negative diarrhea. *Integr Med.* 2000;2(2):79-84.

92. Shan L, Zhao Y, Xiao X, Cai G, He C. Pharmacodynamics study on "tao hua zhi xie granule." *Zhong Yao Cai.* 2003;26(6):420-422.

93. Saitoh K, Kase Y, Ishige A, et al. Effects of Keishi-ka-shakuyaku-to (Gui-Zhi-Jia-Shao-Yao-Tang) on diarrhea and small intestinal movement. *Biol Pharm Bull.* 1999;22(1):87-89.

94. Takasuna K, Kasai Y, Kitano Y, et al. Protective effects of kampo medicines and baicalin against intestinal toxicity of a new anticancer camptothecin derivative, irinotecan hydrochloride (CPT-11), in rats. *Jpn J Cancer Res.* 1995;86(10):978-984.

95. Biradar YS, Singh R, Sharma K, et al. Evaluation of anti-diarrhoeal property and acute toxicity of Triphala Mashi, an Ayurvedic formulation. *J Herb Pharmacother.* 2007;7(3-4):203-212.

96. Jagetia GC, Rao SK, Baliga MS, S Babu K. The evaluation of nitric oxide scavenging activity of certain herbal formulations in vitro: a preliminary study. *Phytother Res.* 2004;18(7):561-565.

97. Zhang WD, Zhou QS, Yang ZL. Clinical and experimental study on wenchangning oral liquor in treating infantile autumn diarrhea. *Zhongguo Zhong Xi Yi Jie He Za Zhi.* 1996;16(8):454-458.

98. Yang S. Application of xiang cheng san in treatment of chronic protracted diarrhea in children. *J Tradit Chin Med.* 1995;15(3):214-219.

99. Bo MQ, Zhang FR. Xi xie ting in the treatment of infantile diarrhea. *Zhongguo Zhong Xi Yi Jie He Za Zhi.* 1993;13(6):343-344,324.

100. Yang Y, Yan HM. Clinical research on effects of yunpi zhixie granule in children with diarrhea. *Zhongguo Zhong Xi Yi Jie He Za Zhi.* 2006;26(10):899-902.

101. Zhu J, Zhong C, Sun D. Clinical and experimental study on zhixie buye mixture in treating infantile diarrhea complicated with dehydration. *Zhongguo Zhong Xi Yi Jie He Za Zhi.* 1999;19(3):137-140.

102. Yamamoto K, Takase H, Abe K, Saito Y, Suzuki A. Pharmacological studies on antidiarrheal effects of a preparation containing berberine and geranii herba. *Nippon Yakurigaku Zasshi.* 1993;101(3):169-175.

103. Kim HY, Shin HS, Park H, et al. In vitro inhibition of coronavirus replications by the traditionally used medicinal herbal extracts, *Cimicifuga rhizoma, Meliae cortex, Coptidis rhizoma,* and *Phellodendron cortex. J Clin Virol.* 2008;41(2):122-128.

104. Park ES, Jo S, Seong JK, et al. Effect of acupuncture in the treatment of young pigs with induced *Escherichia coli* diarrhea. *J Vet Sci.* 2003;4(2):125-128.

105. Lin JH, Lo YY, Shu NS, et al. Control of preweaning diarrhea in piglets by acupuncture and Chinese medicine. *Am J Chin Med.* 1988;16(1-2):75-80.

106. Lin Y, Zhou Z, Shen W, et al. Clinical and experimental studies on shallow needling technique for treating childhood diarrhea. *J Tradit Chin Med.* 1993;13(2):107-114.

107. Anastasi JK, McMahon DJ. Testing strategies to reduce diarrhea in persons with HIV using traditional Chinese medicine: acupuncture and moxibustion. *J Assoc Nurses AIDS Care.* 2003;14(3):28-40.

108. Jump VK, Fargo JD, Akers JF. Impact of massage therapy on health outcomes among orphaned infants in Ecuador: results of a randomized clinical trial. *Fam Community Health.* 2006;29(4):314-319.

109. Silva LM, Cignolini A, Warren R, Budden S, Skowron-Gooch A. Improvement in sensory impairment and social interaction in young children with autism following treatment with an original Qigong massage methodology. *Am J Chin Med.* 2007;35(3):393-406.

110. Wang XF, Teng X. Comparison and analysis on therapeutic effects of acupuncture plus massage therapy and drug on infantile diarrhea. *Zhongguo Zhen Jiu.* 2005;25(2):92-94.

111. Altunç U, Pittler MH, Ernst E. Homeopathy for childhood and adolescence ailments: systematic review of randomized clinical trials. *Mayo Clin Proc.* 2007;82(1):69-75.

112. Simakachorn N, Tongpenyai Y, Tongtan O, Varavithya W. Randomized, double-blind clinical trial of a lactose-free and a lactose-containing formula in dietary management of acute childhood diarrhea. *J Med Assoc Thai.* 2004;87(6):641-649.

113. Walker CL, Black RE. Zinc for the treatment of diarrhoea: effect on diarrhoea morbidity, mortality and incidence of future episodes. *Int J Epidemiol.* 2010;39(Suppl 1):i63-69.

114. Yakoob MY, Theodoratou E, Jabeen A, et al. Preventive zinc supplementation in developing countries: impact on mortality and morbidity due to diarrhea, pneumonia and malaria. *BMC Public Health.* 2011;11(Suppl 3):S23.

115. Bhandari N, Bhan MK, Sazawal S. Impact of massive dose of vitamin A given to preschool children with acute diarrhoea on subsequent respiratory and diarrhoeal morbidity. *BMJ.* 1994;309(6966):1404-1407.

116. Humphreys EH, Smith NA, Azman H, McLeod D, Rutherford GW. Prevention of diarrhoea in children with HIV infection or exposure to maternal HIV infection. *Cochrane Database Syst Rev.* 2010;(6):CD008563.

Chapter

49 *Antibiotic-* and Clostridium *difficile-Associated Diarrhea*

KEY POINTS

○ Probiotics appear to be effective in preventing antibiotic-associated diarrhea (AAD).

○ Probiotics do not have a role in acute treatment of *C difficile*-associated diarrhea (CDAD).

○ Total fecal flora transplant is effective for recurrent CDAD.

○ Hyperimmune bovine colostrum has potential for benefit in recurrent CDAD.

The pathogenesis of AAD and CDAD remains to be fully elucidated, and dysbiosis has been implicated. Literature indicates that the use of proton pump indicators significantly increases the risk of CDAD.[1] There is little evidence for antibiotic treatment of severe CDAD, as many studies excluded these patients.[2]

PROBIOTICS

Probiotics for the Primary Prevention of Antibiotic-Associated Diarrhea in Adults

Numerous studies have shown positive results.[3-8] Probiotics studied include *S boulardii*, *L acidophilus Cl1285* and *L casei*, *L bulgaricus*, *S thermophilus*, etc. However, not all studies have been positive.[9-11]

McFarland's meta-analysis concluded that probiotics significantly reduce the relative risk of AAD (RR = 0.43, p<0.001). *S boulardii*, *L rhamnosus GG*, or probiotic mixtures are effective.[12] The meta-analysis also revealed that probiotics have significant efficacy for *C difficile* disease (RR = 0.59, p<0.01). However, only *S boulardii* was found to be helpful for *C difficile* disease.[12]

> An expert panel led by Floch et al made an A-grade recommendation for use of probiotics for the prevention of antibiotic-induced diarrhea.[13]

Probiotics for the Primary Prevention of Antibiotic-Associated Diarrhea in Children

Numerous studies have examined the effect of probiotics for AAD in children, and the majority have yielded positive results.[14-17] A Cochrane database meta-analysis examined the role of probiotics in preventing pediatric AAD.[18] The per protocol analysis showed the incidence of diarrhea to be statistically significant, favoring probiotics overactive/nonactive controls (RR = 0.49). However, intention-to-treat analysis showed nonsignificant results overall. The authors found data to be promising for *Lactobacillus GG*, *L sporogenes*, and *S boulardii* at 5 to 40 billion CFUs per day.

Probiotics for the Treatment of Antibiotic- and C difficile-Associated Diarrhea

A Cochrane database review examined the efficacy of probiotics in the treatment of antibiotic-associated *C difficile* colitis in adults.[19] The authors concluded that there is insufficient evidence to recommend probiotics as an adjunct to antibiotic therapy for *C difficile* colitis. In addition, the authors found no evidence to support the use of probiotics alone in the treatment of *C difficile* colitis.

Probiotics for the Prevention of Recurrences of C difficile-Associated Diarrhea[20-22]

A systematic review found 2 RCTs examining the effectiveness of *S boulardii* in the prevention of recurrent *C difficile* infection.[22] Two studies have demonstrated a reduction of relapses with recurrent *C difficile* disease (RR = 0.53, p<0.05 and RR = 0.33, p = 0.05).

FECAL BACTERIOTHERAPY OR FLORA REPLACEMENT

About 25% of *C difficile* does not produce toxins. Anecdotal evidence suggests a beneficial role for oral administration of such nontoxic strains for treatment of recurrences.[23]

Fecal bacteriotherapy involves the transfer of the entire bacterial flora from a healthy donor to the sick recipient. It has been used successfully to treat refractory, as well as severe, cases of *C difficile*-associated diarrhea[24] and irritable bowel disease.

Protocol
○ Protocols vary
○ Single as well as multiple sessions have been used
○ Enema administration of blenderized fresh stool
○ Both colonoscopic and nasogastric administration are options[25,26]

Prerequisite Studies in Donor
○ Healthy donor with normal formed stools
○ Should not be a close relative and/or living in the same household
○ No antibiotic use for at least 6 months prior
○ Screen donor stool for bacterial, protozoal, and viral pathogens
○ Complete blood count and comprehensive metabolic profile
○ Exclude hepatitis A, B, and C; HIV; and syphilis

Pre-Enema Preparation of Recipient Patient
○ Administer vancomycin 250 mg tid to 500 mg bid for 7 days.
○ Administer 1 gallon polyethylene glycol solution the day before therapy.

Example of a Representative Protocol

○ Mix 200 to 300 g of donor stool in 250 mL of normal saline. Homogenize briefly and gently in blender.

○ Administer blended product within 10 minutes via retention enema with buttocks slightly raised by pillow to facilitate retention.

○ Encourage the patient to change position every 15 minutes.

○ Administer enema daily for 5 to 7 days.

○ First administration may be undertaken via colonoscope into the cecum, and even the terminal ileum, to potentially enhance efficacy.

BOVINE COLOSTRUM

Bovine immunoglobulin concentrate-*C difficile* retains *C difficile* toxin neutralizing activity after passage through the stomach and small intestine.[27] A prospective, randomized, double-blind study compared *C difficile* immune whey to metronidazole for the treatment of recurrent, mild-to-moderate episodes of CDAD.[28] Both treatments were equally effective in preventing CDAD recurrences.

BERBERINE

Berberine has antimicrobial activity against a variety of pathogens. It has antidiarrheal actions mediated at least in part by its anti-inflammatory effects. As such, it has the potential to have a role in *C difficile*-associated disease.

REFERENCES

1. Pant C, Madonia P, Minocha A. Does PPI therapy predispose to *Clostridium difficile* infection? *Nat Rev Gastroenterol Hepatol.* 2009;6(9): 555-557.

2. Nelson RL, Kelsey P, Leeman H, et al. Antibiotic treatment for *Clostridium difficile*-associated diarrhea in adults. *Cochrane Database Syst Rev.* 2011;9:CD004610.

3. Can M, Besirbellioglu BA, Avci IY, Beker CM, Pahsa A. Prophylactic *Saccharomyces boulardii* in the prevention of antibiotic-associated diarrhea: a prospective study. *Med Sci Monit.* 2006;12(4):PI19-22.

4. Beausoleil M, Fortier N, Guénette S, et al. Effect of a fermented milk combining *Lactobacillus acidophilus* Cl1285 and *Lactobacillus casei* in the prevention of antibiotic-associated diarrhea: a randomized, double-blind, placebo-controlled trial. *Can J Gastroenterol.* 2007;21(11):732-736.

5. Hickson M, D'Souza AL, Muthu N, et al. Use of probiotic *Lactobacillus* preparation to prevent diarrhoea associated with antibiotics: randomised double blind placebo controlled trial. *BMJ*. 2007;335(7610):80.

6. Gao XW, Mubasher M, Fang CY, Reifer C, Miller LE. Dose-response efficacy of a proprietary probiotic formula of *Lactobacillus acidophilus CL1285* and *Lactobacillus casei LBC80R* for antibiotic-associated diarrhea and *Clostridium difficile*-associated diarrhea prophylaxis in adult patients. *Am J Gastroenterol*. 2010;105(7):1636-1641.

7. Koning CJ, Jonkers DM, Stobberingh EE, et al. The effect of a multispecies probiotic on the intestinal microbiota and bowel movements in healthy volunteers taking the antibiotic amoxycillin. *Am J Gastroenterol*. 2008103(1):178-189.

8. Wenus C, Goll R, Loken EB, Biong AS, Halvorsen DS, Florholmen J. Prevention of antibiotic-associated diarrhoea by a fermented probiotic milk drink. *Eur J Clin Nutr*. 2008;62(2):299-301.

9. Conway S, Hart A, Clark A, Harvey I. Does eating yogurt prevent antibiotic-associated diarrhoea? A placebo-controlled randomised controlled trial in general practice. *Br J Gen Pract*. 2007;57(545):953-959.

10. Bravo MV, Bunout D, Leiva L, et al. Effect of probiotic *Saccharomyces boulardii* on prevention of ntibiotic-associated diarrhea in adult outpatients with amoxicillin treatment. *Rev Med Chil*. 2008;136(8):981-988.

11. Stein GY, Nanim R, Karniel E, Moskowitz I, Zeidman A. Probiotics as prophylactic agents against antibiotic-associated diarrhea in hospitalized patients. *Harefuah*. 2007;146(7):520-522,575.

12. McFarland LV. Meta-analysis of probiotics for the prevention of antibiotic associated diarrhea and the treatment of *Clostridium difficile* disease. *Am J Gastroenterol*. 2006;101(4):812-822.

13. Floch MH, Walker WA, Guandalini S, et al. Recommendations for probiotic use—2008. *J Clin Gastroenterol*. 2008;42(Suppl 2):S104-108.

14. Ruszczyński M, Radzikowski A, Szajewska H. Clinical trial: effectiveness of *Lactobacillus rhamnosus* (strains E/N, Oxy and Pen) in the prevention of antibiotic-associated diarrhoea in children. *Aliment Pharmacol Ther*. 2008;28(1):154-161.

15. Szymański H, Armańska M, Kowalska-Duplaga K, Szajewska H. *Bifidobacterium longum PL03*, *Lactobacillus rhamnosus KL53A*, and *Lactobacillus plantarum PL02* in the prevention of antibiotic-associated diarrhea in children: a randomized controlled pilot trial. *Digestion*. 2008;78(1):13-17.

16. Kale-Pradhan PB, Jassal HK, Wilhelm SM. Role of *Lactobacillus* in the prevention of antibiotic-associated diarrhea: a meta-analysis. *Pharmacotherapy*. 2010;30(2):119-126.

17. Szajewska H, Skórka A, Dylag M. Meta-analysis: *Saccharomyces boulardii* for treating acute diarrhoea in children. *Aliment Pharmacol Ther*. 2007;25(3):257-264.

18. Johnston BC, Supina AL, Ospina M, Vohra S. Probiotics for the prevention of pediatric antibiotic-associated diarrhea. *Cochrane Database Syst Rev*. 2007;(2):CD004827.

19. Pillai A, Nelson R. Probiotics for treatment of *Clostridium difficile*-associated colitis in adults. *Cochrane Database Syst Rev*. 2008;(1):CD004611.

20. McFarland LV, Surawicz CM, Greenberg RN, et al. Prevention of beta-lactam-associated diarrhea by *Saccharomyces boulardii* compared with placebo. *Am J Gastroenterol*. 1995;90(3):439-448.

21. Wullt M, Hagslätt ML, Odenholt I. *Lactobacillus plantarum 299v* for the treatment of recurrent *Clostridium difficile*-associated diarrhoea: a double-blind, placebo-controlled trial. *Scand J Infect Dis*. 2003;35(6-7):365-367.

22. Tung JM, Dolovich LR, Lee CH. Prevention of *Clostridium difficile* infection with *Saccharomyces boulardii*: a systematic review. *Can J Gastroenterol*. 2009;23(12):817-821.

23. Seal D, Borriello SP, Barclay F, et al. Treatment of relapsing *Clostridium difficile* diarrhoea by administration of a non-toxigenic strain. *Eur J Clin Microbiol*. 1987;6(1):51-53.

24. Pant C, Sferra TJ, Deshpande A, Minocha A. Clinical approach to severe *Clostridium difficile* infection: update for the hospital practitioner. *Eur J Intern Med*. 2011;22(6):561-568.

25. Persky SE, Brandt LJ. Treatment of recurrent *Clostridium difficile*-associated diarrhea by administration of donated stool directly through a colonoscope. *Am J Gastroenterol*. 2000;95(11):3283-3285.

26. Aas J, Gessert CE, Bakken JS. Recurrent *Clostridium difficile* colitis: case series involving 18 patients treated with donor stool administered via a nasogastric tube. *Clin Infect Dis*. 2003;36(5):580-585.

27. Warny M, Fatimi A, Bostwick EF, et al. Bovine immunoglobulin concentrate-*Clostridium difficile* retains *C difficile* toxin neutralising activity after passage through the human stomach and small intestine. *Gut*. 1999;44(2):212-217.

28. Mattila E, Anttila VJ, Broas M, et al. A randomized, double-blind study comparing *Clostridium difficile* immune whey and metronidazole for recurrent *Clostridium difficile*-associated diarrhoea: efficacy and safety data of a prematurely interrupted trial. *Scand J Infect Dis*. 2008;40(9):702-708.

Chapter

50 *Constipation*

KEY POINTS

○ Interventions like dietary changes, fluid intake changes, bowel retraining regimen, massage, toilet posture, physical exercise, and relaxation exercises provide safe and low-cost options for most patients—at least in the early phases of management.

○ All fibers are not similar in metabolic actions and efficacy in bowel health.

○ All probiotics are not created equal in efficacy.

○ Biofeedback is effective in pelvic floor dyssynergia.

Constipation is a symptomatic disorder and not a single disease, per say. Experts do not always agree on what constipation really means or what is currently defined by ROME III criteria. The prevalence rate of chronic constipation is 15% to 20% in North America. Constipation costs the health care system about $235 million per year, with the majority of it incurred (55%) from inpatient care. Surprisingly, the emergency room visits' cost component is 23%, whereas 16% and 6% of the expenses involve outpatient physicians and outpatient hospital settings, respectively.[1]

MANAGEMENT STRATEGY

The first step in managing constipation is to exclude a secondary cause for constipation. Both the patient and the physician need to be realistic in their expectations since a condition that may have evolved over several years and decades may only be partially amenable to any therapeutic strategy. Patients whose disorder is complicated by numerous diverse neurologic, biologic, psychological, and social factors present a bigger challenge.

ROLE OF LIFESTYLE

Exercise

While evidence linking a lack of physical activity to constipation is conflicting,[2] observational data from across cultures suggest that physical activity and exercise may promote bowel activity. Decreased mobility contributes to the development of constipation at least in a subset of cases. Exercise results in an increase in the number of propagated contractions, which may accelerate colonic transit.[3] Sedentary people are 3 times more likely to report constipation.[4]

Regular Bowel Habit

○ Initiation of defecation is, in part, a conditioned reflex.

○ Establishing a consistent bowel habit may help in establishing a regular pattern of bowel movements.

○ Attempt a bowel movement at least twice a day, usually 30 minutes after meals. The best time is in the morning after breakfast and within 2 hours of waking up.

○ Strain for no more than 5 minutes.

Toileting Posture

Toileting posture is a modifiable factor that should be used as part of an overall management strategy. The use of traditional toilet seats has a potential to make the recto-anal angle more acute, contributing to difficult passage of stools and constipation. Toileting posture is especially of concern in children who sit with their legs dangling in the air. Constipation as a child has the potential to persist throughout life.

Physically challenged subjects need to use higher chairs in order to be able to get up after defecation, and as such use posture changes as described previously for children. Appropriate toilet posture, coupled with abdominal exercises and other lifestyle changes, helps many patients.

SIMPLE WAYS TO MIMIC SQUATTING POSTURE

- ○ Bend forward with elbows resting on thighs
- ○ Support feet on a foot stool while seated on the toilet so that the angle at the thighs is acute

> Regular physical activity, along with appropriate toileting posture (bending forward), support of the feet while seated on toilet, and simple pelvic floor exercises, should be used as part of an overall treatment plan for constipation.

ROLE OF DIET

All Fibers Are Not Created Equal

Dietary fiber affects bowel habits, as well as GI morphology and function. A high-fiber diet increases stool weight and hastens intestinal transit. Lack of response to increasing fiber in diet may indicate colonic inertia or dysfunctional defecation.[5]

FIBER CONSUMPTION

A study from Hong Kong found that insufficient dietary fiber intake is common in Hong Kong preschool children.[6] Constipated children had significantly lower intakes of dietary fiber and micronutrients, including vitamin C, folate, and magnesium, than nonconstipated counterparts—which was attributable to underconsumption of plant foods.

Current recommendations suggest consumption of 20 to 35 g of dietary fiber per day, although the average American's daily intake of dietary fiber is about half of that. Always consume a variety of fiber-rich foods. The dose of fiber in children may be based on the formula (age in years + 5) g/day. It can take 4 to 8 weeks before the effects of the fiber become clearly evident. Always ensure an adequate amount of water intake as well.

SOLUBLE AND INSOLUBLE FIBER

Although neither type is absorbed by the body, they have different properties when mixed with water; hence the designation. A 3:1 ratio of insoluble to soluble fiber in diet is typically used. Wheat bran is one of the more effective fiber laxatives. There is an overlap in function between the 2 types of fibers.

ALL FIBERS ARE NOT THE SAME

Patients need to take fiber for 2 to 3 months before they experience significant symptom relief. Examples of insoluble fiber include cellulose, lignins, and some other hemicelluloses. Pectins, gums, mucilage, and some hemicellulose are soluble fibers.

Fiber Supplements

FIBER 7

Regularity Plus (Nutritional Design ND Lab, Lynbrook NY; formerly known as Fiber 7) is a natural powder fiber. A dose of 7 g bid is helpful in alleviating constipation in nursing home residents.

PSYLLIUM HUSK

It is derived from the seeds of *P ovata* and used as a bulk-forming laxative. Metamucil (Procter & Gamble, Cincinnati, OH) is the commercial prototype. Psyllium can easily be stirred into juices or foods. Psyllium is superior to wheat bran with respect to stool frequency and abdominal distension.[7]

A systematic review indicated that while psyllium is effective, there was insufficient evidence to recommend methyl cellulose, bran, and calcium polycarbophil. A Latin-American consensus on chronic constipation gave psyllium a grade B recommendation.[8]

Caution: Adequate fluid intake is essential when using psyllium. Prescription medications should be taken either 1 hour before or 2 hours after psyllium ingestion.

MISCELLANEOUS FIBERS

Vegetable gum fibers include guar gum, acacia gum, and wheat dextrin (ie, Benefiber [Novartis, Parsippany, NJ]). Hydrolyzed guar gum and galactomannan produce one of the highest amounts of SCFAs.[9]

Methylcellulose is a nonfermentable soluble fiber derived from cellulose (ie, Citrucel [GlaxoSmithKline, Middlesex, UK]) and is believed to produce less bloating and gas than psyllium. Polycarbophil is a synthetic agent and is less likely to cause bloating than psyllium. Soy polysaccharide fiber may be superior to oat fiber or soy oligosaccharide fiber.[10] Cocoa husk and glucomannan (konjac) are also effective.[11-14]

Fiber in Elderly Subjects

Daily intake of yogurt containing galactooligosaccharides, prunes, and linseed reduce the severity of constipation in elderly subjects with mild constipation.[15] Fiber supplementation in the form of a cake allows discontinuation of laxatives and increases the seniors' well being in a nursing home.[16]

Fiber Plus Probiotics

Simultaneous consumption of LGG yogurt (Valio Ltd, Riihimaki, Finland) with additional fiber helps relieve the adverse GI effects associated with an increased intake of fiber.[17]

Effect of Fluid Intake

While this issue may be overblown to some extent, it remains biologically plausible that adequate fluid intake is likely to be a significant factor in normal bowel function.

The precise amount of adequate fluid intake remains unknown. There is a high degree of interindividual variability. Extra fluid intake in normal healthy volunteers does not produce a significant increase in stool output.[18] However, the same may not apply to the not-so-healthy, as well as those who may represent borderline cases of hydration. There is a paucity of literature documenting the benefits of increasing fluid intake in states other than overt dehydration. A daily fiber intake of 25 g can increase stool frequency in patients with chronic functional constipation, and this effect can be significantly enhanced by increasing fluid intake to 1.5 to 2.0 L/day.[19]

PREBIOTICS

Prebiotics are substances that provide substrate for the preferential growth of desirable bacteria, thus shifting the balance in favor of good bacteria. Many of the fibers may be considered prebiotic.

Inulin occurs naturally in plants as oligosaccharides and promotes an increase in the stool mass and healthy intestinal bacteria (ie, *Lactobacillus* and *Bifidobacterium*).

Fructooligosaccharides (FOS) have soluble dietary fiber-like properties that relieve constipation, while stimulating the growth of *bifidobacteria* type of bacteria.[20] Consumption of isomaltooligosaccharides improves stool output and microbial fermentation in the colon in elderly subjects.[21]

Barley is a good source of fiber. The aleurone and scutellum fractions of germinated barley are used to produce GBF. Spent grain is the crude fiber obtained from the fermented distillate of barley. Its safety and efficacy in constipated subjects has been well documented.

PROBIOTICS

Dysbiosis is present in children who have chronic constipation.[22] Lactic acid bacteria have shown promise for treatment.[23,24] Many but not all probiotics[25-33] studied have beneficial results; these include *L reuteri (DSM 17938)*,[25] *L casei rhamnosus*,[26] Lcr35, *L casei Shirota*,[27] *B lactis DN-173-010*,[29,30] *B longum*,[31] *L rhamnosus/P freudenreichii*,[32] and Ecologic Relief (Winclove BV, Amsterdam, The Netherlands).[33] Probiotics with negative results include *Lactobacillus GG*.[28]

Similar positive results have been seen with synbiotics like zir fos (Alfa Wassermans R.L., Bucharest, Romania; *B longum W11* + FOS Actilight [Tereos Syral—Beghin Meiji, Marckolsheim, France]), *L paracasei*-enriched artichokes, as well as Activia (Dannon Inc, White Plains, NY; 10^8 CFU/g of *B animalis* [*DN-173 010*], and FOS).[34,35]

Limited evidence suggests beneficial effects of probiotics for preventing recurrent diverticulitis (including *L acidophilus* and *Bifidobacterium spp*) and as part of colonoscopy preparation (*Bacillus subtilis* and *Streptococcus faecium*).[36,37]

A systematic review on the use of probiotics for functional constipation reported that there is a favorable effect of treatment with *B lactis DN-173 010*, *L casei Shirota*, and *E coli Nissle 1917* in adults.[38] On the other hand, in children, *L casei rhamnosus Lcr35* (but not *L rhamnosus GG*) showed a beneficial effect.

MIND-BODY THERAPIES

Biofeedback

Biofeedback is an effective tool for the treatment of pelvic floor dyssynergia, and its effects are mediated via modification of physiologic behavior as well as colorectal function.[39] It is of benefit in 75% to 100% of the patients.[40] The beneficial response does not depend on the treatment protocol itself.[41] Biofeedback is not just for pelvic floor dyssynergia but is also effective in slow transit constipation.[42,43]

Biofeedback is more effective than diazepam or placebo for patients with pelvic floor dyssynergia-type constipation.[44] Muscular coordination training using instruction and encouragement without a visual display is also effective and may be suitable for use in outpatients.[45]

Gut-directed biofeedback is also effective for the treatment of patients with solitary rectal ulcer syndrome. Successful biofeedback therapy is associated with an increased rectal mucosal blood flow.[46] Patients with multiple sclerosis have abnormalities on anorectal physiology, and biofeedback is effective in some of these patients with constipation.[47] Biofeedback is beneficial for some children with chronic constipation and dyssynergic defecation; however, supplemental home biofeedback does not improve long-term outcomes.[48]

Stress Management

Chronic stress causes a dysfunction of the neuro-humoral-immune system. Severe constipation may be a defense mechanism, where normal physiological and normal emotional responses to stress are replaced by altered bowel patterns.[49] Breaking the vicious cycle of stress by appropriate stress management may help many patients.

Art Therapy

One study examined the effects of modeling clay to treat 6 children, aged 4 to 12 years, with a history of intractable constipation with encopresis refractory to treatment.[50] Clay for art therapy was chosen as a metaphor for feces. Of the 6 children studied, 4 children had no symptoms during 2 months of therapy.

Miscellaneous Mind-Body Therapies

Other mind-body–based therapies, such as hypnotherapy, relaxation techniques, and mental imagery, have the potential to be of benefit in functional constipation; however, data are lacking.

Phytobotanicals

While most of the knowledge has been handed down by word of mouth, much of it can also be found in texts written thousands of years ago. Absence of scientific studies does not necessarily equate with lack of efficacy. Others not on this list may be used for their relaxing and/or antispasmodic effects (eg, chamomile, lavender, and peppermint).

Aloe

Cathartic effect of oral aloe occurs via its components (anthraquinone glycosides) contained in aloe latex. Experts recommend that aloe gel may be taken as 1 to 2 tablespoons each day, whereas *A vera* juice may be taken as one-third of a glass mixed with two-thirds of a glass of juice of your choice per day.

Caution: In 2002, the US Food and Drug Administration (FDA) required that all over-the-counter aloe laxative products be removed from the US market or reformulated because the companies that manufactured them did not provide the necessary safety data.

Auricularia *(Ear Mushroom)*

A double-blind study showed that fiber supplements using ear mushrooms significantly improved constipation-related symptoms.[51]

Buckwheat (Polygonaceae)

Buckwheat acts as a dietary fiber. Buckwheat flour improves diabetes, obesity, hypercholesterolemia, and constipation in animal models.[52]

Cascara Sagrada (Rhamnus purshiana)

Aged bark of cascara is widely used as a mild laxative. *Caution:* The US FDA has banned the use of aloe and cascara sagrada as ingredients in over-the-counter laxative remedies. Currently, it is available only as a dietary supplement.

Cassia alata Linn

Eighty-six percent of patients taking *Cassia* have a stool within 24 hours, compared to only 18% taking the placebo.[53]

Croton

Croton penduliflorus seeds induce bowel movements in mice. *Croton macrostachyus* seeds are used as a laxative.[54]

Flaxseed (Linum usitatissimum)[55]

It is a rich source of fiber and omega-3 fatty acids and has been used as a laxative.

Ginger (Zingiber officinale)

Ginger is a widely used medicinal plant. It relaxes the colon in animals. There is a lack of data on its use in constipation.

Rhubarb

Rhubarb has strong laxative effects. There is a lack of studies documenting efficacy when used by itself in humans.[56]

Yumijangquebo

Yumijangquebo is an herbal laxative used in Korea (Table 50-1).

Herbal Combinations

DAI-KENCHU-TO, OR TJ-100

Dai-kenchu-to hastens GI transit in mice treated with morphine,[57] and may be helpful in postoperative ileus.[58] Dai-kenchu-to stimulates peristalsis and regulates bowel habits.[59]

MISRAKASNEHAM

Liquid Ayurvedic (herbal) preparation (Misrakasneham; a generic mixture of multiple herbs) is equal in efficacy to a conventional senna laxative tablet in the management of opioid-induced constipation in patients with advanced cancer.[60]

PADMA LAX

Padma Lax (Padma AG, Schwerzenbach, Switzerland), an herbal preparation based on Tibetan Medicine, is effective in severe constipation seen in some physically handicapped patients.[61] It contains aloe, calumba root, cascara, chebulic myrobalan fruit, condurango, frangula bark, gentian root, ginger, long pepper, rhubarb, etc.

SMOOTH MOVE

Smooth Move tea (Traditional Medicinals, Sebastopol, CA) is made from the *Senna* leaf and contains stimulant laxative active constituents known as hydroxyanthracene glycosides (sennosides A and B). It induces more bowel movements in nursing home patients with constipation, compared to placebo.[62]

MISCELLANEOUS COMBINATIONS

Matev et al treated constipated subjects with a combination of *Rhamnus frangula*, C *aurantium*, and C *carvi*.[63] The laxative herb combination was effective in all the patients, with a daily defecation seen in

Table 50-1. Some Phytobotanicals Used for
Constipation Across Cultures

Plant	Comment
Calotropis procera[65]	Induces contractions in isolated animal small intestine
C papaya	Reputed to be anti-inflammatory, there is a lack of studies documenting use in constipation
Cynomorium songaricum[66]	Facilitates catharsis
Colocynth (aka bitter apple; in Sanskrit it is called Gavakshi or Indravaruni)[67]	Increases bowel movements in constipated subjects, along with reduced discomfort
F vulgare[68] (fennel seeds)	Used for constipation as part of polyherbal formulations like Smooth Move, etc
Fumaria indica[69]	Used for both diarrhea and constipation; different constituents have spasmolytic and spasmogenic properties
H rosa-sinensis[70]	Used for constipation as well as diarrhea. The contractile and spasmolytic actions are mediated via activation of cholinergic receptors and activation and inhibition of calcium influx, respectively.
Kiwi fruit, aka Chinese gooseberry[71] (edible berry of genus Actinidia)	Improves spontaneous bowel movements in constipated patients
Naringenin flavonoid present in grapefruit and oranges, etc[72]	Stimulates fluid and chloride secretion in colon

(continued)

Table 50-1 *(continued)*. Some Phytobotanicals Used for Constipation Across Cultures

Plant	Comment
P boldus (Boldo)[73]	Data supporting its use in constipation are lacking
Prunus persica (peach)[74]	Contains both cholinomimetic as well as spasmolytic components; cholinergic properties dominate
Radish seeds[75]	Stimulates intestines in animals
Saussurea lappa[76]	Crude extract has cholinergic actions
Senna	Conclusive evidence for its clinical efficacy remains elusive[77,78]

90.6%. Bakera, a traditional steam bath prepared with numerous plants, is popular in Indonesia and is effective against constipation.[64]

MANIPULATIVE AND BODY-BASED PRACTICES

Massage

The term *massage* is very generic and includes a variety of techniques. Aromatherapy massage is complementary to the conventional nursing and medical treatment of constipation in patients with Guillain-Barré syndrome.[79] Aromatherapy massage is superior to placebo for relieving constipation in the elderly.[80]

Physical therapy incorporating abdominal massage appears to be effective in medically refractory constipation in elderly subjects.[81] Abdominal massage in the morning before breakfast in patients with spinal cord injuries results in improvement in frequency and duration of defecation.[82] Others have described similar success with abdominal massage.[83-86] Not-so-promising results were documented in Klauser's trial, which found that massage had no effect on parameters of colonic function to a clinically relevant degree.[87]

MISCELLANEOUS MASSAGE

Baduanjin (Eight-Treasured Exercises) is one of the many health-promoting ancient Chinese exercises. It is thought to be helpful in indigestion, constipation, arthritis, and obesity.[88] Dolk et al could not document any beneficial effect of yogic techniques for constipation due to puborectalis dysfunction.[89] Use of original Qigong massage technique is effective in young children with autism.

Chiropractic and Osteopathic Manipulation

Although chiropractic and osteopathic manipulation techniques are popular, the literature to support their use is scarce.

These are performed in conjunction with external massage of the abdomen, starting in the right lower quadrant and following the course of the large intestine in a clockwise direction. Such a therapy has been reported to be effective over the long term in chronic constipation.[90]

Reflexology

Reflexology is based on the premise that manual pressure to specific areas or zones of the feet correspond to different areas of the body and provide healing benefits accordingly. Early data appear promising.[91,92]

ENERGY-BASED MEDICINE

Electrogalvanic stimulation represents a useful adjunct to the therapeutic armamentarium for pelvic floor dyssynergia in normal transit constipation.[93]

Transcutaneous Electrical Nerve Stimulation Treatment

Transcutaneous electrical nerve stimulation treatment results in amelioration of soiling, along with increase in the frequency of spontaneous defecation in children with chronic treatment-resistant constipation.[94] A comparison of electrical stimulation therapy to biofeedback therapy for treatment of constipated patients with impaired rectal sensation showed that while both are equally effective for improving overall symptoms, only electrical stimulation therapy improves the frequency of wanting to defecate.[95] Other energy-based therapies in use for constipation include Reiki and healing touch; however, there is a paucity of published literature on their effectiveness.

WHOLE-BODY SYSTEMS

Acupuncture

Acupuncture has been used successfully for a wide spectrum of disorders, including functional bowel diseases. This may also be considered part of the broader traditional Chinese medicine. Multiple studies have documented its efficacy against constipation in adults as well as in children.[96,97]

Beneficial acupoints used include Zhigou (TE 6), ST25, CV6, CV4, Tianshu (ST 25), Qihai (CV 6), and Guanyuan (CV 4). Acupuncture at Di4 (He Gu), Ma25 (Tian Shu), Le3 (Yuan), and B125 (Da Chang Yu) is not effective.[98] Abdominal electroacupuncture is superior to cisapride in patients with constipation after stroke.[99] Acupuncture is also effective in children with constipation.[100]

Traditional Chinese Medicine

Traditional Chinese medicine considers constipation in terms of a variety of pathologic dysfunctions, including spleen Qi deficiency, liver Qi stagnation, and yin deficiency. While some of the therapies and studies are outlined here, others are mentioned in other sections because of overlap.

CHENG-CHI-TANG DECOCTIONS

Three Cheng-Chi-Tang decoctions[101,102] are used to treat internal heat and induce purgation.

1. Ta-Cheng-Chi-Tang contains *R palmatum L* (*Polygonaceae*), *Magnolia officinalis Rehd et Wils* (*Magnoliaceae*), *C aurantium L* (*Rutaceae*), and *Mirabilitum* (mirabilite, crystals of sodium sulfate, Na2SO4)

2. Xiao-Chen-Chi-Tang contains *R palmatum, M officinalis*, and *C aurantium*

3. Tiao-Wei-Chen-Chi-Tang contains *R palmatum, Mirabilitum*, and *Glycyrrhiza uralensis Fisch* (*Leguminosae*)

Maren soft capsules contain magnolia bark, rhubarb root, hemp seed, apricot seed, and bitter orange immature fruit. It increases the amount and weight of the stool of normal mice and enhances the movement of stool along the intestines.[103] Animal studies suggest that Yiqi Kaimi Recipe promotes colon motility by increasing the contraction frequency and amplitude of the smooth muscle.[104] Reinforcing Qi and moistening intestine oral liquid is effective in improving anorectal dynamic abnormalities in constipation.[105]

Shenshen Wan is made up of *Radix Pseudostellariae heterophylla, Fructus mori albae, Radix Polygoni multiflori, Semen persicae, Fructus lycii chinensis*, and *Herba cistanches* mixed in honey. It relieves constipation in 98% of elderly patients with dementia.[106] Likewise, Sini powder improves constipation by hastening colonic transit.

Homeopathy

This health system is based on the law of similars. Despite the lack of studies examining their efficacy, a variety of homeopathic medications are popular. These include bryonia for hard, dry stools; nux vomica for incomplete evacuation; silica for large, hard stools; and sulfur for hard stools with painful defecation.

REFERENCES

1. Martin BC, Barghout V, Cerulli A. Direct medical costs of constipation in the United States. *Manag Care Interface.* 2006;19(12):43-49.

2. Stewart RB, Moore MT, Marks RG, Hale WE. Correlates of constipation in an ambulatory elderly population. *Am J Gastroenterol.* 1992;87(7):859-864.

3. Rao KA, Yazaki E, Evans DF, Carbon R. Objective evaluation of small bowel and colonic transit time using pH telemetry in athletes with gastrointestinal symptoms. *Br J Sports Med.* 2004;38(4):482-487.

4. Whitehead WE, Drinkwater D, Cheskin LJ, Heller BR, Schuster MM. Constipation in the elderly living at home. Definition, prevalence, and relationship to lifestyle and health status. *J Am Geriatr Soc.* 1989;37(5):423-429.

5. Voderholzer WA, Schatke W, Mühldorfer BE, et al. Clinical response to dietary fiber treatment of chronic constipation. *Am J Gastroenterol.* 1997;92(1):95-98.

6. Lee WT, Ip KS, Chan JS, Lui NW, Young BW. Increased prevalence of constipation in pre-school children is attributable to under-consumption of plant foods: a community-based study. *J Paediatr Child Health.* 2008;44(4):170-175.

7. Hotz J, Plein K. Effectiveness of *Plantago* seed husks in comparison with wheat brain on stool frequency and manifestations of irritable colon syndrome with constipation. *Med Klin (Munich).* 1994;89(12):645-651.

8. Schmulson Wasserman M, Francisconi C, Olden K, et al. The Latin-American Consensus on chronic constipation. *Gastroenterol Hepatol.* 2008;31(2):59-74.

9. Pylkas AM, Juneja LR, Slavin JL. Comparison of different fibers for in vitro production of short chain fatty acids by intestinal microflora. *J Med Food.* 2005;8(1):113-116.

10. Kapadia SA, Raimundo AH, Grimble GK, Aimer P, Silk DB. Influence of three different fiber-supplemented enteral diets on bowel function and short-chain fatty acid production. *J Paren Enteral Nutr.* 1995;19(1):63-68.

11. Castillejo G, Bulló M, Anguera A, Escribano J, Salas-Salvadó J. A controlled, randomized, double-blind trial to evaluate the effect of a supplement of cocoa husk that is rich in dietary fiber on colonic transit in constipated pediatric patients. *Pediatrics.* 2006;118(3):e641-648.

12. Loening-Baucke V, Miele E, Staiano A. Fiber (glucomannan) is beneficial in the treatment of childhood constipation. *Pediatrics.* 2004;113(3 Pt 1):e259-264.

13. Chen HL, Cheng HC, Liu YJ, Liu SY, Wu WT. Konjac acts as a natural laxative by increasing stool bulk and improving colonic ecology in healthy adults. *Nutrition.* 2006;22(11-12):1112-1119.

14. Chen HL, Cheng HC, Wu WT, Liu YJ, Liu SY. Supplementation of konjac glucomannan into a low-fiber Chinese diet promoted bowel movement and improved colonic ecology in constipated adults: a placebo-controlled, diet-controlled trial. *J Am Coll Nutr.* 2008;27(1):102-108.

15. Sairanen U, Piirainen L, Nevala R, Korpela R. Yoghurt containing galacto-oligosaccharides, prunes and linseed reduces the severity of mild constipation in elderly subjects. *Eur J Clin Nutr.* 2007;61(12):1423-1428.

16. Sturtzel B, Elmadfa I. Intervention with dietary fiber to treat constipation and reduce laxative use in residents of nursing homes. *Ann Nutr Metab.* 2008;52(Suppl 1):54-56.

17. Hongisto SM, Paajanen L, Saxelin M, Korpela R. A combination of fibre-rich rye bread and yoghurt containing *Lactobacillus GG* improves bowel function in women with self-reported constipation. *Eur J Clin Nutr.* 2006;60(3):319-324.

18. Chung BD, Parekh U, Sellin JH. Effect of increased fluid intake on stool output in normal healthy volunteers. *J Clin Gastroenterol.* 1999;28(1):29-32.

19. Anti M, Pignataro G, Armuzzi A, et al. Water supplementation enhances the effect of high-fiber diet on stool frequency and laxative consumption in adult patients with functional constipation. *Hepatogastroenterology.* 1998;45(21):727-732.

20. Moore N, Chao C, Yang LP, et al. Effects of fructo-oligosaccharide-supplemented infant cereal: a double-blind, randomized trial. *Br J Nutr.* 2003;90(3):581-587.

21. Chen HL, Lu YH, Lin JJ, Ko LY. Effects of isomalto-oligosaccharides on bowel functions and indicators of nutritional status in constipated elderly men. *J Am Coll Nutr.* 2001;20(1):44-49.

22. Zoppi G, Cinquetti M, Luciano A, et al. The intestinal ecosystem in chronic functional constipation. *Acta Paediatr.* 1998;87(8):836-841.

23. An HM, Baek EH, Jang S, et al. Efficacy of lactic acid bacteria (LAB) supplement in management of constipation among nursing home residents. *Nutr J.* 2010;9:5.

24. Higashikawa F, Noda M, Awaya T, Nomura K, Oku H, Sugiyama M. Improvement of constipation and liver function by plant-derived lactic acid bacteria: a double-blind, randomized trial. *Nutrition.* 2010;26(4):367-374.

25. Coccorullo P, Strisciuglio C, Martinelli M, et al. *Lactobacillus reuteri* (*DSM 17938*) in infants with functional chronic constipation: a double-blind, randomized, placebo-controlled study. *J Pediatr.* 2010;157(4):598-602.

26. Bu LN, Chang MH, Ni YH, Chen HL, Cheng CC. *Lactobacillus casei rhamnosus Lcr35* in children with chronic constipation. *Pediatr Int.* 2007;49(4):485-490.

27. Koebnick C, Wagner I, Leitzmann P, Stern U, Zunft HJ. Probiotic beverage containing *Lactobacillus casei Shirota* improves gastrointestinal symptoms in patients with chronic constipation. *Can J Gastroenterol.* 2003;17(11):655-659.

28. Banaszkiewicz A, Szajewska H. Ineffectiveness of *Lactobacillus GG* as an adjunct to lactulose for the treatment of constipation in children: a double-blind, placebo-controlled randomized trial. *J Pediatr.* 2005;146(3): 364-369.

29. Agrawal A, Houghton LA, Lea R, et al. Bloating and distention in irritable bowel syndrome: the role of visceral sensation. *Gastroenterology.* 2008;134(7):1882-1889.

30. Yang YX, He M, Hu G, et al. Effect of a fermented milk containing *Bifidobacterium lactis DN-173010* on Chinese constipated women. *World J Gastroenterol.* 2008;14(40):6237-6243.

31. Pitkala KH, Strandberg TE, Finne Soveri UH, et al. Fermented cereal with specific *bifidobacteria* normalizes bowel movements in elderly nursing home residents. A randomized, controlled trial. *J Nutr Health Aging.* 2007;11(4):305-511.

32. Ouwehand AC, Lagström H, Suomalainen T, Salminen S. Effect of probiotics on constipation, fecal azoreductase activity and fecal mucin content in the elderly. *Ann Nutr Metab.* 2002;46(3-4):159-162.

33. Bekkali NL, Bongers ME, Van den Berg MM, Liem O, Benninga MA. The role of a probiotics mixture in the treatment of childhood constipation: a pilot study. *Nutr J.* 2007;6:17.

34. Amenta M, Cascio MT, Di Fiore P, Venturini I. Diet and chronic constipation. Benefits of oral supplementation with symbiotic zir fos (*Bifidobacterium longum* W11 + FOS Actilight). *Acta Biomed.* 2006;77(3): 157-162.

35. De Paula JA, Carmuega E, Weill R. Effect of the ingestion of a symbiotic yogurt on the bowel habits of women with functional constipation. *Acta Gastroenterol Latinoam.* 2008;38(1):16-25.

36. Lamiki P, Tsuchiya J, Pathak S, et al. Probiotics in diverticular disease of the colon: an open label study. *J Gastrointestin Liver Dis.* 2010;19(1):31-36.

37. Lee H, Kim YH, Kim JH, et al. A feasibility study of probiotics pretreatment as a bowel preparation for colonoscopy in constipated patients. *Dig Dis Sci.* 2010;55(8):2344-2351.

38. Chmielewska A, Szajewska H. Systematic review of randomised controlled trials: probiotics for functional constipation. *World J Gastroenterol.* 2010;16(1):69-75.

39. Rao SS, Seaton K, Miller M, et al. Randomized controlled trial of biofeedback, sham feedback, and standard therapy for dyssynergic defecation. *Clin Gastroenterol Hepatol.* 2007;5(3):331-338.

40. Chiarioni G, Whitehead WE, Pezza V, Morelli A, Bassotti G. Biofeedback is superior to laxatives for normal transit constipation due to pelvic floor dyssynergia. *Gastroenterology.* 2006;130(3):657-664.

41. Heymen S, Wexner SD, Vickers D, Nogueras JJ, Weiss EG, Pikarsky AJ. Prospective, randomized trial comparing four biofeedback techniques for patients with constipation. *Dis Colon Rectum*. 1999;42(11):1388-1393.

42. Brown SR, Donati D, Seow-Choen F, Ho YH. Biofeedback avoids surgery in patients with slow-transit constipation: report of four cases. *Dis Colon Rectum*. 2001;44(5):737-739, discussion 739-740.

43. Wang J, Luo MH, Qi QH, Dong ZL. Prospective study of biofeedback retraining in patients with chronic idiopathic functional constipation. *World J Gastroenterol*. 2003;9(9):2109-2113.

44. Heymen S, Scarlett Y, Jones K, et al. Randomized, controlled trial shows biofeedback to be superior to alternative treatments for patients with pelvic floor dyssynergia-type constipation. *Dis Colon Rectum*. 2007;50(4):428-441.

45. Koutsomanis D, Lennard-Jones JE, Roy AJ, Kamm MA. Controlled randomised trial of visual biofeedback versus muscle training without a visual display for intractable constipation. *Gut*. 1995;37(1):95-99.

46. Jarrett ME, Emmanuel AV, Vaizey CJ, Kamm MA. Behavioural therapy (biofeedback) for solitary rectal ulcer syndrome improves symptoms and mucosal blood flow. *Gut*. 2004;53(3):368-370.

47. Munteis E, Andreu M, Martinez-Rodriguez J, et al. Manometric correlations of anorectal dysfunction and biofeedback outcome in patients with multiple sclerosis. *Mult Scler*. 2008;14(2):237-242.

48. Croffie JM, Ammar MS, Pfefferkorn MD, et al. Assessment of the effectiveness of biofeedback in children with dyssynergic defecation and recalcitrant constipation/encopresis: does home biofeedback improve long-term outcomes. *Clin Pediatr (Phila)*. 2005;44(1):63-71.

49. Devroede G, Girard G, Bouchoucha M, et al. Idiopathic constipation by colonic dysfunction. Relationship with personality and anxiety. *Dig Dis Sci*. 1989;34(9):1428-1433.

50. Feldman PC, Villanueva S, Lanne V, Devroede G. Use of play with clay to treat children with intractable encopresis. *J Pediatr*. 1993;122(3):483-488.

51. Kim TI, Park SJ, Choi CH, Lee SK, Kim WH. Effect of ear mushroom (*Auricularia*) on functional constipation. *Korean J Gastroenterol*. 2004;44(1):34-41.

52. Li SQ, Zhang QH. Advances in the development of functional foods from buckwheat. *Crit Rev Food Sci Nutr*. 2001;41(6):451-464.

53. Thamlikitkul V, Bunyapraphatsara N, Dechatiwongse T, et al. Randomized controlled trial of *Cassia alata Linn.* for constipation. *J Med Assoc Thai*. 1990;73(4):217-222.

54. Mazzanti G, Bolle P, Martinoli L, et al. *Croton macrostachys*, a plant used in traditional medicine: purgative and inflammatory activity. *J Ethnopharmacol*. 1987;19(2):213-219.

55. Trepel F. Dietary fiber: more than a matter of dietetics. II. Preventative and therapeutic uses. *Wien Klin Wochenschr*. 2004;116(15-16):511-522.

56.   Kadake K, Fukumoto K, Chikayasu I, Kawai K, Ida K. Clinical effect of rhubarb and glycyrrhiza extract tablets on constipation. *Nippon Rinsho*. 1973;31(10):3069-3073.

57.   Nakamura T, Sakai A, Isogami I, et al. Abatement of morphine-induced slowing in gastrointestinal transit by Dai-kenchu-to, a traditional Japanese herbal medicine. *Jpn J Pharmacol*. 2002;88(2):217-221.

58.   Fukuda H, Chen C, Mantyh C, et al. The herbal medicine, Dai-Kenchu-to, accelerates delayed gastrointestinal transit after the operation in rats. *J Surg Res*. 2006;131(2):290-295.

59.   Iwai N, Kume Y, Kimura O, Ono S, Aoi S, Tsuda T. Effects of herbal medicine Dai-Kenchu-to on anorectal function in children with severe constipation. *Eur J Pediatr Surg*. 2007;17(2):115-118.

60.   Ramesh PR, Kumar KS, Rajagopal MR, Balachandran P, Warrier PK. Managing morphine-induced constipation: a controlled comparison of an Ayurvedic formulation and senna. *J Pain Symptom Manage*. 1998;16(4):240-244.

61.   Feldhaus S. Treatment of a tetraplegic patient with chronic constipation with the Tibetan remedy Padma Lax—a case report. *Forsch Komplementmed*. 2006;13(Suppl 1):31-32.

62.   Bub S, Brinckmann J, Cicconetti G, Valentine B. Efficacy of an herbal dietary supplement (Smooth Move) in the management of constipation in nursing home residents: a randomized, double-blind, placebo-controlled study. *J Am Med Dir Assoc*. 2006;7(9):556-561.

63.   Matev M, Chakurski I, Stefanov G, Koichev A, Angelov I. Use of an herbal combination with laxative action on duodenal peptic ulcer and gastroduodenitis patients with a concomitant obstipation syndrome. *Vutr Boles*. 1981;20(6):48-51.

64.   Zumsteg IS, Weckerle CS. Bakera, a herbal steam bath for postnatal care in Minahasa (Indonesia): documentation of the plants used and assessment of the method. *J Ethnopharmacol*. 2007;111(3):641-650.

65.   Mossa JS, Tariq M, Mohsin A, et al. Pharmacological studies on aerial parts of *Calotropis procera*. *Am J Chin Med*. 1991;19(3-4):223-231.

66.   Tao J, Tu P, Xu W, Chen D. Studies on chemical constituents and pharmacological effects of the stem of *Cynomorium songaricum Rupr*. *Zhongguo Zhong Yao Za Zhi*. 1999;24(5):292-294,318-319.

67.   Lorenz PR, Lippmann F, Dürrling K, Solf M, Geissler J. Pharmaco-toxicological and clinical studies with colocynth pulp extracts (Extr. colocynthidis fructus). *Arzneimittelforschung*. 2005;55(11):621-663.

68.   Picon PD, Picon RV, Costa AF, et al. Randomized clinical trial of a phytotherapic compound containing *Pimpinella anisum*, *Foeniculum vulgare*, *Sambucus nigra*, and *Cassia augustifolia* for chronic constipation. *BMC Complement Altern Med*. 2010;10:17.

69.   Gilani AH, Bashir S, Janbaz KH, Khan A. Pharmacological basis for the use of *Fumaria indica* in constipation and diarrhea. *J Ethnopharmacol*. 2005;96(3):585-589.

70. Gilani AH, Bashir S, Janbaz KH, Shah AJ. Presence of cholinergic and calcium channel blocking activities explains the traditional use of *Hibiscus rosasinensis* in constipation and diarrhoea. *J Ethnopharmacol.* 2005;102(2):289-294.

71. Chan AO, Leung G, Tong T, Wong NY. Increasing dietary fiber intake in terms of kiwifruit improves constipation in Chinese patients. *World J Gastroenterol.* 2007;13(35):4771-4775.

72. Yang ZH, Yu HJ, Pan A, et al. Cellular mechanisms underlying the laxative effect of flavonol naringenin on rat constipation model. *PLoS One.* 2008;3(10):e3348.

73. Piscaglia F, Leoni S, Venturi A, Graziella F, Donati G, Bolondi L. Caution in the use of boldo in herbal laxatives: a case of hepatotoxicity. *Scand J Gastroenterol.* 2005;40(2):236-239.

74. Gilani AH, Aziz N, Ali SM, Saeed M. Pharmacological basis for the use of peach leaves in constipation. *J Ethnopharmacol.* 2000;73(1-2):87-93.

75. Ghayur MN, Gilani AH, Houghton PJ. Species differences in the gut stimulatory effects of radish seeds. *J Pharm Pharmacol.* 2005;57(11):1493-1501.

76. Gilani AH, Shah AJ, Yaeesh S. Presence of cholinergic and calcium antagonist constituents in *Saussurea lappa* explains its use in constipation and spasm. *Phytother Res.* 2007;21(6):541-544.

77. Ramkumar D, Rao SS. Efficacy and safety of traditional medical therapies for chronic constipation: systematic review. *Am J Gastroenterol.* 2005;100(4):936-971.

78. Candy B, Jones L, Goodman ML, Drake R, Tookman A. Laxatives or methylnaltrexone for the management of constipation in palliative care patients. *Cochrane Database Syst Rev.* 2011;(1):CD003448.

79. Shirreffs CM. Aromatherapy massage for joint pain and constipation in a patient with Guillian Barré. *Complement Ther Nurs Midwifery.* 2001;7(2):78-83.

80. Kim MA, Sakong JK, Kim EJ, Kim EH, Kim EH. Effect of aromatherapy massage for the relief of constipation in the elderly. *Taehan Kanho Hakhoe Chi.* 2005;35(1):56-64.

81. Harrington KL, Haskvitz EM. Managing a patient's constipation with physical therapy. *Phys Ther.* 2006;86(11):1511-1519.

82. Albers B, Cramer H, Fischer A, et al. Abdominal massage as intervention for patients with paraplegia caused by spinal cord injury—a pilot study. *Pflege Z.* 2006;59(3):2-8.

83. Ayas S, Leblebici B, Sözay S, Bayramoglu M, Niron EA. The effect of abdominal massage on bowel function in patients with spinal cord injury. *Am J Phys Med Rehabil.* 2006;85(12):951-955.

84. Jeon SY, Jung HM. The effects of abdominal meridian massage on constipation among CVA patients. *Taehan Kanho Hakhoe Chi.* 2005;35(1):135-142.

85. Lämås K, Lindholm L, Stenlund H, Engström B, Jacobsson C. Effects of abdominal massage in management of constipation—a randomized controlled trial. *Int J Nurs Stud.* 2009;46(6):759-767.

86. Lämås K, Lindholm L, Engström B, Jacobsson C. Abdominal massage for people with constipation: a cost utility analysis. *J Adv Nurs.* 2010;66(8):1719-1729.

87. Klauser AG, Flaschenträger J, Gehrke A, Müller-Lissner SA. Abdominal wall massage: effect on colonic function in healthy volunteers and in patients with chronic constipation. *Z Gastroenterol.* 1992;30(4):247-251.

88. Koh TC. Baduanjin—an ancient Chinese exercise. *Am J Chin Med.* 1982;10(1-4):14-21.

89. Dolk A, Holmström B, Johansson C, Frostell C, Nilsson BY. The effect of yoga on puborectalis paradox. *Int J Colorectal Dis.* 1991;6(3):139-142.

90. Quist DM, Duray SM. Resolution of symptoms of chronic constipation in an 8-year-old male after chiropractic treatment. *J Manipulative Physiol Ther.* 2007;30(1):65-68.

91. Bishop E, McKinnon E, Weir E, Brown DW. Reflexology in the management of encopresis and chronic constipation. *Paediatr Nurs.* 2003;15(3):20-21.

92. Woodward S, Norton C, Barriball KL. A pilot study of the effectiveness of reflexology in treating idiopathic constipation in women. *Complement Ther Clin Pract.* 2010;16(1):41-46.

93. Chiarioni G, Chistolini F, Menegotti M, et al. One-year follow-up study on the effects of electrogalvanic stimulation in chronic idiopathic constipation with pelvic floor dyssynergia. *Dis Colon Rectum.* 2004;47(3):346-353.

94. Chase J, Robertson VJ, Southwell B, Hutson J, Gibb S. Pilot study using transcutaneous electrical stimulation (interferential current) to treat chronic treatment-resistant constipation and soiling in children. *J Gastroenterol Hepatol.* 2005;20(7):1054-1061.

95. Chang HS, Myung SJ, Yang SK, et al. Effect of electrical stimulation in constipated patients with impaired rectal sensation. *Int J Colorectal Dis.* 2003;18(5):433-438.

96. Zhang ZL, Ji XQ, Zhao SH, et al. Multi-central randomized controlled trials of electroacupuncture at Zhigou (TE 6) for treatment of constipation induced by stagnation or deficiency of qi. *Zhongguo Zhen Jiu.* 2007;27(7):475-478.

97. Li YH, Yin LL, Wang SX, Wang LH. Observation on the therapeutic effect of acupoint application on constipation. *Zhongguo Zhen Jiu.* 2007;27(3):189-190.

98. Klauser AG, Rubach A, Bertsche O, Müller-Lissner SA. Body acupuncture: effect on colonic function in chronic constipation. *Z Gastroenterol.* 1993;31(10):605-608.

99. Wang DS, Wang S, Kong LL, Wang WY, Cui XM. Clinical observation on abdominal electroacupuncture for treatment of poststroke constipation. *Zhongguo Zhen Jiu.* 2008;28(1):7-9.

100. Broide E, Pintov S, Portnoy S, Barg J, Klinowski E, Scapa E. Effectiveness of acupuncture for treatment of childhood constipation. *Dig Dis Sci.* 2001;46(6):1270-1275.

101. Tseng SH, Chien TY, Chen JR, Lin IH, Wang CC. Hypolipidemic effects of three purgative decoctions. *Evid Based Complement Alternat Med.* 2011;2011:249-254.

102. Tseng SH, Lee HH, Chen LG, Wu CH, Wang CC. Effects of three purgative decoctions on inflammatory mediators. *J Ethnopharmacol.* 2006;105(1-2):118-124.

103. Guo JH, Jiang ML, Peng ZP, et al. Studies on laxative function of maren soft capsule. *Zhongguo Zhong Yao Za Zhi.* 1993;18(4):236-239,256.

104. He CM, Lu JG, Cao YQ. Effects of Yiqi Kaimi Recipe on gastrointestinal-motility and neuropeptides in rats with colonic slow transit constipation. *Zhong Xi Yi Jie He Xue Bao.* 2007;5(2):160-164.

105. Yu S, Wang Y, Wu J. Effect of reinforcing qi and moistening intestine oral liquid on anorectal manometry of asthenia type constipation patients. *Zhongguo Zhong Xi Yi Jie He Za Zhi.* 2000;20(5):325-327.

106. Zhang S, Chang Y, Wang N, Xu D, Liu Z. Clinical and experimental studies on the treatment of senile constipation with shenshen wan. *J Trad Chin Med.* 1996;16(3):182-185.

FEEDING DISORDERS

Chapter

51 *Anorexia Nervosa*

KEY POINTS

- ○ Behavioral therapy aims to empower patients to learn to refrain from potentially harmful eating behaviors.
- ○ Cognitive behavioral therapy (CBT) is effective for patients with eating disorders.
- ○ Family therapy is effective.
- ○ Hypnotherapeutic techniques can help uncover the origin of the disrupted cognition and emotional conflicts, and empower patients to develop control over their thoughts and actions.

Anorexia nervosa is a multifactorial, convoluted complex of learned behaviors. Current pharmacotherapy of anorexia nervosa raises more questions than answers.[1] A focused approach addressing the diverse areas of pathophysiology is likely to achieve better response to therapy than a nonspecific therapeutic strategy.[2]

Studies testing pharmacotherapeutic agents show that the core symptoms of anorexia nervosa are refractory to currently available psychotropic medication.[3] Antidepressants are helpful in patients with depressive symptoms and may help prevent relapse. Even electroconvulsive therapy has been used.

Minocha A. *A Guide to Alternative Medicine and the Digestive System* (pp 291-300).
© 2013 Taylor & Francis Group.

PSYCHOTHERAPIES[4,5]

Behavioral Modification

Eating behaviors are learned behaviors and, as such, have the potential to be unlearned. However, the success is gradual at best. Behavioral approaches alone or combined with CBT may be used. Indirect and permissive suggestions are more effective since they serve to enhance rather than challenge the patient's need to have control. A lenient approach is likely to be more acceptable to patients than a punitive one.

Components of behavioral modification may include the following:

❍ Relearning normal eating habits

❍ Gaining insight into the eating behavior and reasons for persisting

❍ Diet and nutrition counseling

❍ Lifestyle modifications

❍ Shopping style modifications (eg, avoiding certain stores and purchase of trigger foods)

❍ Modification of eating behavior (eg, not watching television at the same time as eating)

Cognitive Behavioral Therapy[6]

CBT improves the outcome and prevents relapse in weight-restored anorexia nervosa.[7] Combined CBT and weight restoration reduces eating disorder symptoms, depression, and general psychopathology during hospitalization.[8] Outpatient CBT is effective.[9]

CBT administered through partially-structured guidance and education achieves higher success by rectifying the interconnected maladaptive and distorted cognitions and behaviors.[10] However, CBT designed specifically to manipulate both attitudes and behavior may not be superior to other types of behavioral treatments.[11]

Nonspecific supportive clinical management is superior to interpersonal psychotherapy, while CBT is intermediate.[12] Self-psychological treatment may be superior to cognitive orientation treatment.[13]

CBT is the leading therapeutic strategy. A new "enhanced" version of the treatment is more effective and provides additional advantages as being suitable for all eating disorders.[6]

Biofeedback Relaxation System

Electrodermal response biofeedback ameliorates eating disorders.[14]

Manualized Guided Self-Help Versus Waiting List Control

Guided self-help reduces the duration of inpatient treatment significantly, along with an improved body image and general psychopathology.[15]

Effect of Type of Psychotherapy

A randomized, controlled trial (RCT) assessed the effectiveness of various outpatient psychotherapies for the treatment of patients with anorexia nervosa.[16] Three specific psychotherapies studied included a year of focal psychoanalytic psychotherapy, 7 months of cognitive-analytic therapy, and family therapy for 1 year. A low contact, "routine" treatment for 1 year served as control. While everyone improved at the end of 1 year, superior results were seen in the patients receiving psychoanalytic psychotherapy and family therapy.

SELF-HELP VERSUS GUIDED SELF-HELP PSYCHOTHERAPY

A Cochrane database review concluded that there are no significant differences in outcome between pure self-help (self-help material only) or guided self-help (self-help material with therapist guidance).[17]

FAMILY THERAPY[18]

Behavioral family systems therapy produces faster results compared to ego-oriented individual therapy.[19] While much of the improvements of family therapy at a 5-year follow-up can be attributed to the natural outcome of the illness, significant benefits attributable to previous psychological treatments are still evident.[20] While both conjoint and separated family therapy are essentially similar in outcome at 5 years, the use of conjoint family meetings should be avoided, at least in earlier stages when parental criticism is quite evident.[21]

> Family therapy may be more effective than usual treatment; however, it is not superior to other forms of psychological interventions.[18]

HYPNOSIS

Hypnosis[22] can help establish a reality-based body image in patients. Children as young as 3 years of age can effectively apply self-hypnosis techniques. While hypnosis plays an important role in improving self-confidence, self-esteem, etc, patients with anorexia nervosa have an extreme need for control, and as such they tend to be poor subjects for hypnosis.

ART-BASED THERAPIES

A therapeutic approach combining art therapy, psychodrama, and verbal therapy has a greater potential for success.[23] Music therapy can also be effective in anorectic patients who are concurrently mentally challenged.[24] Art-based therapies are being increasingly used in combination with other therapies, especially as part of inpatient programs.[25]

SPIRITUALITY

An RCT compared the effectiveness of a spirituality group with cognitive and emotional support groups in subjects receiving inpatient eating disorder treatment for anorexia nervosa.[26] Patients in the spirituality group scored lower on psychological disturbance and eating disorder symptoms compared to others.

TRADITIONAL CHINESE MEDICINE

Nano-Amoni Paste

Sticking 1.5 mL of nano-Amoni paste (nmAP) on the acupoint of Shenque (Ren 8) results in an effective rate of 95% and is superior to placebo.[27]

Acupuncture

Acupuncture, as an adjunct treatment for treating eating disorders, results in an improvement in quality of life, along with improvement in anxiety and perfectionism.[28]

INPATIENT, OUTPATIENT, OR OUTPATIENT SPECIALIST TREATMENT

Results of studies have been conflicting.[29,30] Inpatient treatment may be an option for use in selected patients for long-term rehabilitation.[29] In contrast, a multicenter RCT of adolescents comparing inpatient, outpatient specialist, and general child and adolescent mental health service found that inpatient psychiatric treatment does not provide advantages over outpatient managements.[30] Provision of outpatient specialist services for adolescents with anorexia nervosa may be the most cost effective.

REFERENCES

1. Hebebrand J. Pharmacotherapy of anorexia nervosa: more questions than answers. *J Am Acad Child Adolesc Psychiatry.* 2011;50(9):854-856.

2. Fundudis T. Anorexia nervosa in a pre-adolescent girl: a multimodal behaviour therapy approach. *J Child Psychol Psychiatry.* 1986;27(2):261-273.

3. Casper RC. How useful are pharmacological treatments in eating disorders? *Psychopharmacol Bull.* 2002;36(2):88-104.

4. Hay PP, Bacaltchuk J, Stefano S, Kashyap P. Psychological treatments for bulimia nervosa and binging. *Cochrane Database Syst Rev.* 2009;(4):CD000562.

5. Lock J, Fitzpatrick KK. Advances in psychotherapy for children and adolescents with eating disorders. *Am J Psychother.* 2009;63(4):287-303.

6. Murphy R, Straebler S, Cooper Z, Fairburn CG. Cognitive behavioral therapy for eating disorders. *Psychiatr Clin North Am.* 2010;33(3):611-627.

7. Carter JC, McFarlane TL, Bewell C, et al. Maintenance treatment for anorexia nervosa: a comparison of cognitive behavior therapy and treatment as usual. *Int J Eat Disord.* 2009;42(3):202-207.

8. Bowers WA, Ansher LS. The effectiveness of cognitive behavioral therapy on changing eating disorder symptoms and psychopathology of 32 anorexia nervosa patients at hospital discharge and one year follow-up. *Ann Clin Psychiatry.* 2008;20(2):79-86.

9. Fernández-Aranda F, Bel M, Jiménez S, et al. Outpatient group therapy for anorexia nervosa: a preliminary study. *Eat Weight Disord.* 1998;3(1):1-6.

10. Yeh HW, Tzeng NS, Lai TJ, Chou KR. Cognitive behavioral therapy for eating disorders. *Hu Li Za Zhi.* 2006;53(4):65-73.

11. Channon S, de Silva P, Hemsley D, Perkins R. A controlled trial of cognitive-behavioural and behavioural treatment of anorexia nervosa. *Behav Res Ther.* 1989;27(5):529-535.

12. McIntosh VV, Jordan J, Carter FA, et al. Three psychotherapies for anorexia nervosa: a randomized, controlled trial. *Am J Psychiatry.* 2005;162(4):741-747.

13. Bachar E, Latzer Y, Kreitler S, Berry EM. Empirical comparison of two psychological therapies. Self psychology and cognitive orientation in the treatment of anorexia and bulimia. *J Psychother Pract Res.* 1999;8(2):115-128.

14. Pop-Jordanova N. Psychological characteristics and biofeedback mitigation in preadolescents with eating disorders. *Pediatr Int.* 2000;42(1):76-81.

15. Fichter M, Cebulla M, Quadflieg N, Naab S. Guided self-help for binge eating/purging anorexia nervosa before inpatient treatment. *Psychother Res.* 2008;18(5):594-603.

16. Dare C, Eisler I, Russell G, Treasure J, Dodge L. Psychological therapies for adults with anorexia nervosa: randomised controlled trial of out-patient treatments. *Br J Psychiatry.* 2001;178:216-221.

17. Perkins SJ, Murphy R, Schmidt U, Williams C. Self-help and guided self-help for eating disorders. *Cochrane Database Syst Rev.* 2006;3:CD004191.

18. Fisher CA, Hetrick SE, Rushford N. Family therapy for anorexia ner-vosa. *Cochrane Database Syst Rev.* 2010;(4):CD004780.

19. Robin AL, Siegel PT, Moye AW, Gilroy M, Dennis AB, Sikand A. A con-trolled comparison of family versus individual therapy for adolescents with anorexia nervosa. *J Am Acad Child Adolesc Psychiatry.* 1999;38(12):1482-1489.

20. Eisler I, Dare C, Russell GF, Szmukler G, le Grange D, Dodge E. Family and individual therapy in anorexia nervosa. A 5-year follow-up. *Arch Gen Psychiatry.* 1997;54(11):1025-1030.

21. Eisler I, Simic M, Russell GF, Dare C. A randomised controlled treat-ment trial of two forms of family therapy in adolescent anorexia ner-vosa: a five-year follow-up. *J Child Psychol Psychiatry.* 2007;48(6):552-560.

22. Barabasz M. Efficacy of hypnotherapy in the treatment of eating disor-ders. *Int J Clin Exp Hypn.* 2007;55(3):318-335.

23. Diamond-Raab L, Orrell-Valente JK. Art therapy, psychodrama, and verbal therapy. An integrative model of group therapy in the treatment of adolescents with anorexia nervosa and bulimia nervosa. *Child Adolesc Psychiatr Clin N Am.* 2002;11(2):343-364.

24. Heal M, O'Hara J. The music therapy of an anorectic mentally handi-capped adult. *Br J Med Psychol.* 1993;66(Pt 1):33-41.

25. Frisch MJ, Herzog DB, Franko DL. Residential treatment for eating disorders. *Int J Eat Disord.* 2006;39(5):434-442.

26. Richards PS, Berrett ME, Hardman RK, Eggett DL. Comparative effica-cy of spirituality, cognitive, and emotional support groups for treating eating disorder inpatients. *Eat Disord.* 2006;14(5):401-415.

27. Wu M, Li Z, Yu JE, Lu WW, Ni JX, Xia YL. Multi-centered clinical study on effects of nano-amomi paste in treating children's anorexia. *Chin J Integr Med.* 2007;13(1):55-58.

28. Fogarty S, Harris D, Zaslawski C, McAinch AJ, Stojanovska L. Acupuncture as an adjunct therapy in the treatment of eating disorders: a randomised cross-over pilot study. *Complement Ther Med.* 2010;18(6):233-240.

29. Rø O, Martinsen EW, Hoffart A, Rosenvinge JH. Short-term follow-up of adults with long standing anorexia nervosa or non-specified eating disorder after inpatient treatment. *Eat Weight Disord.* 2004;9(1):62-68.

30. Gowers SG, Clark A, Roberts C, et al. Clinical effectiveness of treat-ments for anorexia nervosa in adolescents: randomised controlled trial. *Br J Psychiatry.* 2007;191:427-435.

Chapter

52 *Bulimia Nervosa*

KEY POINTS

- ○ Bulimia nervosa occurs in up to 1% of young women.
- ○ Prognosis of bulimia nervosa is better than for anorexia nervosa.
- ○ Cognitive behavioral therapy (CBT) is the treatment of choice and is superior to pharmacological treatment.
- ○ Combined psychological plus pharmacological treatment is not superior to psychological treatment alone.

GENERAL STRATEGIES

- ○ Nutritional counseling
- ○ Food diaries
- ○ Advance planning for meals a day in advance

PSYCHOLOGICAL TREATMENTS

Psychotherapy, including CBT and antidepressants, is effective for the treatment of bulimia, especially when employed in combination.[1]

Cognitive Behavioral Therapy

Multiple RCTs have confirmed the effectiveness of CBT compared to no therapy, nondirective therapy, psychodynamic therapy, stress therapy, and pharmacological treatments.

A meta-analysis of randomized placebo-controlled drug and psychosocial studies concluded that CBT provides superior relief of binge eating, purging, and eating behaviors.[1]

An Internet-based self-help therapeutic approach utilizing CBT is a viable option compared to waiting list controls.[2] Group treatment, prefaced by a short individual therapy, may be a cost effective alternative to purely individual treatment utilizing CBT.[3] A large number of bulimic patients also suffer from a substance use disorder. CBT can be adapted as an integrated treatment for such patients since it is effective for both disorders independently.[4]

Self-guided CBT provides a faster relief and is less costly than family therapy. Pure or unguided CBT is not effective in inducing remission.

Motivational Enhancement Therapy

Motivational enhancement therapy is as effective as CBT.[5] This form of therapy is more frequently used for anorexia nervosa rather than bulimia.

Interpersonal Psychotherapy

Individuals with eating disorders have low sensitivity for interpersonal stressors. Interpersonal psychotherapy provides a beneficial short-term intervention, especially in patients with associated depression. It is inferior to CBT.

Dialectical Behavioral Therapy

It represents a modified form of behavioral therapy that focuses on emotional dysfunction underlying the abnormal eating behavior. Dialectical behavioral therapy for 20 weeks results in a significant decrease in binge/purge behavior, compared to controls.[6]

Hypnobehavioral Therapy

Griffiths et al compared pre- and post-findings from a controlled evaluation of hypnobehavioral treatment compared to waiting list controls over a period of 8 weeks.[7] Hypnobehavioral therapy resulted in a significant decrease in bulimic behavior compared to controls.

Family Therapy

Family-based therapy is more effective than individual therapy in patients whose illness is not chronic and onset is prior to the age of 19.[8] It accomplishes abstinence in 40% of cases at the end of treatment and 30% follow up compared to 18% and 10%, respectively, with individual therapy. Family therapy is similar in efficacy to CBT guided self-care,[9] although CBT provides faster relief at a lower cost.[10]

Guided Imagery Therapy

The effect of individual guided imagery therapy designed to enhance self-comforting was examined in an RCT of 50 subjects with bulimia nervosa over 6 weeks.[11] Individual guided imagery therapy treatment groups demonstrated a 74% reduction of binges and 73% of vomiting, along with improvement of attitudes about eating, dieting, and body weight.

Results of meta-analysis indicate that bulimia nervosa-targeted CBT is effective for bulimia nervosa. Other psychotherapies, especially interpersonal psychotherapy, are also effective. Self-help protocols using structured CBT treatment manuals may be helpful. Psychotherapy alone is not likely to be very effective.[1]

MISCELLANEOUS THERAPIES

The role of light therapy is controversial. Individualized yoga treatment may have the potential for efficacy as an adjunct treatment. Attention to spiritual growth and well-being of patients may help in improvement of psychological manifestations, as well as eating behavior.

A Cochrane database review[12] evaluated controlled trials to examine the efficacy of pure self-help (self-help material only) or guided self-help (with therapist guidance) in eating disorders. The authors found that pure/guided self-help was as equally effective as other formal psychological therapies and may have a role as initial step-in treatment—perhaps in lieu of therapist-delivered psychological therapy.

Application of high-frequency, repetitive transcranial magnetic stimulation of the dorsolateral prefrontal cortex reduces cue-induced food cravings in people with bulimia nervosa and may reduce binge eating.

DRUG TREATMENT

Medications are an option in patients refractory to CBT and include treatment with antidepressants, especially selective serotonin reuptake inhibitors. Antiepileptic agents (eg, topiramate) and selective serotonin antagonists (eg, ondansetron) have shown promise. Severe cases may need inpatient treatment.

REFERENCES

1. Hay PP, Bacaltchuk J, Stefano S, et al. Psychological treatments for bulimia nervosa and binging. *Cochrane Database Syst Rev.* 2009;(4):CD000562.
2. Fernández-Aranda, Núñez A, Martínez C, et al. Internet-based cognitive-behavioral therapy for bulimia nervosa: a controlled study. *Cyberpsychol Behav.* 2009;12(1):37-41.
3. Katzman MA, Bara-Carril N, Rabe-Hesketh S, et al. A randomized controlled two-stage trial in the treatment of bulimia nervosa, comparing CBT versus motivational enhancement in Phase 1 followed by group versus individual CBT in Phase 2. *Psychosom Med.* 2010;72(7):656-663.

4. Sysko R, Hildebrandt T. Cognitive-behavioural therapy for individuals with bulimia nervosa and a co-occurring substance use disorder. *Eur Eat Disord Rev*. 2009;17(2):89-100.

5. Treasure JL, Katzman M, Schmidt U, et al. Engagement and outcome in the treatment of bulimia nervosa: first phase of a sequential design comparing motivation enhancement therapy and cognitive behavioural therapy. *Behav Res Ther*. 1999;37(5):405-418.

6. Safer DL, Telch CF, Agras WS. Dialectical behavior therapy for bulimia nervosa. *Am J Psychiatry*. 2001;158(4):632-634.

7. Griffiths RA, Hadzi-Pavlovic D, Channon-Little L. A controlled evaluation of hypnobehavioural treatment for bulimia nervosa: immediate pre-post treatment effects. *Eur Eat Dis*. 1994;2:202–220.

8. Russell GF, Szmukler GI, Dare C, Eisler I. An evaluation of family therapy in anorexia nervosa and bulimia nervosa. *Arch Gen Psychiatry*. 1987;44(12):1047-1056.

9. Paxton SJ. Family therapy does not improve outcomes in adolescents with bulimia nervosa compared to CBT guided self-care. *Evid Based Ment Health*. 2007;10(4):122.

10. Schmidt U, Lee S, Beecham J, et al. A randomized controlled trial of family therapy and cognitive behavior therapy guided self-care for adolescents with bulimia nervosa and related disorders. *Am J Psychiatry*. 2007;164(4):591-598.

11. Esplen MJ, Garfinkel PE, Olmsted M, et al. A randomized controlled trial of guided imagery in bulimia nervosa. *Psychol Med*. 1998;28(6):1347-1357.

12. Perkins SJ, Murphy R, Schmidt U, Williams C. Self-help and guided self-help for eating disorders. *Cochrane Database Syst Rev*. 2006;3:CD004191.

CANCER

Chapter

53 *Diet and Cancer*

KEY POINTS

○ A diet high in fruit and vegetables is protective.
○ Mediterranean diet offers significant protective benefits.
○ Garlic and fish help against cancer.
○ Fiber protects against cancer.
○ Excessive cooking/frying increases the risk of cancer.

Dietary factors have the potential to modulate the development of several cancers of the gastrointestinal (GI) tract.[1,2]

GENERAL CONSIDERATIONS

Vegetarian Versus Nonvegetarian

A prospective comparative investigation of vegetarians and nonvegetarians, in a cohort of 10,998 men and women, found 95 cases of colorectal cancer over a period of 17 years.[3] Smoking, alcohol, and white bread consumption increased the risk, whereas the risk declined in subjects with frequent consumption of fruit. There was no difference in the risk between vegetarians and nonvegetarians in this study (RR = 0.85; 95% CI: 0.55 to 1.32).

Minocha A. *A Guide to Alternative Medicine and the Digestive System* (pp 301-342).

Red, Processed Meat

Examination of the relationship between recent and long-term meat consumption and the risk of colorectal cancer in a cohort of 148,610 adults found that a high intake of red meat and processed meat carries a greater risk of colon cancer.[4]

A population-based, case-control study of colon cancer found that an intake of red meat increases the risk for colon cancer (odds ratio = 2.0, CI: 1.3 to 3.2). Associations were strongest for pan-fried red meat and well- to very well-done red meat.[5]

DIET PATTERNS AND CANCER

Western Versus Prudent Diet

The "Western" dietary pattern is associated with an increased risk of colon cancer.[6] Subjects in the "prudent" dietary lifestyle had high intake of fiber and folate, and this group showed lower risk of colorectal cancer. The "substituters" group (who switch from high-risk to low-risk diet patterns [eg, low-fat products for high-fat products, margarine for butter]) also showed a lower but statistically insignificant instance of colon cancer. The results are consistent with studies showing that fried, preserved, and grilled meat; animal fats; and sugar, as well as obesity, increase the risk for colorectal polyps.[7]

Gerson Regimen

Diet is composed of low sodium, high potassium lactovegetarian foods and fruit juices. There is a lack of effect of this diet in cancer.[8]

Macrobiotic Diet

This low-fat, high complex carbohydrate vegetarian diet improves the quality of life in patients with pancreatic cancer.

Kelly-Gonzalez Regimen

The program involves dietary restrictions, use of digestive aids, and a detoxification regimen including coffee enemas. A 2-year, non-blinded pilot study reported that such an aggressive nutritional regimen, plus high doses of pancreatic enzymes, resulted in increased survival in patients with advanced pancreatic cancer.[9]

Dietary Fat and Cholesterol

The Mobile Clinic Health Examination Survey found that high cholesterol intake is associated with an increased risk for colorectal cancer.[10] In contrast, ingestion of total fat and intake of saturated, monounsaturated, or polyunsaturated fatty acids appeared to have no effect.

Vegetables and Fruit

Results from the Prostate, Lung, Colorectal, and Ovarian (PLCO) Cancer Screening Trial show that diets rich in fruit and deep-yellow vegetables, dark-green vegetables, onions, and garlic are modestly associated with a reduced risk of colorectal adenoma.[11] The effect was mainly seen with high intakes of deep-yellow vegetables, onions, and garlic. The Nurses' Health Study and the Health Professionals' demonstrated that, although fruits and vegetables protect against certain chronic diseases, their frequent consumption does not appear to confer protection from colon or rectal cancer.[12]

Allium *Vegetables*

Allium vegetables,[13] like garlic, onions, leeks, shallots, and chives, may protect against stomach and colorectal cancers.[14] There is an inverse correlation between consumption of garlic, onions, Welsh onions, and Chinese chives and the risk of esophageal and stomach cancer.

Cruciferous *Vegetables*

Cabbage, broccoli, and Brussels sprouts are rich in indole-3-carbinol, which has cancer-preventive effects against liver, colon, and mammary cancer when given before or concurrent with exposure to a carcinogen.[15]

Role of Fiber

A Cochrane database review in 2002 concluded that there was no evidence from randomized, controlled trials (RCTs) to suggest that increased dietary fiber intake for 2 to 4 years would reduce the incidence or recurrence of adenomatous polyps.[16]

Comparison of fiber intake from the PLCO Cancer Screening Trial reported that a high intake of dietary fiber is associated with a lower risk of colorectal adenoma, after adjustment for potential dietary and nondietary risk factors.[17] Multiple other studies have demonstrated similar results.[18-22] In contrast, a Japanese study reported a lack of correlation with fiber intake.[23]

Fruit Versus Vegetable Fiber

A population-based prospective mammography screening study of women in Sweden (n = 61463) found that total fruit and vegetable consumption was inversely associated with colorectal cancer risk during an average 9.6 years of follow-up.[24] This association was primarily related to ingestion of fruit.

SPECIFIC COMPONENTS OF DIET

Berries

Flavonoid-rich extracts of cranberry (*Vaccinia macrocarpa*) slow the growth of explant tumors of several tumor cell lines, including human oral, breast, colon, and prostate, and may even result in complete regression of tumor explants.[25-28]

Garlic (Allium cepa)

Garlic inhibits cellular proliferation, inhibits angiogenesis,[29] and reduces the incidence of aberrant crypt foci in colon models of carcinogenesis.[30]

Studies show as much as 10-fold difference in the death rate from stomach cancer in 2 Chinese provinces, based on the differences in garlic consumption. While high dietary garlic is linked to reduced cancer risk, garlic supplements do not appear to have the same effect.[31] A systematic review concluded that there is consistent scientific evidence, derived from animal studies, of the protective effects of garlic on colorectal cancer.[32]

Kim et al concluded that there is limited evidence indicating a relationship between garlic consumption and reduced risk of colon, prostate, esophageal, larynx, oral, ovary, or renal cell cancers while there was no beneficial effect against gastric, breast, lung, or endometrial cancer.[33]

MISCELLANEOUS

- ❍ Ginger suppresses colon cancer cell growth while also inhibiting the blood supply of the tumor via angiogenesis.
- ❍ Olives protect against tumors in a chemically induced rat colon cancer model.
- ❍ Most, but not all, studies report a reduction in the risk of cancer with increasing ingestion of Welsh onions, onions, and Chinese chives.

○ Sage has been associated with a decreased risk of lung cancer as part of a Mediterranean diet.

○ Tomato (*Lycopersicon esculentum*) and garlic (*A cepa*), individually as well as together, synergistically combine to inhibit chemical colon carcinogenesis.

REFERENCES

1. Pauwels EK. The protective effect of the Mediterranean diet: focus on cancer and cardiovascular risk. *Med Princ Pract*. 2011;20(2):103-111.

2. Schmid A. The role of meat fat in the human diet. *Crit Rev Food Sci Nutr*. 2011;51(1):50-66.

3. Sanjoaquin MA, Appleby PN, Thorogood M, Mann JI, Key TJ. Nutrition, lifestyle and colorectal cancer incidence: a prospective investigation of 10998 vegetarians and non-vegetarians in the United Kingdom. *Br J Cancer*. 2004;90(1):118-121.

4. Sinha R, Peters U, Cross AJ, et al. Meat, meat cooking methods and preservation, and risk for colorectal adenoma. *Cancer Res*. 2005;65(17):8034-8041.

5. Butler LM, Sinha R, Millikan RC, et al. Heterocyclic amines, meat intake, and association with colon cancer in a population-based study. *Am J Epidemiol*. 2003;157(5):434-445.

6. Slattery ML, Boucher KM, Caan BJ, Potter JD, Ma KN. Eating patterns and risk of colon cancer. *Am J Epidemiol*. 1998;148(1):4-16.

7. Kotzev I, Mirchev M, Manevska B, Ivanova I, Kaneva M. Risk and protective factors for development of colorectal polyps and cancer (Bulgarian experience). *Hepatogastroenterology*. 2008;55(82-83):381-387.

8. Cassileth B. Gerson regimen. *Oncology (Williston Park)*. 2010;24(2):201.

9. Gonzalez NJ, Isaacs LL. Evaluation of pancreatic proteolytic enzyme treatment of adenocarcinoma of the pancreas, with nutrition and detoxification support. *Nutr Cancer*. 1999;33(2):117-124.

10. Järvinen R, Knekt P, Hakulinen T, Rissanen H, Heliövaara M. Dietary fat, cholesterol and colorectal cancer in a prospective study. *Br J Cancer*. 2001;85(3):357-361.

11. Millen AE, Subar AF, Graubard BI, et al; PLCO Cancer Screening Trial Project Team. Fruit and vegetable intake and prevalence of colorectal adenoma in a cancer screening trial. *Am J Clin Nutr*. 2007;86(6):1754-1764.

12. Michels KB, Giovannucci E, Joshipura KJ, et al. Prospective study of fruit and vegetable consumption and incidence of colon and rectal cancers. *J Natl Cancer Inst*. 2000;92(21):1740-1752. Erratum in: 2001;93(11):879.

13. Sengupta A, Ghosh S, Bhattacharjee S. *Allium* vegetables in cancer prevention: an overview. *Asian Pac J Cancer Prev*. 2004;5(3):237-245.

14. Bianchini F, Vainio H. *Allium* vegetables and organosulfur compounds: do they help prevent cancer? *Environ Health Perspect*. 2001;109(9):893-902.

15. Kim DJ, Shin DH, Ahn B, et al. Chemoprevention of colon cancer by Korean food plant components. *Mutat Res.* 2003;523-524:99-107.

16. Asano T, McLeod RS. Dietary fibre for the prevention of colorectal adenomas and carcinomas. *Cochrane Database Syst Rev.* 2002;(2):CD003430.

17. Peters U, Sinha R, Chatterjee N, et al; Prostate, Lung, Colorectal, and Ovarian Cancer Screening Trial Project Team. Dietary fibre and colorectal adenoma in a colorectal cancer early detection programme. *Lancet.* 2003;361(9368):1491-1495.

18. Bingham SA, Day NE, Luben R, et al. European Prospective Investigation into Cancer and Nutrition. Dietary fibre in food and protection against colorectal cancer in the European Prospective Investigation into Cancer and Nutrition (EPIC): an observational study. *Lancet.* 2003;361(9368):1496-501. Erratum in: 2003;362(9388):1000.

19. Park Y, Hunter DJ, Spiegelman D, et al. Dietary fiber intake and risk of colorectal cancer: a pooled analysis of prospective cohort studies. *JAMA.* 2005;294(22):2849-2857.

20. Egeberg R, Olsen A, Loft S, et al. Intake of wholegrain products and risk of colorectal cancers in the Diet, Cancer and Health cohort study. *Br J Cancer.* 2010;103(5):730-734.

21. Larsson SC, Giovannucci E, Bergkvist L, Wolk A. Whole grain consumption and risk of colorectal cancer: a population-based cohort of 60,000 women. *Br J Cancer.* 2005;92(9):1803-1807.

22. Dahm CC, Keogh RH, Spencer EA, et al. Dietary fiber and colorectal cancer risk: a nested case-control study using food diaries. *J Natl Cancer Inst.* 2010;102(9):614-626.

23. Uchida K, Kono S, Yin G, et al. Dietary fiber, source foods and colorectal cancer risk: the Fukuoka Colorectal Cancer Study. *Scand J Gastroenterol.* 2010;45(10):1223-1231.

24. Terry P, Giovannucci E, Michels KB, et al. Fruit, vegetables, dietary fiber, and risk of colorectal cancer. *J Natl Cancer Inst.* 2001;93(7):525-533.

25. Ferguson PJ, Kurowska EM, Freeman DJ, Chambers AF, Koropatnick J. In vivo inhibition of growth of human tumor lines by flavonoid fractions from cranberry extract. *Nutr Cancer.* 2006;56(1):86-94.

26. Boateng J, Verghese M, Shackelford L, et al. Selected fruits reduce azoxymethane (AOM)-induced aberrant crypt foci (ACF) in Fisher 344 male rats. *Food Chem Toxicol.* 2007;45(5):725-732.

27. Seeram NP, Adams LS, Zhang Y, et al. Blackberry, black raspberry, blueberry, cranberry, red raspberry, and strawberry extracts inhibit growth and stimulate apoptosis of human cancer cells in vitro. *J Agric Food Chem.* 2006;54(25):9329-9339.

28. Seeram NP. Berry fruits: compositional elements, biochemical activities, and the impact of their intake on human health, performance, and disease. *J Agric Food Chem.* 2008;56(3):627-629.

29. Matsuura N, Miyamae Y, Yamane K, et al. Aged garlic extract inhibits angiogenesis and proliferation of colorectal carcinoma cells. *J Nutr.* 2006;136(Suppl 3):842S-846S.

30. Sengupta A, Ghosh S, Bhattacharjee S, Das S. Indian food ingredients and cancer prevention - an experimental evaluation of anticarcinogenic effects of garlic in rat colon. *Asian Pac J Cancer Prev.* 2004;5(2):126-132.

31. Fleischauer AT, Arab L. Garlic and cancer: a critical review of the epidemiologic literature. *J Nutr.* 2001;131(3s):1032S-1040S.

32. Ngo SN, Williams DB, Cobiac L, Head RJ. Does garlic reduce risk of colorectal cancer? A systematic review. *J Nutr.* 2007;137(10):2264-2269.

33. Kim JY, Kwon O. Garlic intake and cancer risk: an analysis using the Food and Drug Administration's evidence-based review system for the scientific evaluation of health claims. *Am J Clin Nutr.* 2009;89(1):257-264.

Chapter

54 *Lifestyle Factors and Cancer*

KEY POINTS

○ Obesity increases the risk for many digestive cancers including colorectal cancer.

○ Smoking and alcohol intake increase the risk for cancer.

○ The role of coffee in cancer protection is controversial.

○ Physical activity is protective against colon cancer but not gastric or rectal cancer.

Lifestyle factors have the potential to modulate the development of several cancers of the GI tract, including colorectal cancer.

OBESITY

Obesity confers an increased risk of digestive tract cancers, including colorectal cancer.[1] Insulin resistance may play a role since insulin is an important growth factor for colonocytes and it also increases proliferation of colonic tumors.

Coffee[2]

Coffee has no effect on colorectal cancer risk.[3] In contrast, the risk of oral, pharyngeal, and esophageal cancers is inversely associated with coffee consumption.[4]

Tea[5-9]

Tea, especially green tea, exhibits antineoplastic effects in vitro.[6] Whether green tea is better than black tea is controversial.[7] The antimutagenic activity of tea is not affected by the presence of skim milk.[8] There may be a modest positive association with higher tea consumption (900 g/d or four 8-oz cups) and colon cancer.[10] Green tea does not protect against esophageal cancer, while drinking tea at high temperatures increases esophageal cancer risk.[11]

Alcohol

Alcohol intake of 30 g/d or greater increases the risk of colorectal cancer[12]; the risk is higher for rectal cancer.[13] Alcohol drinking also increases the risk for oropharyngeal and squamous cell esophageal cancers.[14] The role of different types of alcoholic beverages is unclear.

Smoking

Most data suggest that smoking increases the risk of both upper and lower GI cancers in addition to making the patients a higher risk for major surgeries. However, a population-based, case-unaffected sibling study in the Colon Cancer Family Registry found that although there was no overall association between smoking and the risk for colon cancer, smoking did increase the risk of rectal cancer.[13]

Carbonated Beverages

There is no correlation between sweetened carbonated beverages and a risk for cancer of the colon or other sites.[10,15]

Physical Exercise

Multiple studies have shown that physical activity is protective against cancer. Increased physical activity is associated with a 25% reduction in colon cancer risk. Subjects who are consistently active throughout life have greater risk reductions than those who have been only active in recent years. There is no effect of activity and rectal cancer.[16]

REFERENCES

1. Charette N, Leclercq IA. Why should the gastroenterologist bother about obesity? An oncologic point of view. *Acta Gastroenterol Belg.* 2010;73(4):504-509.

2. Butt MS, Sultan MT. Coffee and its consumption: benefits and risks. *Crit Rev Food Sci Nutr.* 2011;51(4):363-373.

3. Je Y, Liu W, Giovannucci E. Coffee consumption and risk of colorectal cancer: a systematic review and meta-analysis of prospective cohort studies. *Int J Cancer.* 2009;124(7):1662-1668.

4. Naganuma T, Kuriyama S, Kakizaki M, et al. Coffee consumption and the risk of oral, pharyngeal, and esophageal cancers in Japan: the Miyagi Cohort Study. *Am J Epidemiol.* 2008;168(12):1425-1432.

5. Khan N, Mukhtar H. Cancer and metastasis: prevention and treatment by green tea. *Cancer Metastasis Rev.* 2010;29(3):435-445.

6. Santana-Rios G, Orner GA, Amantana A, Provost C, Wu SY, Dashwood RH. Potent antimutagenic activity of white tea in comparison with green tea in the Salmonella assay. *Mutat Res.* 2001;495(1-2):61-74.

7. Gupta S, Saha B, Giri AK. Comparative antimutagenic and anticlasto-genic effects of green tea and black tea: a review. *Mutat Res.* 2002;512(1):37-65.

8. Catterall F, Kassimi AI, Clifford MN, Ioannides C. Influence of milk on the antimutagenic potential of green and black teas. *Anticancer Res.* 2003;23(5A):3863-3867.

9. Dashwood RH, Xu M, Hernaez JF, Hasaniya N, Youn K, Razzuk A. Cancer chemopreventive mechanisms of tea against heterocyclic amine mutagens from cooked meat. *Proc Soc Exp Biol Med.* 1999;220(4):239-243.

10. Zhang X, Albanes D, Beeson WL, et al. Risk of colon cancer and coffee, tea, and sugar-sweetened soft drink intake: pooled analysis of prospective cohort studies. *J Natl Cancer Inst.* 2010;102(11):771-783.

11. Wu M, Liu AM, Kampman E, et al. Green tea drinking, high tea temperature and esophageal cancer in high- and low-risk areas of Jiangsu Province, China: a population-based case-control study. *Int J Cancer.* 2009;124(8):1907-1913.

12. Cho E, Smith-Warner SA, Ritz J, et al. Alcohol intake and colorectal cancer: a pooled analysis of 8 cohort studies. *Ann Intern Med.* 2004;140(8):603-613.

13. Poynter JN, Haile RW, Siegmund KD, et al. Colon Cancer Family Registry. Associations between smoking, alcohol consumption, and colorectal cancer, overall and by tumor microsatellite instability status. *Cancer Epidemiol Biomarkers Prev.* 2009;18(10):2745-2750.

14. Turati F, Garavello W, Tramacere I, et al. A meta-analysis of alcohol drinking and oral and pharyngeal cancers. Part 2: results by subsites. *Oral Oncol.* 2010;46(10):720-726.

15. Gallus S, Turati F, Tavani A, et al. Soft drinks, sweetened beverages and risk of pancreatic cancer. *Cancer Causes Control.* 2011;22(1):33-39.

16. Wolin KY, Yan Y, Colditz GA. Physical activity and risk of colon adenoma: a meta-analysis. *Br J Cancer.* 2011;104(5):882-825.

Chapter

55 *Micronutrients and Cancer*

KEY POINTS

- ○ Omega-3 fatty acids, calcium, and vitamin D have protective effects against cancer.[1]
- ○ Zinc, magnesium, and vitamin B_6 (pyridoxine) play a beneficial role against cancer.[2]
- ○ The effect of folic acid supplementation in cancer is controversial.[3]
- ○ Vitamin A supplementation has no beneficial effects and may be harmful.
- ○ The role of antioxidants and micronutrients (ie, folic acid, selenium, and omega-3 fatty acids) in cancer is coming under increasing scrutiny.[4,5]

MICRONUTRIENTS

Fish Oil and Omega-3 Fatty Acids

Fish oil derived from tuna inhibits experimental colon cancer.[6] A meta-analysis concluded that relative risks for the highest, compared with the lowest, fish ingestion are 0.88 (CI: 0.78 to 1.00) for colorectal cancer incidence.[7]

Alpha Lipoic Acid

It is effective against several cancer cell lines, including breast and lung, in vitro. Combination of intravenous alpha lipoic acid and oral low-dose naltrexone has also been successfully used in advanced pancreatic cancer.[8]

Antineoplastons

These are naturally occurring peptide fractions with activity against cancer. Targeted therapy with antineoplastons contributed to an over 5-year survival rate in recurrent diffuse intrinsic glioblastomas and anaplastic astrocytomas.[9] Antineoplastons may increase survival in metastatic colon cancer.[10]

Arginine

It has been used as part of immune-enhanced nutritional support. Some data indicate that such therapy reduces postoperative morbidity, mortality, and infectious complications in cancer patients and may affect outcome.

Vitamin A

Studies on the role of carotenoids/vitamin A in cancer have yielded mixed results in digestive cancer. The laboratory data appear to be more promising than the human data.[11-16] Some RCTs on the use of vitamin A supplementation to prevent lung cancer in high-risk patients show that vitamin A actually increases the risk.

A Food and Drug Administration (FDA) evidence-based review reported no credible evidence of the protective effect of lycopene against prostate, lung, colorectal, gastric, breast, ovarian, endometrial, or pancreatic cancer.[17] Similarly, there was no effect of tomato intake.

Calcium[18-25]

A paired sample study found that concentrations of copper, iron, and nickel in cancerous tissue samples are higher than those in the noncancerous samples, while the calcium levels are lower in cancerous tissues.[18]

A meta-analysis of 26,335 cases of colorectal cancer concluded that a high intake of dietary/supplemental calcium decreases the risk of colorectal cancer. Combined evidence from 2 RCTs suggested that calcium supplementation (1200 mg/d) results in a decrease in occurrence of colorectal adenoma.[25] These data need to be taken in context of reports that calcium supplementation is associated with increased cardiovascular risk.

Vitamin D[26,27]

Actions of vitamin D in colorectal adenomas are mediated via vitamin D receptors. Risk of advanced colorectal neoplasia is decreased in subjects with vitamin D intake greater than 645 IU/d.[27] However, an updated 2011 meta-analysis for the US Preventive Services Task Force concluded that data are not strong enough to draw conclusions regarding the benefits versus risks of vitamin D supplementation for the prevention of cancer.[28]

Calcium Plus Vitamin D[29-32]

A meta-analysis from 60 epidemiological studies concluded that high milk and dairy product intake reduces the risk of colon cancer.[29] Calcium and vitamin D act together to reduce the risk of colorectal adenoma recurrence, and the protective effects last for at least 5 years after discontinuation of supplementation.[32]

> The Institute of Medicine has concluded that existing evidence that vitamin D or calcium supplementation reduces cancer risk is inconclusive.[33]

Folate[34-40]

Data on the risk of folate and colon cancer have been somewhat mixed, though a temporal association between folic acid fortification and an increase in colorectal cancer rates has been documented by epidemiologic data. However, this does not prove causality.[34,35] A larger meta-analysis of 27 studies indicated a protective effect of folate against colon cancer. This offers reassurance to women taking folic acid during the preconception period in order to prevent neural tube defects.[40]

Pyridoxine or Vitamin B_6

Vitamin B_6 is critical for DNA synthesis. The Nurses' Health Study concluded that total vitamin B_6 intake is significantly inversely associated with colon cancer risk.[41] Recent meta-analysis showing the inverse relationship between vitamin B_6 levels and the risk of colorectal cancer confirms this protective effect against colorectal cancer.[2]

Vitamin C

Studies like the Physicians' Health Study II and the Women's Antioxidant Cardiovascular Study have not shown any beneficial effects of vitamin C in preventing cancer.[42,43]

Selenium

Epidemiological studies suggest an inverse relationship between selenium intake and the incidence of certain cancers. Most of the trials in humans on the effect of selenium on cancer incidence/biomarkers have found beneficial effects. A prospective randomized trial found that the mean concentration of selenium in colorectal cancer is higher than in the case of polyps.

Magnesium

The Swedish Mammography Cohort from 1987 to 1990 reported an inverse association of magnesium intake and the risk of colorectal cancer.[44]

Zinc

Decreased zinc levels are associated with the development of pre-neoplastic lesions in the colonic mucosa in a colon cancer model in rats. Zinc treatment to rats in a chemically induced rat model of colon cancer significantly restored normalcy in the colonic histology.[45]

An ecological study for White Americans for 1970 to 1994 found that zinc dietary index is inversely correlated with bladder, breast, colon, esophageal, gastric, rectal, laryngeal, nasopharyngeal, oral, skin, and vulvar cancer, as well as Hodgkin's lymphoma.[46] Relative risks for proximal colon cancer decrease more than 50% across categories for zinc intake. In contrast, one comparative study found a lack of relationship between zinc and colorectal cancer.[47]

Antioxidants

A meta-analysis of 8 randomized trials (n = 17,620) reported that there is a lack of convincing evidence that antioxidant supplements (beta-carotene; vitamins A, C, E; and selenium, alone or in combination) have significant beneficial effects on the primary or secondary prevention of colorectal adenoma.[48]

A recent meta-analysis examined the effect of antioxidants for the prevention of cancer. Twenty-two RCTs of 161,045 total subjects were included in the analysis. Antioxidants did not have any effect on the primary or secondary prevention of cancer.[49] In fact, their use increased the risk of bladder cancer.

Miscellaneous Micronutrients

Trace element levels and activity of related enzymes are variable, depending upon the neoplastic process. A meta-analysis and systematic review on the efficacy and safety of multivitamin and mineral supplement use concluded that evidence is insufficient to prove the presence or absence of benefits from the use of multivitamin and mineral supplements to prevent cancer and chronic disease.[50]

REFERENCES

1. Toner CD, Davis CD, Milner JA. The vitamin D and cancer conundrum: aiming at a moving target. *J Am Diet Assoc.* 2010;110(10):1492-1500.
2. Larsson SC, Orsini N, Wolk A. Vitamin B_6 and risk of colorectal cancer: a meta-analysis of prospective studies. *JAMA.* 2010;303(11):1077-1083.

3. Hubner RA, Houlston RS. Folate and colorectal cancer prevention. *Br J Cancer*. 2009;100(2):233-239.

4. Muecke R, Schomburg L, Buentzel J, et al. Selenium or no selenium—that is the question in tumor patients: a new controversy. *Integr Cancer Ther*. 2010;9(2):136-141.

5. Bjelakovic G, Nikolova D, Simonetti RG, Gluud C. Antioxidant supplements for preventing gastrointestinal cancers. *Cochrane Database Syst Rev*. 2008;(3):CD004183.

6. Kohno H, Yamaguchi N, Ohdoi C, Nakajima S, Odashima S, Tanaka T. Modifying effect of tuna orbital oil rich in docosahexaenoic acid and vitamin D_3 on azoxymethane-induced colonic aberrant crypt foci in rats. *Oncol Rep*. 2000;7(5):1069-1074.

7. Geelen A, Schouten JM, Kamphuis C, et al. Fish consumption, n-3 fatty acids, and colorectal cancer: a meta-analysis of prospective cohort studies. *Am J Epidemiol*. 2007;166(10):1116-1125.

8. Berkson BM, Rubin DM, Berkson AJ. Revisiting the ALA/N (alpha-lipoic acid/low-dose naltrexone) protocol for people with metastatic and nonmetastatic pancreatic cancer: a report of 3 new cases. *Integr Cancer Ther*. 2009;8(4):416-422.

9. Burzynski SR, Janicki TJ, Weaver RA, Burzynski B. Targeted therapy with antineoplastons A10 and AS2-1 of high-grade, recurrent, and progressive brainstem glioma. *Integr Cancer Ther*. 2006;5(1):40-47.

10. Ogata Y, Tsuda H, Matono K, et al. Long-term survival following treatment with antineoplastons for colon cancer with unresectable multiple liver metastases: report of a case. *Surg Today*. 2003;33(6):448-453.

11. Tang FY, Shih CJ, Cheng LH, Ho HJ, Chen HJ. Lycopene inhibits growth of human colon cancer cells via suppression of the Akt signaling pathway. *Mol Nutr Food Res*. 2008;52(6):646-654.

12. Tang FY, Cho HJ, Pai MH, Chen YH. Concomitant supplementation of lycopene and eicosapentaenoic acid inhibits the proliferation of human colon cancer cells. *J Nutr Biochem*. 2009;20(6):426-434.

13. Schnäbele K, Briviba K, Bub A, et al. Effects of carrot and tomato juice consumption on faecal markers relevant to colon carcinogenesis in humans. *Br J Nutr*. 2008;99(3):606-613.

14. Dorjgochoo T, Gao YT, Chow WH, et al. Plasma carotenoids, tocopherols, retinol and breast cancer risk: results from the Shanghai Women Health Study (SWHS). *Breast Cancer Res Treat*. 2009;117(2):381-389.

15. Walfisch S, Walfisch Y, Kirilov E, et al. Tomato lycopene extract supplementation decreases insulin-like growth factor-I levels in colon cancer patients. *Eur J Cancer Prev*. 2007;16(4):298-303.

16. Alabaster O, Tang Z, Frost A, Shivapurkar N. Effect of beta-carotene and wheat bran fiber on colonic aberrant crypt and tumor formation in rats exposed to azoxymethane and high dietary fat. *Carcinogenesis*. 1995;16(1):127-132.

17. Kavanaugh CJ, Trumbo PR, Ellwood KC. The U.S. Food and Drug Administration's evidence-based review for qualified health claims: tomatoes, lycopene, and cancer. *J Natl Cancer Inst*. 2007;99(14):1074-1085.

18. Yaman M, Kaya G, Yekeler H. Distribution of trace metal concentrations in paired cancerous and non-cancerous human stomach tissues. *World J Gastroenterol.* 2007;13(4):612-618.

19. Holt PR, Atillasoy EO, Gilman J, et al. Modulation of abnormal colonic epithelial cell proliferation and differentiation by low-fat dairy foods: a randomized controlled trial. *JAMA.* 1998;280(12):1074-1079.

20. Baron JA, Beach M, Mandel JS, et al. Calcium supplements for the prevention of colorectal adenomas. Calcium Polyp Prevention Study Group. *N Engl J Med.* 1999;340(2):101-107.

21. Wu K, Willett WC, Fuchs CS, Colditz GA, Giovannucci EL. Calcium intake and risk of colon cancer in women and men. *J Natl Cancer Inst.* 2002;94(6):437-446.

22. Cho E, Smith-Warner SA, Spiegelman D, et al. Dairy foods, calcium, and colorectal cancer: a pooled analysis of 10 cohort studies. *J Natl Cancer Inst.* 2004;96(13):1015-1022. Erratum: 2004;96(22):1724.

23. Shaukat A, Scouras N, Schünemann HJ. Role of supplemental calcium in the recurrence of colorectal adenomas: a metaanalysis of randomized controlled trials. *Am J Gastroenterol.* 2005;100(2):390-394.

24. Pufulete M. Intake of dairy products and risk of colorectal neoplasia. *Nutr Res Rev.* 2008;21(1):56-67.

25. Weingarten MA, Zalmanovici A, Yaphe J. Dietary calcium supplementation for preventing colorectal cancer and adenomatous polyps. *Cochrane Database Syst Rev.* 2008;(1):CD003548.

26. Kim HS, Newcomb PA, Ulrich CM, et al. Vitamin D receptor polymorphism and the risk of colorectal adenomas: evidence of interaction with dietary vitamin D and calcium. *Cancer Epidemiol Biomarkers Prev.* 2001;10(8):869-874.

27. Lieberman DA, Prindiville S, Weiss DG, Willett W; VA Cooperative Study Group 380. Risk factors for advanced colonic neoplasia and hyperplastic polyps in asymptomatic individuals. *JAMA.* 2003;290(22):2959-2967.

28. Chung M, Lee J, Terasawa T, Lau J, Trikalinos TA. Vitamin D with or without calcium supplementation for prevention of cancer and fractures: an updated meta-analysis for the U.S. Preventive Services Task Force. *Ann Intern Med.* 2011;155(12):827-838.

29. Huncharek M, Muscat J, Kupelnick B. Colorectal cancer risk and dietary intake of calcium, vitamin D, and dairy products: a meta-analysis of 26,335 cases from 60 observational studies. *Nutr Cancer.* 2009;61(1):47-69.

30. Wactawski-Wende J, Kotchen JM, Anderson GL, et al. Women's Health Initiative Investigators. Calcium plus vitamin D supplementation and the risk of colorectal cancer. *N Engl J Med.* 2006;354(7):684-96. Erratum: 2006;354(10):1102.

31. Grau MV, Baron JA, Sandler RS, et al. Vitamin D, calcium supplementation, and colorectal adenomas: results of a randomized trial. *J Natl Cancer Inst.* 2003;95(23):1765-1771.

32. Grau MV, Baron JA, Sandler RS, et al. Prolonged effect of calcium supplementation on risk of colorectal adenomas in a randomized trial. *J Natl Cancer Inst*. 2007;99(2):129-136.

33. Ross AC, Manson JE, Abrams SA, et al. The 2011 report on dietary reference intakes for calcium and vitamin D from the Institute of Medicine: what clinicians need to know. *J Clin Endocrinol Metab*. 2011;96(1):53-8.

34. Mason JB, Dickstein A, Jacques PF, et al. A temporal association between folic acid fortification and an increase in colorectal cancer rates may be illuminating important biological principles: a hypothesis. *Cancer Epidemiol Biomarkers Prev*. 2007;16(7):1325-1329.

35. Lee JE, Willett WC, Fuchs CS, et al. Folate intake and risk of colorectal cancer and adenoma: modification by time. *Am J Clin Nutr*. 2011;93(4):817-825.

36. Giovannucci E, Stampfer MJ, Colditz GA, et al. Multivitamin use, folate, and colon cancer in women in the Nurses' Health Study. *Ann Intern Med*. 1998;129(7):517-524.

37. Sanjoaquin MA, Allen N, Couto E, Roddam AW, Key TJ. Folate intake and colorectal cancer risk: a meta-analytical approach. *Int J Cancer*. 2005;113(5):825-828.

38. Logan RF, Grainge MJ, Shepherd VC, Armitage NC, Muir KR; ukCAP Trial Group. Aspirin and folic acid for the prevention of recurrent colorectal adenomas. *Gastroenterology*. 2008;134(1):29-38.

39. Cole BF, Baron JA, Sandler RS, et al. Polyp Prevention Study Group. Folic acid for the prevention of colorectal adenomas: a randomized clinical trial. *JAMA*. 2007;297(21):2351-2359.

40. Kennedy DA, Stern SJ, Moretti M, et al. Folate intake and the risk of colorectal cancer: a systematic review and meta-analysis. *Cancer Epidemiol*. 2011;35(1):2-10.

41. Wei EK, Giovannucci E, Selhub J, et al. Plasma vitamin B6 and the risk of colorectal cancer and adenoma in women. *J Natl Cancer Inst*. 2005;97(9):684-692.

42. Gaziano JM, Glynn RJ, Christen WG, et al. Vitamins E and C in the prevention of prostate and total cancer in men: the Physicians' Health Study II randomized controlled trial. *JAMA*. 2009;301(1):52-62.

43. Lin J, Cook NR, Albert C, et al. Vitamins C and E and beta carotene supplementation and cancer risk: a randomized controlled trial. *J Natl Cancer Inst*. 2009;101(1):14-23.

44. Larsson SC, Bergkvist L, Wolk A. Magnesium intake in relation to risk of colorectal cancer in women. *JAMA*. 2005;293(1):86-89.

45. Dani V, Goel A, Vaiphei K, Dhawan DK. Chemopreventive potential of zinc in experimentally induced colon carcinogenesis. *Toxicol Lett*. 2007;171(1-2):10-18.

46. Grant WB. An ecological study of cancer mortality rates including indices for dietary iron and zinc. *Anticancer Res*. 2008;28(3B):1955-1963.

47. Sorribes Carreras P, Torres Feced P. Zinc intake deficiency and colorectal cancer: what is the situation in our population? *Nutr Hosp*. 2000;15(4):153-155.

48. Bjelakovic G, Nagorni A, Nikolova D, Simonetti RG, Bjelakovic M, Gluud C. Meta-analysis: antioxidant supplements for primary and secondary prevention of colorectal adenoma. *Aliment Pharmacol Ther.* 2006;24(2):281-291.

49. Myung SK, Kim Y, Ju W, Choi HJ, Bae WK. Effects of antioxidant supplements on cancer prevention: meta-analysis of randomized controlled trials. *Ann Oncol.* 2010;21(1):166-179.

50. Huang HY, Caballero B, Chang S, et al. The efficacy and safety of multivitamin and mineral supplement use to prevent cancer and chronic disease in adults: a systematic review for a National Institutes of Health state-of-the-science conference. *Ann Intern Med.* 2006;145(5):372-385.

Chapter
56 *Complementary and Alternative Therapies for Cancer*

KEY POINTS

○ Many phytobotanicals have been shown to be effective in the prevention and treatment of neoplasia.

○ Acupuncture is effective for reducing chemotherapy-induced nausea and vomiting.

○ Patients on touch therapy, especially Reiki, suffered significantly less pain compared to controls.

○ Massage therapy alleviates nausea, anxiety, depression, anger, stress, and fatigue.

This chapter primarily covers the role of complementary and alternative therapies, especially phytobotanicals and traditional Chinese medicine. Because of the overlap, some factors like fiber, garlic, etc have been discussed in chapters on the effect of diet, lifestyles, micronutrients, etc.

PHYTOBOTANICALS

Aloe

Oral administration of aloe reduces the number and size of papillomas, as well as tumor incidence, when compared to control mice.[1]

Angelica keiskei

A keiskei is rich in chalcones. It suppresses tumor promotion in an in vivo 2-stage model of mouse carcinogenesis.[2]

Arabinoxylan

A prebiotic with antioxidant properties, it protects against colon cancer in experimental cancer models.[3]

Artemisia annua

Artesunate, derived from artemisinin, is the active principle from Chinese herb *A annua*. It is active against leukemia and colon cancer cell lines.[4]

Asimina triloba *(Pawpaw)*[5,6]

The pawpaw (*A triloba, Annonaceae*) is a small tree native to eastern North America. The botanical extract exhibits cytotoxicity against human colon, lung, and breast cancer.[6]

Astragalus

Astragalus has been called the "senior of all herbs." Immune-adjuvant activity is seen after subcutaneous injection of *Astragalus* extract.[7] *Radix Astragali* inhibits gastric cancer cells in vitro. *Astragalus* injection plus chemotherapy may improve the survival and quality of life in certain cancers.[8]

Azadirachta indica *(Neem)*

This reduces the average number of papillomas per mouse, as well as the percentage of tumor-bearing animals in experimental models of carcinogenesis.[9]

Basil

Basil, or sweet basil (*O basilicum*), is grown throughout India and is widely known for its medicinal value. It reduces carcinogen-induced tumor incidence in tumor models at the peri-initiation stage.[10]

Beta-Glucan

Lentinan is a beta-glucan and suppresses the toxic effects of chemotherapy and improves quality of life in colorectal cancer patients. Adding it to standard chemotherapy improves prognosis in gastric cancer patients.[11]

Black Cohosh **(Cimicifuga)**

Cycloartane triterpenoids derived from *Cimicifuga yunnanensis* inhibit tumor cells and induce apoptosis in breast and gastric cancer cells. Paradoxically, one animal study indicated that black cohosh increases the risk of lung metastases in tumor-bearing animals.

Black Seed (Nigella sativa)

Black seed (*N sativa*)[12] contains the bioactive component thymoquinone. It inhibits the growth of colon cancer cells in vitro.

Boswellia

B serrata[13] is a traditional Ayurvedic medicinal plant. It inhibits angiogenesis and induces apoptosis in various cancer lines. Its bioactive components inhibit tumor growth in the human prostate tumor xenograft in mice.

Brassica campestris (Mustard)[14]

It enhances antioxidant defenses and inhibits experimental tumorigenesis.[15]

Bromelain

Bromelain is a proteolytic digestive enzyme obtained from the pineapple plant (*A comosus*). Bromelain treatment results in a significantly increased survival in experimental animal tumor models, along with a reduced number of lung metastasis.[16] It improves quality of life and may improve survival in colorectal cancer.[17-20]

Bromelia

Bromelia is a rich source of resistant fiber. Fastuosain is a cysteine proteinase obtained from *Bromelia fastuosa*. It has antitumor effects against melanoma in mice.[21]

Bupleurum

It inhibits tumor cell growth of lung and liver cancer in vitro and in vivo.

Catalpa ovata (Catalpa)

It inhibits experimental colon carcinogenesis in rats.[22]

Chaparral

Native Americans have traditionally used chaparral for tea, as well as medicinal purposes. The FDA does not include it in its list of "generally recognized as safe."[23]

Chlorophyll

Chlorophyll binds to dietary mutagens and prevents DNA damage. It is known as one of the preventive elements in a cancer prevention diet.[24]

Chrysanthemum

It has proapoptotic and antineoplastic actions. It is contained in several anticancer multiherbal formulations, including PC-SPES and hua-sheng-ping.

Cocklebur (Xanthium strumarium)

Lactones from cocklebur demonstrate cytotoxic activity against human colon, breast, and lung cancer cells in vitro.[25]

Coriolus

It demonstrates significant immune-adjuvant activity after subcutaneous vaccination.[7] Human studies in cancer are lacking.

Cumin

Cumin modulates carcinogen metabolism and inhibits experimental tumorigenesis in mice.[26]

Curcuma longa *(Turmeric)*[27-29]

Curcumin is the bioactive polyphenolic chemical component of the popular herbal spice turmeric, also known as yellow curry powder. It affects carcinogenesis at both the initiation and promotion stage and induces apoptosis in various cancer lines.[30] It inhibits the incidence and tumor load of papillomas and squamous cell carcinomas of the GI tract.[31]

Animal studies suggest that a daily dose of 1.6 g of curcumin is required for chemopreventive effect in humans.[32,33] A dose of turmeric is 2 to 4 g/d, and some experts argue that up to 12 g/d is safe.

Cymbopogon citratus Stapf *(Lemon Grass)*

It acts at both the initiation stage and the promotion stage[34] and inhibits colon carcinogenesis in animals.

Devil's Claw (Harpagophytum procumbens)

It has anti-inflammatory and analgesic properties. It may be useful in cancer-related pain.

Echinacea[35-38]

Daily ingestion of *Echinacea* attenuates leukemia and extends the life span of leukemic mice.[35,36] *Echinacea purpurea* administration to human subjects results in attenuation of intestinal bacteria.[38]

Fagopyrum cymosum

F cymosum inhibits growth of cancer cells from lung, liver, colon, leukocytes, and bone.

Flaxseed

An RCT found that flaxseed supplementation inhibits prostate cancer proliferation in men prior to surgery.[39]

Ganoderma lucidum *(Reishi Mushroom)*

It is a component of several multiherbal, anticancer formulations. It prevents cancer invasion and metastasis in tumor-bearing mice. Ingesting 1.5 g/d suppresses the development of colorectal adenomas.[40]

Geum quellyon Sweet

G quellyon Sweet is rich in tannins. It inhibits human colon cancer cells in vitro.

Ginger

Ginger exerts anticarcinogenic effects in the human colon, as well as in liver cancer.[41,42]

Ginkgo

G biloba exocarp polysaccharides inhibit gastric cancer cells in vitro and have been used in humans.[43] Phase II studies indicate that ginkgo extract, when combined with 5-fluorouracil, may be useful in advanced colorectal cancer.[44] Preliminary data suggest it may be a valuable adjunct in pancreatic cancer.

Ginseng

Ginseng has various types. Ginseng in diet suppresses colon carcinogenesis in rats.[45] *Ginseng saponins* inhibits the lung metastasis of melanoma, as well as colon cancer cells. A comparison of white and red ginseng showed that white ginseng, and not its red counterpart, reduces the risk of adenocarcinoma of the small intestine and colon without any effect on the number of aberrant crypt foci.[46]

Greater Celandine (Chelidonium majus)

Ukrain is a semi-synthetic derivative of *C majus* alkaloids. A systematic review of 7 RCTs concluded that Ukrain has curative effects on a range of cancers, although the methodological quality of most studies was poor.[47]

Hibiscus sabdariffa Linn *(Roselle)*

Roselle (*H sabdariffa*) has antimutagenic actions and inhibits experimental colon carcinogenesis.

Huanglian

Huanglian is a Chinese herb that is effective against gastric, colon, and breast cancer cells in vitro.[48]

Jiaogulan (Gynostemma pentaphyllum)

It inhibits DNA repair genes of cancer cells along with the invasion of tumor cells. It inhibits experimental esophageal cancer in mice.

Lawsonia inermis (Henna Leaf)

Henna leaf (*L inermis*), also known as *Mehndi* in India, is a popular natural dye. It inhibits experimental cancers in animals.[49]

Litchi chinensis (Litchi or Lychee Fruit)

Litchi fruit pericarp extract is rich in polyphenolic compounds. It causes a 41% decrease in tumor mass in rodent models.

Magnolol (Hou p'u of Magnolia officinalis)

Magnolol, isolated from the Chinese herb Hou p'u of *M officinalis*, inhibits cultured human colon cancer cells.

Maitake

Injection of Maitake acts as an immune-adjuvant and may help in cancer.[7]

Mastic Oil

Mastic oil, derived from *P lentiscus*, inhibits tumor growth associated with apoptosis and reduced angiogenesis.

Mistletoe

Standardized mistletoe extract augments immune response and down-regulates metastatic tumor growth in murine cancer.[50]

Modified Citrus Pectin

Ingestion of modified citrus pectin protects against liver metastasis in a colon cancer model in mice.

Momordica (Bitter Melon or Bitter Gourd, Gac Fruit)[51-54]

It enhances lymphocyte activity in vitro and in vivo in mice,[52] and decreases the incidence and total tumor burden in experimental colon carcinogenesis.[53,54]

Moringa oleifera

Topical application of *M oleifera* extract inhibits papillomas in mice.

Murdannia loriformis

M loriformis extracts exert antimutagenic action against several mutagens and inhibit chemical colon carcinogenesis.

Paeonia lactiflora *(Peony)*

It is used in a variety of multiherbal, anticancer preparations. It inhibits tumor growth, including hepatoma, and has a synergistic action with cis-platinum against cancer cells.

Panax notoginseng

P notoginseng, also known as *Panax pseudoginseng*, is a commonly used Chinese herb. *Notoginseng* flower extract enhances the antiproliferative effect of 5-fluorouracil on human colorectal cancer and may decrease the dosage of chemotherapeutic agents.[55]

Perilla Oil

Perilla oil is rich in alpha-linolenic acid. It inhibits azoxymethane-induced aberrant crypt foci in rats.

Podophyllum hexandrum[56]

It has cytotoxic properties and enhances radiation-induced apoptosis.

Poria cocos

Triterpene acids from *P cocos* inhibit skin tumor promotion in vivo.

Punica granatum *(Pomegranate)*

Pomegranate seed oil decreases the incidence and burden of colon cancer in rats.[57] These actions are mediated via increasing conjugated linoleic acid in the colon.

Resistant Starch

A randomized, placebo-controlled trial compared the effects of aspirin and resistant starch Novelose in patients with Lynch syndrome. Results showed a lack of effect of aspirin or resistant starch on the incidence of colorectal adenoma or carcinoma.[58]

Rhubarb (Genus Rheum)

It inhibits tumor invasion, proliferation, and migration. Rhubarb extract reduces the radiation-induced lung toxicity and pulmonary function in patients with lung cancer.[59]

Scutellaria barbata[60] *(Baikal Skullcap)*

The major bioactive components are wogonin, baicalein, and baicalin. It inhibits carcinogenesis in a variety of cancers, including liver and pancreas.

Shiitake Mushroom Extract

It induces apoptosis and inhibits tumor growth. Clinical data are lacking.

Taraxacum officinale *(Dandelion)*

It has antioxidant, proapoptotic, and antiproliferative properties.

Uncaria tomentosa *(Cat's Claw)*

The Amazonian vine *U tomentosa* (cat's claw) has multiple medicinal properties. Pteropodine and isomitraphylline are 2 of the medical cat's claw preparations.[61] It induces apoptosis in proliferating acute lymphoblastic leukemia cells, breast cancer cell lines, etc. Oral pretreatment of rats with *U tomentosa* protects against gastritis and prevents apoptosis.[62]

HERBAL COMBINATIONS

Chinese Herbal Medicine[63-66]

A meta-analysis concluded that Chinese herbal medicine (combined with chemotherapy) improved survival at 1, 2, and 3 years, compared to chemotherapy alone.[65] Similar results were seen in the treatment of gastric cancer.[66]

Chinese Red Yeast Rice

Chinese red yeast rice is produced by fermentation of *M purpureus Went* yeast with white rice. It reduces cellular proliferation and inhibits tumor growth in vitro.

Chi-Shen Extract

It is made from *S miltiorrhiza* and *R Paeoniae*. It induces apoptosis and cell death in a hepatoma cell line.

Essiac[67-70]

Essiac (Canadian Health Products, New Brunswick, Canada) is an herbal combination of burdock root (*Arctium lappa*), sheep sorrel (*Rumex acetosella*), slippery elm inner bark (*Ulmus fulva*), and Turkish rhubarb (*R palmatum*). While it is widely used by patients with breast cancer, Essiac does not have a significant effect on mood or quality of life.[69] In fact, Essiac users fared worse on some parameters. A case of a 64-year-old man with hormone-refractory prostate cancer responding to Essiac tea has been described.[70]

Flor-Essence

Effects of Flor-Essence herbal tonic (Flora Inc, Lynden, WA) are controversial. Flor-Essence can actually stimulate the growth of human breast cancer cells.[71]

HemoHIM

HemoHIM (Atomy Inc, Federal Way, WA) is a mixture of 3 herbs: *R Angelicae*, *Cnidium rhizome*, and *R Paeoniae*. It enhances the antineoplastic activity of radiation and chemotherapy in tumor-bearing mice.

Huachansu

Huachansu treatment improves leukopenia in gastric cancer, without changing the remission rates.

Lectin-Mistletoe

Lectin-standardized mistletoe extract treatment results in a significant reduction of chemotherapy-induced toxicity, as well as prolonged relapse-free intervals in breast cancer.[72]

MycoPhyto Complex

MycoPhyto Complex (EcoNugenics, Santa Rosa, CA) is a mixture of mycelia from *Agaricus blazei*, *Cordyceps sinensis*, *Coriolus versicolor*, *G lucidum*, *Grifola frondosa*, and *Polyporus umbellatus*, along with β-1, 3-glucan isolated from the *S cerevisiae*. It exhibits antiproliferative and antimetastatic properties.

PHY906

PHY906 (800 mg bid) is a Chinese herbal formulation. It is cytoprotective and may be useful as adjunct anticancer treatment against advanced pancreatic and hepatocellular cancer.

PC-SPES[73]

PC-SPES is a mixture of 8 herbs with antitumor effects in prostate cancer and colon cancer. The herbs are *Chrysanthemum morifolium*, *G lucidum* (a root fungus), *G glabra* (Spanish liquorice), *Isatis indigotica*, *P pseudoginseng*, *Rabdosia rubescens*, *S baicalensis*, and *S repens* (saw palmetto). It inhibits colon cancer growth in vitro, as well as in vivo, in mice.[74]

Caution: The FDA recalled the product from the market in 2002 because of concerns of adulteration and toxicity.

Shen-Qi (Ginseng-Astragalus)

Shen-Qi (*Ginseng-Astragalus*) injection, used in conjunction with chemotherapy, is superior to chemotherapy alone for treatment of GI cancers.[75]

Shikunshito-Kamiho

Shikunshito-Kamiho is a Chinese herbal combination of 8 drugs (*R Ginseng, Hoelen, Atractylodis rhizoma, R Glycyrrhizae, Prunellae spica, Ostreae testa, Laminaria thallus,* and *Sargassum*). Shikunshito-Kamiho reduces aberrant crypts foci in animal models of carcinogenesis.[76]

Shi-Quan-Da-Bu-Tang or SQT[77-79]

Shi-Quan-Da-Bu-Tang (Ten Significant Tonic Decoction), or SQT (Juzentaihoto, TJ-48), is a mixture of 10 herbs (*Rehmannia glutinosa, P lactiflora, Liqusticum wallichii, A sinensis, G uralensis, P cocos, Atractylodes macrocephala, P ginseng, A membranaceus,* and *Cinnamomum cassia*). It increases recurrence-free survival in patients with liver cancer.[78] It enhances the therapeutic efficacy of several chemotherapeutic agents, as well as radiotherapy agents.[79]

Sho-Saiko-To

It is a traditional Chinese herbal mixture of 7 herbs. It induces apoptosis and inhibits tumor proliferation. Administration of sho-saiko-to to patients with viral hepatitis B reduces the risk of hepatocellular cancer and improves survival.[80]

Triphala

Triphala is a popular herbal combination of 3 different plants, namely *T chebula, Terminalia belerica,* and *E officinalis*. It reduces the chemically induced forestomach papillomagenesis in mice.[81]

Wobenzym

Wobenzym is composed of pancreatin, papain, bromelain, trypsin, and chymotrypsin. Oral ingestion of Wobenzym leads to a significant increases in reactive oxygen species compared to placebo.[82] It enhances the cytotoxic capacity of white blood cells against tumor cells.

Miscellaneous Herbal Combinations

A variety of combinations have been used with variable success.[83-86]

○ A meta-analysis concluded that combined *Astragalus*-based therapies, plus platinum-based chemotherapy, improves response and reduces the risk of death at 12 months.[86]

○ Jin Fu Kang reduces the risk of death at 24 months.

○ Ai Di injection stabilizes or improves performance status.

Herbal Remedy Interactions With Chemotherapeutic Agents

Cheng and colleagues searched scientific literature for evidence of herb-drug interactions in cancer therapy and identified 168 articles. They found little direct evidence for such adverse interactions.[87] Complementary and alternative medicine products that could potentially increase the risk of breast cancer or interact with tamoxifen or aromatase inhibitors include garlic, *Ginkgo biloba*, echinacea, ginseng, valerian, and phytoestrogens, excluding soy.[88] While concerns have been raised about interaction with soy, data indicate that soy food consumption is actually associated with a decreased risk of death and recurrence of breast cancer.[89] See Chapter 33 for more details.

NONBOTANICAL THERAPIES AND SUPPLEMENTS

Bee Pollen[90]

Bee pollen has antioxidant, proapoptotic, and antiangiogenic properties in vitro. It is considered a good source of nutrition and may reduce the side effects of anticancer therapy.

A Cochrane database review concluded that several treatment strategies are beneficial at preventing or reducing the severity of mucositis associated with chemotherapy. Effective treatments included *A vera*, amifostine, cryotherapy, granulocyte-colony stimulating factor, intravenous glutamine, honey, keratinocyte growth factor, laser, polymyxin/tobramycin/amphotericin antibiotic pastille/paste, and sucralfate.[91]

Cartilage[92]

Bovine and shark cartilage have antiangiogenic properties in vitro. RCTs of regimens involving cartilage (AE-941) have shown no benefit in lung and colon cancer.[93] (Just an aside, sharks get cancer too![94])

Chelation Therapy

The role of chelation therapy in cancer is in its infancy. Tetrathiomolybdate is a copper chelator and demonstrates anticancer and antiangiogenic properties in vivo.[95] Ethylenediaminetetraacetic acid has been used for ovarian cancer.[96]

Coenzyme Q10[97]

It is also known as *ubiquinone*, *ubidecarenone*, and *vitamin Q10*. A pilot study showed an improved survival of patients with end-stage cancer treated with coenzyme Q10 and a mixture of other antioxidants for 9 years.[98] Recombinant interferon alpha-2b in combination with coenzyme Q10 reduces recurrence in postoperative cases of melanoma.[99]

Dehydroepiandrosterone[100]

Intravaginal dehydroepiandrosterone promotes regression of cervical cancer with low-grade dysplasia.[101]

Gamma-Linolenic Acid[102-104]

Intravesical gamma-linolenic acid administration in patients with recurrent superficial bladder cancer results in a response rate of 43%, which is similar to conventional intravesical therapies. Preliminary data indicate gamma-linolenic acid's potential for benefit in pancreatic cancer.[104]

Glutamine[105]

Glutamine, given prior to each chemotherapy treatment, reduces the incidence of severe diarrhea and decreases the amount of diarrhea. Glutamine is effective in protecting against chemotherapy-induced mucositis.[91]

Hoxsey Formula[106]

It is not a formula per say, but rather a therapeutic regimen. The components of therapy vary with cancer; however, potassium iodide is part of all regimens. There is a lack of clinical evidence to support its use.

Hydrazine Sulfate

Hydrazine sulfate is believed to prevent cancer cachexia. Scientific data have refuted most of these claims, and it may even make patients worse.[107-109] Adverse events include GI complaints and hepatorenal damage.

Melatonin

It improves the outcome of colon cancer in hamsters. Melatonin plus *A vera* tincture improves response in patients with advanced solid malignancies.[110] A Cochrane database review concluded that the data, although encouraging, are not convincing of the beneficial effect of melatonin in breast cancer.[111]

Perillyl Alcohol[112-114]

It inhibits tumor cell growth in pancreatic cancer. Pilot studies suggest that administration to patients with pancreatic cancer increases survival.[114]

Thymus Factors[115,116]

A Cochrane database review concluded that purified thymic extracts do not enhance a response to anticancer treatment or decrease the risk of death.[116] However, they do reduce the risk of serious infections in patients on chemo- or radiation therapy.

HOMEOPATHY[117-119]

A Cochrane database review concluded that evidence supports the beneficial effects of topical calendula for the prevention of acute dermatitis due to radiation therapy, and of Traumeel S mouthwash in the treatment of chemotherapy-induced stomatitis.[118]

ACUPUNCTURE[120]

Fewer patients undergoing acupuncture-point stimulation suffer from nausea and vomiting compared to controls. A Cochrane database review concluded there is insufficient evidence to determine whether acupuncture is effective for pain control in cancer patients.[121]

MIND-BODY THERAPIES

Hyponotherapy[122-124]

The role of hypnotherapy is primarily in the control of pain, as well as nausea and vomiting associated with cancer care and improving the quality of life.

Lifestyle Modification Counseling and Therapy[125]

Lifestyle modifications may affect disease outcome and survival. This issue has been discussed in more detail in previous chapters.

Behavioral Therapies

Multiple behavioral strategies, individually or in combination, have been used.[126,127] A multidisciplinary approach utilizing cognitive, emotional, physical, social, and spiritual strategies improves the quality of life in patients receiving radiation therapy for advanced cancer.[127]

Relaxation Therapy

Relaxation techniques improve mood and quality of life and reduce pain, nausea, and vomiting. Much depends upon the individual preferences/bias of the patient. If nothing else, the latter can help maximize the placebo benefit while we await more definitive large RCTs.

MISCELLANEOUS THERAPIES

Aromatherapy/Massage

A Cochrane database review found that aromatherapy and massage improve psychosocial well being in cancer patients.[128] Evidence of a beneficial effect of massage on nausea, anxiety, depression, stress, and fatigue is encouraging.

Therapeutic Touch

Patients on touch therapy suffer less pain compared to controls.[129] Greater beneficial effects are seen in those that utilize Reiki, compared to controls.

Yoga[130]

Yoga is a multidimensional program of meditation, exercise, and lifestyle. It improves emotional and cognitive function, as well as social functioning and quality of life.

Spirituality

Religion and spirituality play a pivotal role across cultures, and it is even more increased toward the end of life. Current spiritual well being and past negative religious experiences determine the degree of anxiety and depression.[131]

REFERENCES

1. Chaudhary G, Saini MR, Goyal PK. Chemopreventive potential of *Aloe vera* against 7,12-dimethylbenz(a)anthracene induced skin papillomagenesis in mice. *Integr Cancer Ther.* 2007;6(4):405-412.

2. Akihisa T, Tokuda H, Hasegawa D, et al. Chalcones and other compounds from the exudates of *Angelica keiskei* and their cancer chemopreventive effects. *J Nat Prod.* 2006;69(1):38-42.

3. Femia AP, Salvadori M, Broekaert WF, et al. Arabinoxylan-oligosaccharides (AXOS) reduce preneoplastic lesions in the colon of rats treated with 1,2-dimethylhydrazine (DMH). *Eur J Nutr.* 2010;49(2):127-132.

4. Efferth T, Dunstan H, Sauerbrey A, Miyachi H, Chitambar CR. The antimalarial artesunate is also active against cancer. *Int J Oncol.* 2001;18(4):767-773.

5. McLaughlin JL. Paw paw and cancer: annonaceous acetogenins from discovery to commercial products. *J Nat Prod.* 2008;71(7):1311-1321.

6. Zhao GX, Chao JF, Zeng L, McLaughlin JL. (2,4-cis)-asimicinone and (2,4-trans)-asimicinone: two novel bioactive ketolactone acetogenins from *Asimina triloba* (*Annonaceae*). *Nat Toxins.* 1996;4(3):128-134.

7. Ragupathi G, Yeung KS, Leung PC, et al. Evaluation of widely consumed botanicals as immunological adjuvants. *Vaccine.* 2008;26(37):4860-4865.

8. McCulloch M, See C, Shu XJ, et al. Astragalus-based Chinese herbs and platinum-based chemotherapy for advanced non-small-cell lung cancer: meta-analysis of randomized trials. *J Clin Oncol.* 2006;24(3):419-430.

9. Dasgupta T, Banerjee S, Yadava PK, Rao AR. Chemopreventive potential of *Azadirachta indica* (Neem) leaf extract in murine carcinogenesis model systems. *J Ethnopharmacol.* 2004;92(1):23-36.

10. Dasgupta T, Rao AR, Yadava PK. Chemomodulatory efficacy of basil leaf (*Ocimum basilicum*) on drug metabolizing and antioxidant enzymes, and on carcinogen-induced skin and forestomach papillomagenesis. *Phytomedicine.* 2004;11(2-3):139-151.

11. Yoshino S, Watanabe S, Imano M, et al. Improvement of QOL and prognosis by treatment of superfine dispersed lentinan in patients with advanced gastric cancer. *Hepatogastroenterology.* 2010;57(97):172-177.

12. Gali-Muhtasib H, Diab-Assaf M, Boltze C, et al. Thymoquinone extracted from black seed triggers apoptotic cell death in human colorectal cancer cells via a p53-dependent mechanism. *Int J Oncol.* 2004;25(4):857-866.

13. Poeckel D, Werz O. Boswellic acids: biological actions and molecular targets. *Curr Med Chem.* 2006;13(28):3359-3369.

14. Johnson IT. Phytochemicals and cancer. *Proc Nutr Soc.* 2007;66(2):207-215.

15. Gagandeep, Dhiman M, Mendiz E, Rao AR, Kale RK. Chemopreventive effects of mustard (*Brassica compestris*) on chemically induced tumorigenesis in murine forestomach and uterine cervix. *Hum Exp Toxicol.* 2005;24(6):303-312.

16. Báez R, Lopes MT, Salas CE, Hernández M. In vivo antitumoral activity of stem pineapple (*Ananas comosus*) bromelain. *Planta Med.* 2007;73(13):1377-1383.

17. Sakalová A, Bock PR, Dedík L, et al. Retrolective cohort study of an additive therapy with an oral enzyme preparation in patients with multiple myeloma. *Cancer Chemother Pharmacol.* 2001;47(Suppl):S38-S44.

18. Eckert K, Grabowska E, Stange R, Schneider U, Eschmann K, Maurer HR. Effects of oral bromelain administration on the impaired immunocytotoxicity of mononuclear cells from mammary tumor patients. *Oncol Rep.* 1999;6(6):1191-1199.

19. Beuth J. Proteolytic enzyme therapy in evidence-based complementary oncology: fact or fiction? *Integr Cancer Ther.* 2008;7(4):311-316.

20. Beuth J, Ost B, Pakdaman A, et al. Impact of complementary oral enzyme application on the postoperative treatment results of breast cancer patients—results of an epidemiological multicentre retrolective cohort study. *Cancer Chemother Pharmacol.* 2001;47(Suppl):S45-S54.

21. Guimarães-Ferreira CA, Rodrigues EG, Mortara RA, et al. Antitumor effects in vitro and in vivo and mechanisms of protection against melanoma B16F10-Nex2 cells by fastuosain, a cysteine proteinase from *Bromelia fastuosa. Neoplasia.* 2007;9(9):723-733.

22. Suzuki R, Yasui Y, Kohno H, et al. Catalpa seed oil rich in 9t,11t,13c-conjugated linolenic acid suppresses the development of colonic aberrant crypt foci induced by azoxymethane in rats. *Oncol Rep.* 2006;16(5):989-996.

23. Kauma H, Koskela R, Mäkisalo H, Autio-Harmainen H, Lehtola J, Höckerstedt K. Toxic acute hepatitis and hepatic fibrosis after consumption of chaparral tablets. *Scand J Gastroenterol.* 2004;39(11):1168-1171.

24. Divisi D, Di Tommaso S, Salvemini S, Garramone M, Crisci R. Diet and cancer. *Acta Biomed.* 2006;77(2):118-123.

25. Ramírez-Erosa I, Huang Y, Hickie RA, Sutherland RG, Barl B. Xanthatin and xanthinosin from the burs of *Xanthium strumarium L.* as potential anticancer agents. *Can J Physiol Pharmacol.* 2007;85(11):1160-1172.

26. Gagandeep, Dhanalakshmi S, Méndiz E, Rao AR, Kale RK. Chemopreventive effects of *Cuminum cyminum* in chemically induced forestomach and uterine cervix tumors in murine model systems. *Nutr Cancer.* 2003;47(2):171-180.

27. Qiu X, Du Y, Lou B, et al. Synthesis and identification of new 4-arylidene curcumin analogues as potential anticancer agents targeting nuclear factor-κB signaling pathway. *J Med Chem.* 2010. [Epub ahead of print]

28. Patel VB, Misra S, Patel BB, Majumdar AP. Colorectal cancer: chemopreventive role of curcumin and resveratrol. *Nutr Cancer.* 2010;62(7):958-967.

29. Goel A, Aggarwal BB. Curcumin, the golden spice from Indian saffron, is a chemosensitizer and radiosensitizer for tumors and chemoprotector and radioprotector for normal organs. *Nutr Cancer.* 2010;62(7):919-930.

30. Milacic V, Banerjee S, Landis-Piwowar KR, Sarkar FH, Majumdar AP, Dou QP. Curcumin inhibits the proteasome activity in human colon cancer cells in vitro and in vivo. *Cancer Res.* 2008;68(18):7283-7292.

31. Huang MT, Lou YR, Ma W, Newmark HL, Reuhl KR, Conney AH. Inhibitory effects of dietary curcumin on forestomach, duodenal, and colon carcinogenesis in mice. *Cancer Res.* 1994;54(22):5841-5847.

32. Perkins S, Verschoyle RD, Hill K, et al. Chemopreventive efficacy and pharmacokinetics of curcumin in the min/+ mouse, a model of familial adenomatous polyposis. *Cancer Epidemiol Biomarkers Prev.* 2002;11(6):535-540.

33. Sharma RA, McLelland HR, Hill KA, et al. Pharmacodynamic and pharmacokinetic study of oral *Curcuma* extract in patients with colorectal cancer. *Clin Cancer Res.* 2001;7(7):1894-1900.

34. Suaeyun R, Kinouchi T, Arimochi H, Vinitketkumnuen U, Ohnishi Y. Inhibitory effects of lemon grass (*Cymbopogon citratus Stapf*) on formation of azoxymethane-induced DNA adducts and aberrant crypt foci in the rat colon. *Carcinogenesis.* 1997;18(5):949-955.

35. Miller SC. *Echinacea*: a miracle herb against aging and cancer? Evidence in vivo in mice. *Evid Based Complement Alternat Med.* 2005;2(3):309-314.

36. Hayashi I, Ohotsuki M, Suzuki I, Watanabe T. Effects of oral administration of *Echinacea purpurea* (American herb) on incidence of spontaneous leukemia caused by recombinant leukemia viruses in AKR/J mice. *Nihon Rinsho Meneki Gakkai Kaishi.* 2001;24(1):10-20.

37. Melchart D, Clemm C, Weber B, et al. Polysaccharides isolated from *Echinacea purpurea* herba cell cultures to counteract undesired effects of chemotherapy—a pilot study. *Phytother Res.* 2002;16(2):138-142.

38. Hill LL, Foote JC, Erickson BD, Cerniglia CE, Denny GS. *Echinacea purpurea* supplementation stimulates select groups of human gastrointestinal tract microbiota. *J Clin Pharm Ther.* 2006;31(6):599-604.

39. Demark-Wahnefried W, Polascik TJ, George SL, et al. Flaxseed supplementation (not dietary fat restriction) reduces prostate cancer proliferation rates in men presurgery. *Cancer Epidemiol Biomarkers Prev.* 2008;17(12):3577-3587.

40. Oka S, Tanaka S, Yoshida S, et al. A water-soluble extract from culture medium of *Ganoderma lucidum* mycelia suppresses the development of colorectal adenomas. *Hiroshima J Med Sci.* 2010;59(1):1-6.

41. Brown AC, Shah C, Liu J, Pham JT, Zhang JG, Jadus MR. Ginger's (*Zingiber officinale Roscoe*) inhibition of rat colonic adenocarcinoma cells proliferation and angiogenesis in vitro. *Phytother Res.* 2009;23(5):640-645.

42. Kundu JK, Na HK, Surh YJ. Ginger-derived phenolic substances with cancer preventive and therapeutic potential. *Forum Nutr.* 2009;61:182-192.

43. Chen HS, Zhai F, Chu YF, Xu F, Xu AH, Jia LC. Clinical study on treatment of patients with upper digestive tract malignant tumors of middle and late stage with *Ginkgo biloba* exocarp polysaccharides capsule preparation. *Zhong Xi Yi Jie He Xue Bao.* 2003;1(3):189-191.

44. Hauns B, Häring B, Köhler S, Mross K, Unger C. Phase II study of combined 5-fluorouracil/*Ginkgo biloba* extract (GBE 761 ONC) therapy in 5-fluorouracil pretreated patients with advanced colorectal cancer. *Phytother Res.* 2001;15(1):34-38.

45. Fukushima S, Wanibuchi H, Li W. Inhibition by ginseng of colon carcinogenesis in rats. *J Korean Med Sci.* 2001;16(Suppl):S75-S80.

46. Ichihara T, Wanibuchi H, Iwai S, et al. White, but not red, ginseng inhibits progression of intestinal carcinogenesis in rats. *Asian Pac J Cancer Prev.* 2002;3(3):243-250.

47. Ernst E, Schmidt K. Ukrain—a new cancer cure? A systematic review of randomised clinical trials. *BMC Cancer.* 2005;5:69.

48. Li GH, Sun FJ, Chen F, Yang SB, Zhang J. Effect on mouse S180 MDR tumour cell expression correlated factorial matter by 70% ethanol with Huanglian Jiedu Tang. *Zhongguo Zhong Yao Za Zhi.* 2007;32(18):1906-1908.

49. Dasgupta T, Rao AR, Yadava PK. Modulatory effect of henna leaf (*Lawsonia inermis*) on drug metabolising phase I and phase II enzymes, antioxidant enzymes, lipid peroxidation and chemically induced skin and forestomach papillomagenesis in mice. *Mol Cell Biochem.* 2003;245(1-2):11-22.

50. Braun JM, Ko HL, Schierholz JM, Beuth J. Standardized mistletoe extract augments immune response and down-regulates local and metastatic tumor growth in murine models. *Anticancer Res.* 2002;22(6C):4187-4190.

51. Grover JK, Yadav SP. Pharmacological actions and potential uses of *Momordica charantia*: a review. *J Ethnopharmacol.* 2004;93(1):123-132.

52. Pongnikorn S, Fongmoon D, Kasinrerk W, Limtrakul PN. Effect of bitter melon (*Momordica charantia Linn*) on level and function of natural killer cells in cervical cancer patients with radiotherapy. *J Med Assoc Thai.* 2003;86(1):61-68.

53. Deep G, Dasgupta T, Rao AR, Kale RK. Cancer preventive potential of *Momordica charantia L.* against benzo(a)pyrene induced fore-stomach tumourigenesis in murine model system. *Indian J Exp Biol.* 2004;42(3): 319-322.

54. Tien PG, Kayama F, Konishi F, et al. Inhibition of tumor growth and angiogenesis by water extract of Gac fruit (*Momordica cochinchinensis Spreng*). *Int J Oncol.* 2005;26(4):881-889.

55. Wang CZ, Luo X, Zhang B, et al. Notoginseng enhances anti-cancer effect of 5-fluorouracil on human colorectal cancer cells. *Cancer Chemother Pharmacol.* 2007;60(1):69-79.

56. Giri A, Lakshmi Narasu M. Production of podophyllotoxin from *Podophyllum hexandrum*: a potential natural product for clinically useful anticancer drugs. *Cytotechnology.* 2000;34(1-2):17-26.

57. Kohno H, Suzuki R, Yasui Y, Hosokawa M, Miyashita K, Tanaka T. Pomegranate seed oil rich in conjugated linolenic acid suppresses chemically induced colon carcinogenesis in rats. *Cancer Sci.* 2004;95(6):481-486.

58. Burn J, Bishop DT, Mecklin JP, et al; CAPP2 Investigators. Effect of aspirin or resistant starch on colorectal neoplasia in the Lynch syndrome. *N Engl J Med.* 2008;359(24):2567-2578.

59. Yu HM, Liu YF, Cheng YF, Hu LK, Hou M. Effects of rhubarb extract on radiation induced lung toxicity via decreasing transforming growth factor-beta-1 and interleukin-6 in lung cancer patients treated with radiotherapy. *Lung Cancer.* 2008;59(2):219-226.

60. Li-Weber M. New therapeutic aspects of flavones: the anticancer properties of Scutellaria and its main active constituents Wogonin, Baicalein and Baicalin. *Cancer Treat Rev.* 2009;35(1):57-68.

61. Pilarski R, Poczekaj-Kostrzewska M, Ciesiołka D, Szyfter K, Gulewicz K. Antiproliferative activity of various *Uncaria tomentosa* preparations on HL-60 promyelocytic leukemia cells. *Pharmacol Rep.* 2007;59(5):565-572.

62. Sandoval M, Okuhama NN, Zhang XJ, et al. Anti-inflammatory and antioxidant activities of cat's claw (*Uncaria tomentosa* and *Uncaria guianensis*) are independent of their alkaloid content. *Phytomedicine.* 2002;9(4):325-337.

63. Cha RJ, Zeng DW, Chang QS. Non-surgical treatment of small cell lung cancer with chemo-radio-immunotherapy and traditional Chinese medicine. *Zhonghua Nei Ke Za Zhi.* 1994;33(7):462-466.

64. Mok TS, Yeo W, Johnson PJ, et al. A double-blind placebo-controlled randomized study of Chinese herbal medicine as complementary therapy for reduction of chemotherapy-induced toxicity. *Ann Oncol.* 2007;18(4):768-774.

65. Shu X, McCulloch M, Xiao H, Broffman M, Gao J. Chinese herbal medicine and chemotherapy in the treatment of hepatocellular carcinoma: a meta-analysis of randomized controlled trials. *Integr Cancer Ther.* 2005;4(3):219-229.

66. Gan T, Wu Z, Tian L, Wang Y. Chinese herbal medicines for induction of remission in advanced or late gastric cancer. *Cochrane Database Syst Rev.* 2010;(1):CD005096.

67. Leonard SS, Keil D, Mehlman T, Proper S, Shi X, Harris GK. Essiac tea: scavenging of reactive oxygen species and effects on DNA damage. *J Ethnopharmacol.* 2006;103(2):288-296.

68. Ottenweller J, Putt K, Blumenthal EJ, Dhawale S, Dhawale SW. Inhibition of prostate cancer-cell proliferation by Essiac. *J Altern Complement Med.* 2004;10(4):687-691.

69. Zick SM, Sen A, Feng Y, Green J, Olatunde S, Boon H. Trial of Essiac to ascertain its effect in women with breast cancer (TEA-BC). *J Altern Complement Med.* 2006;12(10):971-980.

70. Al-Sukhni W, Grunbaum A, Fleshner N. Remission of hormone-refractory prostate cancer attributed to Essiac. *Can J Urol.* 2005;12(5):2841-2842.

71. Kulp KS, Montgomery JL, Nelson DO, et al. Essiac and Flor-Essence herbal tonics stimulate the in vitro growth of human breast cancer cells. *Breast Cancer Res Treat.* 2006;98(3):249-259.

72. Schumacher K, Schneider B, Reich G, et al. Influence of postoperative complementary treatment with lectin-standardized mistletoe extract on breast cancer patients. A controlled epidemiological multicentric retrolective cohort study. *Anticancer Res.* 2003;23(6D):5081-5087.

73. Lee CO. Complementary and alternative medicine patients are talking about: PC-SPES. *Clin J Oncol Nurs.* 2005;9(1):113-114.

74. Huerta S, Arteaga JR, Irwin RW, Ikezoe T, Heber D, Koeffler HP. PC-SPES inhibits colon cancer growth in vitro and in vivo. *Cancer Res.* 2002;62(18):5204-5209.

75. Li NQ. Clinical and experimental study on shen-qi injection with chemotherapy in the treatment of malignant tumor of digestive tract. *Zhongguo Zhong Xi Yi Jie He Za Zhi.* 1992;12(10):588-592,579.

76. Yoo BH, Lee BH, Kim JS, Kim NJ, Kim SH, Ryu KW. Effects of Shikunshito-Kamiho on fecal enzymes and formation of aberrant crypt foci induced by 1,2-dimethylhydrazine. *Biol Pharm Bull.* 2001;24(6):638-642.

77. Saiki I. A Kampo medicine "Juzen-taiho-to"—prevention of malignant progression and metastasis of tumor cells and the mechanism of action. *Biol Pharm Bull.* 2000;23(6):677-688.

78. Tsuchiya M, Kono H, Matsuda M, Fujii H, Rusyn I. Protective effect of Juzen-taiho-to on hepatocarcinogenesis is mediated through the inhibition of Kupffer cell-induced oxidative stress. *Int J Cancer.* 2008;123(11):2503-11.

79. Zee-Cheng RK. Shi-quan-da-bu-tang (ten significant tonic decoction), SQT. A potent Chinese biological response modifier in cancer immunotherapy, potentiation and detoxification of anticancer drugs. *Methods Find Exp Clin Pharmacol.* 1992;14(9):725-736.

80. Oka H, Yamamoto S, Kuroki T, et al. Prospective study of chemoprevention of hepatocellular carcinoma with Sho-saiko-to (TJ-9). *Cancer.* 1995;76(5):743-749.

81. Deep G, Dhiman M, Rao AR, Kale RK. Chemopreventive potential of Triphala (a composite Indian drug) on benzo(a)pyrene induced forestomach tumorigenesis in murine tumor model system. *J Exp Clin Cancer Res.* 2005;24(4):555-563.

82. Zavadova E, Desser L, Mohr T. Stimulation of reactive oxygen species production and cytotoxicity in human neutrophils in vitro and after oral administration of a polyenzyme preparation. *Cancer Biother.* 1995;10(2):147-152.

83. Mazzio EA, Soliman KF. In vitro screening for the tumoricidal properties of international medicinal herbs. *Phytother Res.* 2009;23(3):385-398.

84. Volate SR, Davenport DM, Muga SJ, Wargovich MJ. Modulation of aberrant crypt foci and apoptosis by dietary herbal supplements (quercetin, curcumin, silymarin, ginseng and rutin). *Carcinogenesis.* 2005;26(8):1450-1456.

85. Ragupathi G, Yeung KS, Leung PC, et al. Evaluation of widely consumed botanicals as immunological adjuvants. *Vaccine.* 2008;26(37):4860-4865.

86. McCulloch M, See C, Shu XJ, et al. Astragalus-based Chinese herbs and platinum-based chemotherapy for advanced non-small-cell lung cancer: meta-analysis of randomized trials. *J Clin Oncol.* 2006;24(3):419-430.

87. Cheng CW, Fan W, Ko SG, Song L, Bian ZX. Evidence-based management of herb-drug interaction in cancer chemotherapy. *Explore (NY).* 2010;6(5):324-329.

88. Malekzadeh F, Rose C, Ingvar C, Jernström H. Natural remedies and hormone preparations—potential risk for breast cancer patients. A study surveys the use of agents which possibly counteract with the treatment. *Lakartidningen.* 2005;102(44):3226-3228,3230-3231.

89. Shu XO, Zheng Y, Cai H, et al. Soy food intake and breast cancer survival. *JAMA.* 2009;302(22):2437-2443.

90. Izuta H, Shimazawa M, Tsuruma K, Araki Y, Mishima S, Hara H. Bee products prevent VEGF-induced angiogenesis in human umbilical vein endothelial cells. *BMC Complement Altern Med.* 2009;9:45.

91. Worthington HV, Clarkson JE, Bryan G, et al. Interventions for preventing oral mucositis for patients with cancer receiving treatment. *Cochrane Database Syst Rev.* 2011;4:CD000978.

92. Liu N, Lapcevich RK, Underhill CB, et al. Metastatin: a hyaluronan-binding complex from cartilage that inhibits tumor growth. *Cancer Res.* 2001;61(3):1022-1028.

93. Lu C, Lee JJ, Komaki R, Herbst RS, et al. Chemoradiotherapy with or without AE-941 in stage III non-small cell lung cancer: a randomized phase III trial. *J Natl Cancer Inst.* 2010;102(12):859-865.

94. Finkelstein JB. Sharks do get cancer: few surprises in cartilage research. *J Natl Cancer Inst.* 2005;97(21):1562-1563.

95. Tisato F, Marzano C, Porchia M, Pellei M, Santini C. Copper in diseases and treatments, and copper-based anticancer strategies. *Med Res Rev.* 2010;30(4):708-749.

96. Rosenblum MG, Verschraegen CF, Murray JL, et al. Phase I study of 90Y-labeled B72.3 intraperitoneal administration in patients with ovarian cancer: effect of dose and EDTA coadministration on pharmacokinetics and toxicity. *Clin Cancer Res.* 1999;5(5):953-961.

97. Villalba JM, Parrado C, Santos-Gonzalez M, Alcain FJ. Therapeutic use of coenzyme Q10 and coenzyme Q10-related compounds and formulations. *Expert Opin Investig Drugs.* 2010;19(4):535-554.

98. Hertz N, Lister RE. Improved survival in patients with end-stage cancer treated with coenzyme Q(10) and other antioxidants: a pilot study. *J Int Med Res.* 2009;37(6):1961-1971. Erratum: 2010;38(1):293.

99. Rusciani L, Proietti I, Paradisi A, et al. Recombinant interferon alpha-2b and coenzyme Q10 as a postsurgical adjuvant therapy for melanoma: a 3-year trial with recombinant interferon-alpha and 5-year follow-up. *Melanoma Res.* 2007;17(3):177-183.

100. Cameron DR, Braunstein GD. The use of dehydroepiandrosterone therapy in clinical practice. *Treat Endocrinol.* 2005;4(2):95-114.

101. Suh-Burgmann E, Sivret J, Duska LR, Del Carmen M, Seiden MV. Long-term administration of intravaginal dehydroepiandrosterone on regression of low-grade cervical dysplasia—a pilot study. *Gynecol Obstet Invest.* 2003;55(1):25-31.

102. Das UN. Can essential fatty acids reduce the burden of disease(s)? *Lipids Health Dis.* 2008;7:9.

103. Kenny FS, Pinder SE, Ellis IO, et al. Gamma linolenic acid with tamoxifen as primary therapy in breast cancer. *Int Cancer.* 2000;85(5):643-648.

104. Agombar A, Cooper AJ, Johnson CD. An aqueous formulation of gamma-linolenic acid with anti-proliferative action on human pancreatic cancer cell lines. *Anticancer Drugs.* 2004;15(2):157-160.

105. Xue H, Sawyer MB, Wischmeyer PE, Baracos VE. Nutrition modulation of gastrointestinal toxicity related to cancer chemotherapy: from preclinical findings to clinical strategy. *J Parenter Enteral Nutr.* 2011;35(1):74-90.

106. Smith M, Boon HS. Counseling cancer patients about herbal medicine. *Patient Educ Couns.* 1999;38(2):109-120.

107. Yavuzsen T, Davis MP, Walsh D, LeGrand S, Lagman R. Systematic review of the treatment of cancer-associated anorexia and weight loss. *J Clin Oncol.* 2005;23(33):8500-8511.

108. Loprinzi CL, Goldberg RM, Su JQ, et al. Placebo-controlled trial of hydrazine sulfate in patients with newly diagnosed non-small-cell lung cancer. *J Clin Oncol.* 1994;12(6):1126-1129.

109. Loprinzi CL, Kuross SA, O'Fallon JR, et al. Randomized placebo-controlled evaluation of hydrazine sulfate in patients with advanced colorectal cancer. *J Clin Oncol.* 1994;12(6):1121-1125.

110. Lissoni P, Giani L, Zerbini S, Trabattoni P, Rovelli F. Biotherapy with the pineal immunomodulating hormone melatonin versus melatonin plus aloe vera in untreatable advanced solid neoplasms. *Nat Immun.* 1998;16(1):27-33.

111. Ernst E, Schmidt K, Baum M. Complementary/alternative therapies for the treatment of breast cancer. A systematic review of randomized clinical trials and a critique of current terminology. *Breast J.* 2006;12(6):526-530.

112. Garcia DG, Amorim LM, de Castro Faria MV, et al. The anticancer drug perillyl alcohol is a Na/K-ATPase inhibitor. *Mol Cell Biochem.* 2010;345(1-2):29-34.

113. Yeruva L, Hall C, Elegbede JA, Carper SW. Perillyl alcohol and methyl jasmonate sensitize cancer cells to cisplatin. *Anticancer Drugs.* 2010;21(1):1-9.

114. Matos JM, Schmidt CM, Thomas HJ, et al. A pilot study of perillyl alcohol in pancreatic cancer. *J Surg Res.* 2008;147(2):194-199.

115. Lersch C, Zeuner M, Bauer A, et al. Nonspecific immunostimulation with low doses of cyclophosphamide (LDCY), thymostimulin, and *Echinacea purpurea* extracts (echinacin) in patients with far advanced colorectal cancers: preliminary results. *Cancer Invest.* 1992;10(5):343-348.

116. Wolf E, Milazzo S, Boehm K, Zwahlen M, Horneber M. Thymic peptides for treatment of cancer patients. *Cochrane Database Syst Rev.* 2011;2:CD003993.

117. Frenkel M. Homeopathy in cancer care. *Altern Ther Health Med.* 2010;16(3):12-16.

118. Kassab S, Cummings M, Berkovitz S, van Haselen R, Fisher P. Homeopathic medicines for adverse effects of cancer treatments. *Cochrane Database Syst Rev.* 2009;(2):CD004845.

119. Längler A, Spix C, Edelhäuser F, Kameda G, Kaatsch P, Seifert G. Use of homeopathy in pediatric oncology in Germany. *Evid Based Complement Altern Med.* 2011;2011:867151.

120. O'Regan D, Filshie J. Acupuncture and cancer. *Auton Neurosci.* 2010;157(1-2):96-100.

121. Paley CA, Johnson MI, Tashani OA, Bagnall AM. Acupuncture for cancer pain in adults. *Cochrane Database Syst Rev.* 2011;(1):CD007753.

122. Sohl SJ, Stossel L, Schnur JB, Tatrow K, Gherman A, Montgomery GH. Intentions to use hypnosis to control the side effects of cancer and its treatment. *Am J Clin Hypn.* 2010;53(2):93-100.

123. Richardson J, Smith JE, McCall G, Richardson A, Pilkington K, Kirsch I. Hypnosis for nausea and vomiting in cancer chemotherapy: a systematic review of the research evidence. *Eur J Cancer Care (Engl)*. 2007;16(5):402-412.

124. Lotfi-Jam K, Carey M, Jefford M, Schofield P, Charleson C, Aranda S. Nonpharmacologic strategies for managing common chemotherapy adverse effects: a systematic review. *J Clin Oncol*. 2008;26(34):5618-5629.

125. Pekmezi DW, Demark-Wahnefried W. Updated evidence in support of diet and exercise interventions in cancer survivors. *Acta Oncol*. 2011;50(2):167-178.

126. Lapid MI, Rummans TA, Brown PD, et al. Improving the quality of life of geriatric cancer patients with a structured multidisciplinary intervention: a randomized controlled trial. *Palliat Support Care*. 2007;5(2):107-114.

127. Rummans TA, Clark MM, Sloan JA, et al. Impacting quality of life for patients with advanced cancer with a structured multidisciplinary intervention: a randomized controlled trial. *J Clin Oncol*. 2006;24(4):635-642.

128. Fellowes D, Barnes K, Wilkinson S. Aromatherapy and massage for symptom relief in patients with cancer. *Cochrane Database Syst Rev*. 2004;(2):CD002287.

129. So PS, Jiang Y, Qin Y. Touch therapies for pain relief in adults. *Cochrane Database Syst Rev*. 2008;(4):CD006535.

130. Lin KY, Hu YT, Chang KJ, Lin HF, Tsauo JY. Effects of yoga on psychological health, quality of life, and physical health of patients with cancer: a meta-analysis. *Evid Based Complement Altern Med*. 2011;2011:659876.

131. Johnson KS, Tulsky JA, Hays JC, et al. Which domains of spirituality are associated with anxiety and depression in patients with advanced illness? *J Gen Intern Med*. 2011;26(7):751-758.

Chapter

57 *Role of Prebiotics and Probiotics in Cancer*

KEY POINTS

○ Although experimental data in animal models support the potential anticarcinogenic action of probiotics, there is a paucity of direct human data.[1,2]

○ Probiotics are helpful for the treatment and prevention of chemo- and radiation-induced diarrhea.

Potential mechanisms of antitumor effects include alteration of physicochemical conditions in the colon, binding to potential carcinogens, production of short-chain fatty acids, production of anti-tumorigenic or antimutagenic substances, detoxification of carcinogens, enhancement of host immunity, and alteration of the host's physiology.[3-5]

ANIMAL DATA

Daily oral administration of *L acidophilus* in yogurt suppresses colon cancer.[6] The synbiotic combination of resistant starch and *B lactis* promotes the apoptotic response to a genotoxic carcinogen in rat colon.[7] Inulin and oligofructose induce apoptosis and reduce the severity of experimental colon cancer.[8]

HUMAN DATA

Inulin enriched with oligofructose plus *L rhamnosus GG* and *B lactis* after "curative resection" in colon cancer results in minor effects on immune parameters.[9] Synbiotic food (oligofructose-enriched inulin [SYN1] plus *L rhamnosus GG* and *B lactis Bb12*) results in reduced colorectal cell proliferation, along with improved epithelial barrier function.[10] Probiotics decrease the incidence of radiation-induced diarrhea.[11] Probiotic therapy reduces postoperative complications in colon cancer.[12]

REFERENCES

1. Kumar M, Kumar A, Nagpal R, et al. Cancer-preventing attributes of probiotics: an update. *Int J Food Sci Nutr.* 2010;61(5):473-496.

2. Pagnini C, Corleto VD, Hoang SB, Saeed R, Cominelli F, Delle Fave G. Commensal bacteria and "oncologic surveillance": suggestions from an experimental model. *J Clin Gastroenterol.* 2008;42(Suppl 3, Pt 2):S193-S196.

3. Lee do K, Jang S, Kim MJ, et al. Anti-proliferative effects of *Bifidobacterium adolescentis* SPM0212 extract on human colon cancer cell lines. *BMC Cancer.* 2008;8:310.

4. Kanauchi O, Mitsuyama K, Andoh A, Iwanaga T. Modulation of intestinal environment by prebiotic germinated barley foodstuff prevents chemo-induced colonic carcinogenesis in rats. *Oncol Rep.* 2008;20(4):793-801.

5. Yeh SL, Lin MS, Chen HL. Inhibitory effects of a soluble dietary fiber from *Amorphophallus konjac* on cytotoxicity and DNA damage induced by fecal water in Caco-2 cells. *Planta Med.* 2007;73(13):1384-1348.

6. Urbanska AM, Bhathena J, Martoni C, Prakash S. Estimation of the potential antitumor activity of microencapsulated *Lactobacillus acidophilus* yogurt formulation in the attenuation of tumorigenesis in Apc(Min/+) mice. *Dig Dis Sci.* 2009;54(2):264-273.

7. Le Leu RK, Brown IL, Hu Y, et al. A synbiotic combination of resistant starch and *Bifidobacterium lactis* facilitates apoptotic deletion of carcinogen-damaged cells in rat colon. *J Nutr*. 2005;135(5):996-1001.

8. Hughes R, Rowland IR. Stimulation of apoptosis by two prebiotic chicory fructans in the rat colon. *Carcinogenesis*. 2001;22(1):43-47.

9. Roller M, Clune Y, Collins K, Rechkemmer G, Watzl B. Consumption of prebiotic inulin enriched with oligofructose in combination with the probiotics *Lactobacillus rhamnosus* and *Bifidobacterium lactis* has minor effects on selected immune parameters in polypectomised and colon cancer patients. *Br J Nutr*. 2007;97(4):676-684.

10. Rafter J, Bennett M, Caderni G, et al. Dietary synbiotics reduce cancer risk factors in polypectomized and colon cancer patients. *Am J Clin Nutr*. 2007;85(2):488-496.

11. Chitapanarux I, Chitapanarux T, Traisathit P, et al. Randomized controlled trial of live *Lactobacillus acidophilus* plus *Bifidobacterium bifidum* in prophylaxis of diarrhea during radiotherapy in cervical cancer patients. *Radiat Oncol*. 2010;5:31.

12. Liu Z, Qin H, Yang Z, et al. Randomised clinical trial: the effects of perioperative probiotic treatment on barrier function and post-operative infectious complications in colorectal cancer surgery—a double-blind study. *Aliment Pharmacol Ther*. 2011;33(1):50-63.

LIVER

Phytobotanical Treatment of Liver Disorders

KEY POINTS

- ○ *Astragalus* has a beneficial effect in hepatocellular cancer.
- ○ Glycyrrhizin and stronger Neominophagen C (SNMC) have antiviral properties and protect against hepatic carcinogenesis.
- ○ Therapies such as silymarin (milk thistle) and S-adenosylmethionine have great therapeutic rationale for the treatment of liver disorders, especially alcoholic liver disease.[1]
- ○ Matrine from *Sophorae flavescentis* is effective against hepatitis B.

TREATMENTS

There are over 300 preparations used for the treatment of jaundice and chronic liver diseases in Indian systems of medicine alone, and these utilize over 80 Indian medicinal plants.[2] While this chapter focuses primarily on herbs used across cultures, select Chinese herbal concoctions and Ayurvedic remedies are described separately.

Andrographis paniculata *(Kalmegh)*

Also known as *Indian Echinacea*, it is used in traditional Indian medicine for a variety of liver disorders.[3] It has antiviral activity against HIV and increases CD4(+) lymphocyte count in HIV-1 infected

Minocha A. *A Guide to Alternative Medicine and the Digestive System* (pp 343-380).
© 2013 Taylor & Francis Group.

individuals.[4] It is effective against *Herpes simplex* and protects against a variety of toxins, including carbon tetrachloride, ethanol, and acetaminophen.[5-8]

Anoectochilus formosanus Hay

A formosanus Hay is used for treating liver disorders and cancer in China. It has hepatoprotective activity against carbon tetrachloride and acetaminophen-induced liver damage.

Astragalus (Milk-Vetch or Goat's Thorn)

Studies in mice suggest that *Astragalus* has a hepatoprotective effect against acetaminophen-induced hepatotoxicity.[9] The *Astragalus-Polygonum* antifibrosis decoction is effective in reducing hepatic fibrosis and inflammatory activity of chronic hepatitis B.[10]

A systematic review concluded that products containing *Astragalus* have a beneficial effect in the treatment of hepatocellular cancer.[11]

Buddleja

Catapol is found in flowering parts. It has an antihepatotoxic activity comparable to that of silymarin.

Bupleurum

Bupleurum belongs to the *Apiaceae* family, which is composed of almost 200 species. The therapeutic effects are attributed to the bioactive saikosaponins in the plant. Its extracts enhance 5-fluorouracil-induced cytotoxicity in hepatoma cells. Saikosaponins suppress inflammation and fibrogenesis. Human data indicate that it is of benefit in viral hepatitis (ie, both hepatitis B and C).

Capparis spinosa (Capers)

Capers is used as an anti-inflammatory agent. It contains natural anticarcinogens, and its extracts may have potential as anticancer agents.

Cassia fistula

C fistula leaves protect the liver against injury from toxins like acetaminophen and carbon tetrachloride.[12,13]

Centella asiatica (Gotu Kola)

Besides its culinary use, it is used for medicinal purposes in Ayurveda, Chinese, and African medicine.

It protects against acute toxic liver injury in animals. Concerns have been raised about its potential hepatotoxicity.

Cichorium intybus *(Chicory)*

Chicory protects against hepatotoxic effects of nitrosamine compounds. Its cichotyboside extract protects against hepatic injury induced by carbon tetrachloride in animals.[14]

CognoBlend

CognoBlend (UniCity, New Braunfels, TX) is a proprietary formula containing *B monnieri*, *G biloba*, cat's claw, Gotu Kola, and rosemary. It improves neurological function and biochemical parameters in patients with hepatic encephalopathy.[15]

Commiphora wightii *(Commiphora)*[16]

The primary bioactive therapeutic agent in gum resin from *C wightii* (*C mukul*) is guggulsterone. It inhibits tumor initiation, promotion, and metastasis.

Cordyceps

Parasitic *Cordyceps* fungi are composed of about 400 species. It exerts antitumor properties in vitro. Herbal combinations that include *Cordyceps*, such as the Fuzheng Huayu recipe, inhibit fibrosis and improve liver tests in patients with cirrhosis.

Coriolus versicolor

See Protein-Bound Polysaccharide on page 349.

Curcumin

See Turmeric on page 352.

Egyptian Herbal Mixture Formulation

Egyptian herbal mixture formulation (*T chebula*, *Senae*, rhubarb, black cumin, aniseed, fennel, and licorice) ameliorates hepatic abnormalities in rats fed a high-fat diet.

Euphrasia *(Eyebright)*

Eyebright has potential as an antidote for alpha-amanitin poisoning. Aucubin derived from Eyebright protects against liver injury by inhibiting hepatic RNA.[17] It suppresses hepatitis B viral DNA replication in vitro.

Ficus Hispida

In addition to antidiarrheal actions, extract of *F hispida* protects the liver against acetaminophen- and azathioprine-induced hepatotoxicity.[18]

Ganoderma lucidum *(Reishi Mushroom)*[19-21]

It inhibits tumorigenesis and metastasis of human hepatoma cells. Oral administration reduces hepatitis B virus (HBV) surface antigen and HBV e antigen, and protects against chemically induced liver injury.[20] It protects against the recurrence of colorectal adenoma in humans.[21] It inhibits cancer metastasis in vivo.

Geranium carolinianum

It is also known as *Carolina cranesbill* and *Carolina geranium*. Intragastric administration to hepatitis B-infected ducks results in a decrease in HBV DNA level.[22]

Ginseng

Ginseng belongs to the genus *Panax* and family *Araliaceae*. The biotherapeutic components are composed of ginsenosides. It protects against injury induced by various chemicals, including carbon tetrachloride, aflatoxin B1, and thioacetamide. Ginsenosides have benefits against obesity, fatty liver, and hypertriglyceridemia in mice fed a high-fat diet. Brazilian ginseng inhibits tumor proliferation and induces apoptosis in hepatic carcinogenesis. Korean red ginseng accelerates liver regeneration and ameliorates liver injury after partial hepatectomy.

Red ginseng administered over 3 years reduces nonorgan-specific human cancer risk [0.35 (0.13 to 0.96; p = 0.03)], compared to placebo.[23] Case-control studies data suggest that the use of ginseng significantly reduces liver and various gastrointestinal (GI) cancers.[24]

Glycyrrhiza

See Licorice on page 347.

Gynostemma pentaphyllum *(Jiaogulan)*[25-27]

It exerts a hepatoprotective activity in multiple models of experimental liver injury. Gypenoside is a saponins extract, which induces apoptosis in human hepatoma cells. It is a useful adjunct to diet therapy for type 2 diabetes and nonalcoholic fatty liver disease (NAFLD).[26,27]

Hippophae rhamnoides *(Sea Buckthorn)*

Sea buckthorn seed oil protects against carbon tetrachloride-induced hepatotoxicity.

Indian Gooseberry

See *Phyllanthus* on page 349.

Legumes

Commonly ingested legumes, mung bean, adzuki bean, black bean, and rice bean protect against acetaminophen-induced hepatotoxicity in rats. Mung bean has the best effects.

Licorice (Glycyrrhiza)[28]

Ancient manuscripts from China, India, and Greece document the use of *Glycyrrhiza* in health and sickness.

Glycyrrhizin is a constituent of many popular herbal medications worldwide, including Kampo, TJ-9, Herbal Recipe 861, and stronger Neominophagen C (SNMC). Glycyrrhizin protects against hepatotoxicity due to hepatotoxins like carbon tetrachloride. It displays antiviral activity against a variety of viruses, including HIV-1 and vaccinia in vitro.[29]

It improves abnormal biochemical parameters due to hepatitis C virus (HCV) in humans.[30-36] SNMC improves survival in subacute hepatic failure due to viral hepatitis.[32] It improves biochemical parameters as well as liver histology in patients with liver cirrhosis.[33] SNMC combined with interferon is more effective in patients with hepatitis C compared to interferon alone.[34]

A short course of glycyrrhizin before the administration of human lymphoblastoid interferon acts as an immune-modulator and provides beneficial effect in patients with chronic hepatitis B.[37] Combination treatment of chronic hepatitis B in children with Transfer Factor and high-dose SNMC results in 75% of patients becoming HBe-Ag negative within 18 weeks.[38] Glycyrrhizin may be effective for controlling HBV replication and treating chemotherapy-induced HBV hepatitis in chronic HBV carriers with non-Hodgkins lymphoma.[39]

Glycyrrhizin and SNMC reduce the risk of hepatocellular carcinoma (HCC).[40-43] Intravenous glycyrrhizin therapy significantly decreases the hepatic carcinogenesis rate (hazard ratio, 0.49; p = 0.014) in patients with interferon-resistant active chronic hepatitis C.[41]

A 2007 report on the safety assessment of many licorice products found them to be safe for use.[44]

Kumada demonstrated that at 13 years, liver cirrhosis occurred in 28% of patients with hepatitis C on long-term SNMC compared to 40% in controls.[33] At year 15, HCC developed in only 13% of patients on long-term SNMC compared to 25% in controls.

Milk Thistle (Silybum marianum)[45-52]

The active therapeutic extract is silymarin. Milk thistle also contains silybin, which is a potential iron chelator and, as such, has potential to be an adjunct in the treatment of hemochromatosis.

Results on the studies in alcoholic liver disease have been conflicting.[47-50] Silymarin 140 mg tid to patients with cirrhosis results in a superior 4-year survival rate of 58% versus 39% for placebo ($p<0.05$).[47] Other studies have failed to show benefit.[48-50]

It does not appear to have any benefit in hepatitis C.[51,52] Patients with acute hepatitis given silymarin have faster improvement in clinical and laboratory markers, including jaundice, compared to controls.

A systematic review concluded that milk thistle is beneficial in select liver diseases.[45] It is reasonable to employ silymarin as a supportive element in the therapy of *Amanita phalloides* poisoning, as well as for alcoholic and grade Child "A" liver cirrhosis.

Mistletoe (Viscum)

It protects against carbon tetrachloride-induced hepatic injury. Preliminary evidence indicates that it may be of benefit in patients with hepatitis C,[53] HCC,[54] etc.

Paeonia lactiflora (Paeonia)

Paeoniflorin and paeonol are the main active components. The extract from *P lactiflora* and *A membranaceus* combined have better hepatoprotective activity than each herb used individually. It protects against toxin-induced injury, and ameliorates alcoholic steatohepatitis in mice and rats.[55] Paeonol exerts antitumor effects in HepA-hepatoma–bearing mice. A high-dose treatment with *Paeonia rubra* is effective in arresting the development of liver fibrosis in patients with chronic hepatitis.[56]

Pergularia

Pergularia daemia is a perennial herb traditionally used for liver diseases. Its extracts improve biochemical parameters and liver histology in carbon tetrachloride-induced liver damage in rats. The protective effect is significant, compared to the use of silymarin used as a positive control.[57]

Phosphogliv

Phosphogliv is a Russian hepatoprotective formulation. Compared to standard therapy, phosphogliv provides better relief of symptoms and biochemical liver tests.[58]

Phyllanthus *(Amla)*[59-70]

It contains phenolic compounds like tannins, phyllembelic acid, phyllembelin, rutin, curcuminoids, and emblicol that provide therapeutic benefits. It exerts antiviral activity against HBV and woodchuck hepatitis virus in vitro. Examination of 7 preparations revealed Capsule 1 and tuo cha zhen zhu cao were the most potent anti-HBV extracts.[60]

It ameliorates chemically induced injury.[61] It normalizes liver enzymes in diabetic rats. A study of 6 different *Phyllanthus* species (ie, *P hirtellus, P gunnii, P gasstroemii, P similis, P amarus,* and *P tenellus*) revealed that all of them are effective in inhibiting HBV.[62] Its extract induces apoptosis of human HCC cells.

A Cochrane database review concluded that there is no convincing evidence that *Phyllanthus* benefits patients with hepatitis B.[70]

Picrorhiza kurroa[71-74]

P kurroa is part of numerous Indian and Chinese herbal preparations used for liver diseases. Its components include kutkoside and picroside. Kutkin is a mixture of both picroside and kutkoside.

It protects against chemical liver injury as well as carcinogenesis. Mice pretreated with kutkin have improved survival after lethal doses of *A phalloides* or "death cap."[72] It inhibits HBV antigens (HBsAg and HBsAg) in healthy HBsAg carriers.[73] *P. kurroa* root powder treatment for acute viral hepatitis (HBsAg negative) results in a significant biochemical improvement compared to placebo.[74]

Protein-Bound Polysaccharide[75]

Protein-bound polysaccharide is obtained from a mushroom (*C versicolor*) and is reputed for its immune-stimulant properties. It inhibits experimental colon cancer. Neonatal inoculation with protein-bound polysaccharide increases the resistance of adult animals challenged with tumor cells. It decreases thorastat-induced malignant hepatic tumors and increases survival in Syrian hamsters. Protein-bound polysaccharide used as part of adjuvant therapy reduces metastasis in patients with colorectal cancer.

Rhubarb[76-79]

Rhubarb belongs to the genus *Rheum*. Its extracts exert hepatoprotective effects in animal models.

Rhaponticin from rhubarb rhizomes improves steatosis and blood glucose in diabetic animals. Rhubarb prevents liver fibrosis induced by a choline-deficient diet. It has beneficial effects on hepatic encephalopathy in rats with acute liver failure. It induces apoptosis and cell cycle arrest in human liver cancer cells.

Rhubarb has been used for the treatment of viral hepatitis.[78] Rhubarb improves liver function and jaundice in infantile cholestatic hepatitis.[79] Chronic use of *R palmatum* may result in hepatotoxicity.

Safflower

EH0202, a Japanese Kampo herbal mixture of 4 herbs including safflower, induces interferon. EH0202 treatment in chronic hepatitis C reduces HCV-RNA levels in patients with high viral titers.[80] Safflower oil-supplemented diet reduces the risk of acute hepatitis in Long-Evans cinnamon rats.[81]

Salvia

Salvia belongs to the mint family. *S miltiorrhiza* (or Danshen) is also known as *red sage* or *Chinese sage*. It inhibits hepatic fibrosis and induces apoptosis.[82] Its extracts inhibit HBV replication.[83] Tanshinone II-A, an alcohol extract, inhibits metastasis of liver cancer. It improves liver function and inhibits liver fibrosis in patients with chronic hepatitis B.[84,85] *Salvia* injection is more effective in compensated cirrhosis compared to decompensated cases.[86]

Drinking *Salvia officinalis* tea potentiates carbon tetrachloride hepatotoxicity in mice.[87] While the tea by itself is not the likely culprit, herb-drug interactions have been implicated.

Schisandra[88-91]

Schisandra fruit is the most active medicinal component. It stimulates cytoprotective responses in liver and inhibits secretion of HBsAg and HBeAg. Schisandrin B reduces hepatic lipid contents in hypercholesterolemic mice.

Gomisin A from *Schisandra* protects against fulminant hepatic failure induced by D-galactosamine and lipopolysaccharide in mice by inhibiting apoptosis and reducing oxidative stress. It protects against hepatic injury induced by chemicals such as mercuric chloride, carbon tetrachloride, menadione aflatoxin B1, and cadmium chloride in experimental animal models.[89]

Schisandrae lignans, combined with *Astragalus polysaccharides*, have a synergistic protective effect on chronic liver injury in rats. *Fructus schisandrae*-containing compounds (KY88) may affect the elimination of HBV, strengthen the immune system, and stimulate liver cell regeneration. It inhibits secretion of HBsAg and HBeAg.[90] "Eklikit" extract from the *Schisandra chinensis* ameliorates alcohol-induced liver injury.[91]

Scutellaria radix

It induces apoptosis and inhibits chemically induced hepatic carcinogenesis in animals. The wogonin extract inhibits the secretion of the HBV antigens.[92] Use of intravenous wagnonin in HBV-infected ducks decreases HBV-DNA levels. Baicalin from *S radix* suppresses hepatic steatosis in animals fed a high-fat diet.

Sophorae flavescentis[93-96]

Matrine and kurorinone extracts of *S flavescentis* have been used for hepatitis B.[93] It inhibits the replication of HCV-RNA.[94] A systematic review of randomized, controlled trials (RCTs) concluded that matrine has antiviral activity, as evident on liver tests and clinical improvement.[93] The viral and liver biochemical responses are better when it is combined with interferon-alpha, thymosin, or basic treatment.

Spirulina[97-100]

It ameliorates acute fatty liver induced by the administration of simvastatin, ethanol, or hypercholesterolemic diet. It prevents fatty liver (associated with experimental diabetes). *Spirulina* pretreatment prevents experimentally induced chemical liver injury and carcinogenesis in animals. Treatment with spiruline for 1 month has no effect on the aminotransferases in patients with viral hepatitis.[99] A case series found beneficial effects of *Spirulina maxima* in patients with NAFLD.[100]

Taraxacum officinale *(Dandelion)*[101]

Dandelion, also known as *lion's tooth* and *blowball*, has been used to treat liver disorders across cultures. It inhibits hepatic fibrosis in animal models of carbon tetrachloride-induced liver fibrosis.[102] The root extracts protect against alcohol-induced hepatotoxicity. Dietary supplementation with a leafy vegetable mix containing dandelion protects liver cells in mice fed a high-fat diet.

Thunbergia

Various species are known by different names, such as clockvine, Orange clockvine, Black-eyed Susan vine, etc. *Thunbergia laurifolia* protects against alcohol-induced liver injury.

Tinospora

Also known as *Guduchi*, *T cordifolia* has a potential for benefit in diabetes, toxic liver damage, NAFLD, and cancer.[103]

Turmeric (Curcumin)[104-107]

It inhibits HBV as well as HCV replication and attenuates ethanol-induced liver damage.[106] It attenuates liver injury induced by aflatoxin, ethanol, thioacetamide, acetaminophen, iron overdose, and carbon tetrachloride. Curcumin improves sclerosing cholangitis in mice.

SELECT HERBAL COMBINATION THERAPIES

○ Herbal mixture of *G biloba*, *P ginseng*, and *S chinensis* extract protects against carbon tetrachloride-induced liver injury.[108]

○ *A formosanus*, *G lucidum*, and *G pentaphyllum* demonstrate anti-inflammatory and liver-protective effects.

○ Herbal mixtures consisting of puerarin (kudzu root) and either polyenylphosphatidylcholine from soy or curcumin provide protection against alcohol-related disorders in rats.[109]

○ Preparations containing ginseng combined with trace elements and multivitamins improve liver function in the elderly with toxin-induced chronic liver disease.[110]

○ Herbal combination of *S miltiorrhiza* and *A membranaceus* improves portal hypertension and reduces liver fibrosis in liver cirrhosis.[111]

Miscellaneous Herbal Therapies Used Across the World

○ *Ecballium elaterium*, *Luffa echinata*, *Clerodendrum serratum*, and *Momordica dioica* protect against chemically induced liver injury.

○ *A blazei* may be effective in patients with hepatitis B.

REFERENCES

1. Barve A, Khan R, Marsano L, Ravindra KV, McClain C. Treatment of alcoholic liver disease. *Ann Hepatol*. 2008;7(1):5-15.

2. Thyagarajan SP, Jayaram S, Gopalakrishnan V, Hari R, Jeyakumar P, Sripathi MS. Herbal medicines for liver diseases in India. *J Gastroenterol Hepatol*. 2002;17(Suppl 3):S370-376.

3. Trivedi NP, Rawal UM, Patel BP. Hepatoprotective effect of andrographolide against hexachlorocyclohexane-induced oxidative injury. *Integr Cancer Ther*. 2007;6(3):271-280.

4. Calabrese C, Berman SH, Babish JG, et al. A phase I trial of andrographolide in HIV positive patients and normal volunteers. *Phytother Res*. 2000;14(5):333-338.

5. Visen PK, Shukla B, Patnaik GK, Dhawan BN. Andrographolide protects rat hepatocytes against paracetamol-induced damage. *J Ethnopharmacol.* 1993;40(2):131-136.

6. Wiart C, Kumar K, Yusof MY, Hamimah H, Fauzi ZM, Sulaiman M. Antiviral properties of ent-labdene diterpenes of *Andrographis paniculata Nees.*, inhibitors of *herpes simplex* virus type 1. *Phytother Res.* 2005;19(12):1069-1070.

7. Singha PK, Roy S, Dey S. Protective activity of andrographolide and arabinogalactan proteins from *Andrographis paniculata Nees.* against ethanol-induced toxicity in mice. *J Ethnopharmacol.* 2007;111(1):13-21.

8. Kapil A, Koul IB, Banerjee SK, Gupta BD. Antihepatotoxic effects of major diterpenoid constituents of *Andrographis paniculata. Biochem Pharmacol.* 1993;46(1):182-185.

9. Wang DQ, Critchley JA, Ding BG, et al. Protection against paracetamol-induced hepatic damage using total flavonoids of *Astragalus. Zhongguo Zhong Yao Za Zhi.* 2001;26(9):617-620.

10. Chen H, Weng L. Comparison on efficacy in treating liver fibrosis of chronic hepatitis B between *Astragalus polygonum* anti-fibrosis decoction and jinshuibao capsule. *Zhongguo Zhong Xi Yi Jie He Za Zhi.* 2000;20(4):255-257.

11. Wu P, Dugoua JJ, Eyawo O, Mills EJ. Traditional Chinese medicines in the treatment of hepatocellular cancers: a systematic review and meta-analysis. *J Exp Clin Cancer Res.* 2009;28:112.

12. Bhakta T, Banerjee S, Mandal SC, Maity TK, Saha BP, Pal M. Hepatoprotective activity of *Cassia fistula* leaf extract. *Phytomedicine.* 2001;8(3):220-224.

13. Bhakta T, Mukherjee PK, Mukherjee K, et al. Evaluation of hepatoprotective activity of *Cassia fistula* leaf extract. *J Ethnopharmacol.* 1999;66(3):277-282.

14. Ahmed B, Al-Howiriny TA, Siddiqui AB. Antihepatotoxic activity of seeds of *Cichorium intybus. J Ethnopharmacol.* 2003;87(2-3):237-240.

15. Kaziulin AN, Petukhov AB, Kucheriavy IuA. Efficiency of includes of bioactive substances in diet of patient with hepatic encephalopathy. *Vopr Pitan.* 2006;75(2):40-44.

16. Rahimi R, Shams-Ardekani MR, Abdollahi M. A review of the efficacy of traditional Iranian medicine for inflammatory bowel disease. *World J Gastroenterol.* 2010;16(36):4504-4514.

17. Chang IM. Liver-protective activities of aucubin derived from traditional oriental medicine. *Res Commun Mol Pathol Pharmacol.* 1998;102(2):189-204.

18. Mandal SC, Saraswathi B, Kumar CK, Mohana Lakshmi S, Maiti BC. Protective effect of leaf extract of *Ficus hispida Linn.* against paracetamol-induced hepatotoxicity in rats. *Phytother Res.* 2000;14(6):457-459.

19. Xu Z, Chen X, Zhong Z, Chen L, Wang Y. *Ganoderma lucidum* polysaccharides: immunomodulation and potential anti-tumor activities. *Am J Chin Med.* 2011;39(1):15-27.

20. Shi Y, Sun J, He H, Guo H, Zhang S. Hepatoprotective effects of *Ganoderma lucidum* peptides against D-galactosamine-induced liver injury in mice. *J Ethnopharmacol.* 2008;117(3):415-419.

21. Oka S, Tanaka S, Yoshida S, et al. A water-soluble extract from culture medium of *Ganoderma lucidum* mycelia suppresses the development of colorectal adenomas. *Hiroshima J Med Sci.* 2010;59(1):1-6.

22. Li J, Huang H, Feng M, Zhou W, Shi X, Zhou P. In vitro and in vivo anti-hepatitis B virus activities of a plant extract from *Geranium carolinianum L. Antiviral Res.* 2008;79(2):114-120.

23. Yun TK, Zheng S, Choi SY, et al. Non-organ-specific preventive effect of long-term administration of Korean red ginseng extract on incidence of human cancers. *J Med Food.* 2010;13(3):489-494.

24. Yun TK. Experimental and epidemiological evidence on non-organ specific cancer preventive effect of Korean ginseng and identification of active compounds. *MutatRes.* 2003;523-524:63-74.

25. Chen MH, Chen SH, Wang QF, et al. The molecular mechanism of gypenosides-induced G1 growth arrest of rat hepatic stellate cells. *J Ethnopharmacol.* 2008;117(2):309-317.

26. Huyen VT, Phan DV, Thang P, Hoa NK, Ostenson CG. Antidiabetic effect of *Gynostemma pentaphyllum* tea in randomly assigned type 2 diabetic patients. *Horm Metab Res.* 2010;42(5):353-357.

27. Chou SC, Chen KW, Hwang JS, et al. The add-on effects of *Gynostemma pentaphyllum* on nonalcoholic fatty liver disease. *Altern Ther Health Med.* 2006;12(3):34-39.

28. Dhiman RK. Herbal hepatoprotective agents: marketing gimmick or potential therapies? *Trop Gastroenterol.* 2003;24(3):160-162.

29. Fiore C, Eisenhut M, Krausse R, et al. Antiviral effects of *Glycyrrhiza* species. *Phytother Res.* 2008;22(2):141-148.

30. Coon JT, Ernst E. Complementary and alternative therapies in the treatment of chronic hepatitis C: a systematic review. *J Hepatol.* 2004;40(3):491-500.

31. van Rossum TG, Vulto AG, Hop WC, Brouwer JT, Niesters HG, Schalm SW. Intravenous glycyrrhizin for the treatment of chronic hepatitis C: a double-blind, randomized, placebo-controlled phase I/II trial. *J Gastroenterol Hepatol.* 1999;14(11):1093-1099.

32. Acharya SK, Dasarathy S, Tandon A, Joshi YK, Tandon BN. A preliminary open trial on interferon stimulator (SNMC) derived from *Glycyrrhiza glabra* in the treatment of subacute hepatic failure. *Indian J Med Res.* 1993;98:69-74.

33. Kumada H. Long-term treatment of chronic hepatitis C with glycyrrhizin [stronger neo-minophagen C (SNMC)] for preventing liver cirrhosis and hepatocellular carcinoma. *Oncology.* 2002;62(Suppl 1):94-100.

34. Abe Y, Ueda T, Kato T, Kohli Y. Effectiveness of interferon, glycyrrhizin combination therapy in patients with chronic hepatitis C. *Nippon Rinsho.* 1994;52(7):1817-1822.

35. Tsubota A, Kumada H, Arase Y, et al. Combined ursodeoxycholic acid and glycyrrhizin therapy for chronic hepatitis C virus infection: a randomized controlled trial in 170 patients. *Eur J Gastroenterol Hepatol.* 1999;11(10):1077-1083.

36. Tanaka N, Horiuchi A, Yamaura T, et al. Efficacy and safety of addition of minor bloodletting (petit phlebotomy) in hepatitis C virus-infected patients receiving regular glycyrrhizin injections. *J Gastroenterol.* 2009;44(6):577-582.

37. Hayashi J, Kajiyama W, Noguchi A, et al. Glycyrrhizin withdrawal followed by human lymphoblastoid interferon in the treatment of chronic hepatitis B. *Gastroenterol Jpn.* 1991;26(6):742-746.

38. Sumiyama K, Kobayashi M, Miyashiro E, Koike M. Combination therapy with transfer factor and high dose stronger neo-minophagen C in chronic hepatitis B in children (HBe Ag positive). *Acta Paediatr Jpn.* 1991;33(3):327-334.

39. Matsuo K, Takenaka K, Shimomura H, et al. Lamivudine and glycyrrhizin for treatment of chemotherapy-induced hepatitis B virus (HBV) hepatitis in a chronic HBV carrier with non-Hodgkin lymphoma. *Leuk Lymphoma.* 2001;41(1-2):191-195.

40. Morgan TR. Chemoprevention of hepatocellular carcinoma in chronic hepatitis C. *Recent Results Cancer Res.* 2011;188:85-99.

41. Ikeda K. Glycyrrhizin injection therapy prevents hepatocellular carcinogenesis in patients with interferon-resistant active chronic hepatitis C. *Hepatol Res.* 2007;37(Suppl 2):S287-S293.

42. Veldt BJ, Hansen BE, Ikeda K, Verhey E, Suzuki H, Schalm SW. Long-term clinical outcome and effect of glycyrrhizin in 1093 chronic hepatitis C patients with non-response or relapse to interferon. *Scand J Gastroenterol.* 2006;41(9):1087-1094.

43. Arase Y, Ikeda K, Murashima N, et al. The long term efficacy of glycyrrhizin in chronic hepatitis C patients. *Cancer.* 1997;79(8):1494-1500.

44. Cosmetic Ingredient Review Expert Panel. Final report on the safety assessment of glycyrrhetinic acid, potassium glycyrrhetinate, disodium succinoyl glycyrrhetinate, glyceryl glycyrrhetinate, glycyrrhetinyl stearate, stearyl glycyrrhetinate, glycyrrhizic acid, ammonium glycyrrhizate, dipotassium glycyrrhizate, disodium glycyrrhizate, trisodium glycyrrhizate, methyl glycyrrhizate, and potassium glycyrrhizinate. *Int J Toxicol.* 2007;26(Suppl 2):79-112.

45. Saller R, Brignoli R, Melzer J, Meier R. An updated systematic review with meta-analysis for the clinical evidence of silymarin. *Forsch Komplementmed.* 2008;15(1):9-20.

46. Abenavoli L, Capasso R, Milic N, Capasso F. Milk thistle in liver diseases: past, present, future. *Phytother Res.* 2010;24(10):1423-1432.

47. Ferenci P, Dragosics B, Dittrich H, et al. Randomized controlled trial of silymarin treatment in patients with cirrhosis of the liver. *J Hepatol.* 1989;9(1):105-113.

48. Lucena MI, Andrade RJ, de la Cruz JP, Rodriguez-Mendizabal M, Blanco E, Sánchez de la Cuesta F. Effects of silymarin MZ-80 on oxidative stress in patients with alcoholic cirrhosis. Results of a randomized, double-blind, placebo-controlled clinical study. *Int J Clin Pharmacol Ther.* 2002;40(1):2-8.

49. Trinchet JC, Coste T, Lévy VG, et al. Treatment of alcoholic hepatitis with silymarin. A double-blind comparative study in 116 patients. *Gastroenterol Clin Biol.* 1989;13(2):120-124.

50. Parés A, Planas R, Torres M, et al. Effects of silymarin in alcoholic patients with cirrhosis of the liver: results of a controlled, double-blind, randomized and multicenter trial. *J Hepatol.* 1998;28(4):615-621.

51. Gordon A, Hobbs DA, Bowden DS, et al. Effects of *Silybum marianum* on serum hepatitis C virus RNA, alanine aminotransferase levels and well-being in patients with chronic hepatitis C. *J Gastroenterol Hepatol.* 200621(1 Pt 2):275-280.

52. Tanamly MD, Tadros F, Labeeb S, et al. Randomised double-blinded trial evaluating silymarin for chronic hepatitis C in an Egyptian village: study description and 12-month results. *Dig Liver Dis.* 2004;36(11):752-759.

53. Tusenius KJ, Spoek AM, van Hattum J. Exploratory study on the effects of treatment with two mistletoe preparations on chronic hepatitis C. *Arzneimittelforschung.* 2005;55(12):749-753.

54. Mabed M, El-Helw L, Shamaa S. Phase II study of viscum fraxini-2 in patients with advanced hepatocellular carcinoma. *Br J Cancer.* 2004;90(1):65-69.

55. Hu S, Shen G, Zhao W, Wang F, Jiang X, Huang D. Paeonol, the main active principles of *Paeonia moutan*, ameliorates alcoholic steatohepatitis in mice. *J Ethnopharmacol.* 2010;128(1):100-106.

56. Yang DG. Comparison of pre- and post-treatmental hepatohistology with heavy dosage of *Paeonia rubra* on chronic active hepatitis caused liver fibrosis. *Zhongguo Zhong Xi Yi Jie He Za Zhi.* 1994;14(4):207-209,195.

57. Sureshkumar SV, Mishra SH. Hepatoprotective effect of extracts from *Pergularia daemia Forsk. J Ethnopharmacol.* 2006;107(2):164-168.

58. Uchaïkin VF, Luchshev VI, Zharov SN, et al. New domestic phospholipid preparation "Fosfogliv" as an effective treatment for patients with acute viral hepatitis. *Klin Med (Mosk).* 2000;78(5):39-42.

59. Krishnaveni M, Mirunalini S. Therapeutic potential of *Phyllanthus emblica* (amla): the Ayurvedic wonder. *J Basic Clin Physiol Pharmacol.* 2010;21(1):93-105.

60. Liu Z, Fu X, Zhang N, Zhang G, Liu D. The inhibitory effect of Chinese herb *Phyllanthus* on hepatitis B virus in vitro. *Zhonghua Shi Yan He Lin Chuang Bing Du Xue Za Zhi.* 1997;11(3):282-285.

61. Pramyothin P, Ngamtin C, Poungshompoo S, Chaichantipyuth C. Hepatoprotective activity of *Phyllanthus amarus Schum. et. Thonn.* extract in ethanol treated rats: in vitro and in vivo studies. *J Ethnopharmacol.* 2007;114(2):169-173.

62. Shead A, Vickery K, Pajkos A, et al. Effects of *Phyllanthus* plant extracts on duck hepatitis B virus in vitro and in vivo. *Antiviral Res.* 1992;18(2):127-138.

63. Thyagarajan SP, Subramanian S, Thirunalasundari T, Venkateswaran PS, Blumberg BS. Effect of *Phyllanthus amarus* on chronic carriers of hepatitis B virus. *Lancet.* 1988;2(8614):764-766.

64. Thamlikitkul V, Wasuwat S, Kanchanapee P. Efficacy of *Phyllanthus amarus* for eradication of hepatitis B virus in chronic carriers. *J Med Assoc Thai.* 1991;74(9):381-385.

65. Doshi JC, Vaidya AB, Antarkar DS, Deolalikar R, Antani DH. A two-stage clinical trial of *Phyllanthus amarus* in hepatitis B carriers: failure to eradicate the surface antigen. *Indian J Gastroenterol.* 1994;13(1):7-8.

66. Chan HL, Sung JJ, Fong WF, et al. Double-blinded placebo-controlled study of *Phyllanthus urinaris* for the treatment of chronic hepatitis B. *Aliment Pharmacol Ther.* 2003;18(3):339-345.

67. Xin-Hua W, Chang-Qing L, Xing-Bo G, Lin-Chun F. A comparative study of *Phyllanthus amarus* compound and interferon in the treatment of chronic viral hepatitis B. *Southeast Asian J Trop Med Public Health.* 2001;32(1):140-142.

68. Narendranathan M, Remla A, Mini PC, Satheesh P. A trial of *Phyllanthus amarus* in acute viral hepatitis. *Trop Gastroenterol.* 1999;20(4):164-166.

69. Wang MX, Cheng HW, Li YJ, Meng LM, Mai K. Efficacy of *Phyllanthus spp.* in treating patients with chronic hepatitis B. *Zhongguo Zhong Yao Za Zhi.* 1994;19(12):750-751,764.

70. Xia Y, Luo H, Liu JP, Gluud C. *Phyllanthus* species for chronic hepatitis B virus infection. *Cochrane Database Syst Rev.* 2011;4:CD008960.

71. Cao Y, Liu JW, Yu YJ, et al. Synergistic protective effect of picroside II and NGF on PC12 cells against oxidative stress induced by H2O2. *Pharmacol Rep.* 2007;59(5):573-579.

72. Floersheim GL, Bieri A, Koenig R, Pletscher A. Protection against *Amanita phalloides* by the iridoid glycoside mixture of *Picrorhiza kurroa* (kutkin). *Agents Actions.* 1990;29(3-4):386-387.

73. Mehrotra R, Rawat S, Kulshreshtha DK, Patnaik GK, Dhawan BN. In vitro studies on the effect of certain natural products against hepatitis B virus. *Indian J Med Res.* 1990;92:133-138.

74. Vaidya AB, Antarkar DS, Doshi JC, et al. *Picrorhiza kurroa* (Kutaki) Royle ex Benth as a hepatoprotective agent--experimental & clinical studies. *J Postgrad Med.* 1996;42(4):105-108.

75. Matsunaga K, Iijima H, Kobayashi H. Neonatal inoculation with the protein-bound polysaccharide PSK increases resistance of adult animals to challenge with syngeneic tumor cells and reduces azoxymethane-induced precancerous lesions in the colon. *Cancer Epidemiol Biomarkers Prev.* 2000;9(12):1313-1322.

76. Xing XY, Zhao YL, Kong WJ, Wang JB, et al. Investigation of the "dose-time-response" relationships of rhubarb on carbon tetrachloride-induced liver injury in rats. *J Ethnopharmacol.* 2011;135(2):575-581.

77. Sheng X, Wang M, Lu M, Xi B, Sheng H, Zang YQ. Rhein ameliorates fatty liver disease through negative energy balance, hepatic lipogenic regulation, and immunomodulation in diet-induced obese mice. *Am J Physiol Endocrinol Metab.* 2011;300(5):E886-893.

78. Cui X, Wang Y, Kokudo N, Fang D, Tang W. Traditional Chinese medicine and related active compounds against hepatitis B virus infection. *Biosci Trends.* 2010;4(2):39-47.

79. Huang ZH, Dong YS, Ye WY. Clinical observation on treatment of infantile cholestatic hepatitis syndrome by rhubarb. *Zhongguo Zhong Xi Yi Jie He Za Zhi.* 1997;17(8):459-461.

80. Kaji K, Yoshida S, Nagata N, et al. An open-label study of administration of EH0202, a health-food additive, to patients with chronic hepatitis C. *J Gastroenterol.* 2004;39(9):873-878.

81. Shibata T, Nagayasu H, Kawano T, et al. Unsaturated fatty acid feeding prevents the development of acute hepatitis in Long-Evans cinnamon (LEC) rats. *Anticancer Res.* 1999;19(6B):5169-5174.

82. Stickel F, Brinkhaus B, Krähmer N, Seitz HK, Hahn EG, Schuppan D. Antifibrotic properties of botanicals in chronic liver disease. *Hepatogastroenterology.* 2002;49(46):1102-118.

83. Zhou Z, Zhang Y, Ding XR, et al. Protocatechuic aldehyde inhibits hepatitis B virus replication both in vitro and in vivo. *Antiviral Res.* 2007;74(1):59-64.

84. Jin CX, Yang J, Sun HF. Comparative study of the clinical effects of *Salvia miltiorrhiza* injection and shengmai injection on chronic hepatitis B. *Zhongguo Zhong Xi Yi Jie He Za Zhi.* 2006;26(10):936-938.

85. She SF, Huang XZ, Tong GD. Clinical study on treatment of liver fibrosis by different dosages of *Salvia* injection. *Zhongguo Zhong Xi Yi Jie He Za Zhi.* 2004;24(1):17-20.

86. Ye F, Liu Y, Qiu G, Zhao Y, Liu M. Clinical study on treatment of cirrhosis by different dosages of *Salvia* injection. *Zhong Yao Cai.* 2005;28(9):850-854.

87. Lima CF, Fernandes-Ferreira M, Pereira-Wilson C. Drinking of *Salvia officinalis* tea increases CCl(4)-induced hepatotoxicity in mice. *Food Chem Toxicol.* 2007;45(3):456-464.

88. Stacchiotti A, Li Volti G, Lavazza A, Rezzani R, Rodella LF. Schisandrin B stimulates a cytoprotective response in rat liver exposed to mercuric chloride. *Food Chem Toxicol.* 2009;47(11):2834-2840.

89. Ip SP, Mak DH, Li PC, Poon MK, Ko KM. Effect of a lignan-enriched extract of *Schisandra chinensis* on aflatoxin B1 and cadmium chloride-induced hepatotoxicity in rats. *Pharmacol Toxicol.* 1996;78(6):413-416.

90. Loo WT, Cheung MN, Chow LW. *Fructus schisandrae* (Wuweizi)-containing compound inhibits secretion of HBsAg and HBeAg in hepatocellular carcinoma cell line. *Biomed Pharmacother.* 2007;61(9):606-610.

91. Kushnerova NF, Sprygin VG, Rakhmanin IuA. Influence of complex plant polyphenol preparation Eklikit on process of liver functions recovery after alcohol intoxication. *Biomed Khim.* 2004;50(6):605-611.

92. Guo Q, Zhao L, You Q, et al. Anti-hepatitis B virus activity of wogonin in vitro and in vivo. *Antiviral Res.* 2007;74(1):16-24.

93. Liu J, Zhu M, Shi R, Yang M. *Radix Sophorae flavescentis* for chronic hepatitis B: a systematic review of randomized trials. *Am J Chin Med.* 2003;31(3):337-354.

94. Tang ZM, Peng M, Zhan CJ. Screening 20 Chinese herbs often used for clearing heat and dissipating toxin with nude mice model of hepatitis C viral infection. *Zhongguo Zhong Xi Yi Jie He Za Zhi.* 2003;23(6):447-448.

95. Chen C, Guo SM, Liu B. A randomized controlled trial of kurorinone versus interferon-alpha2a treatment in patients with chronic hepatitis B. *J Viral Hepat.* 2000;7(3):225-229.

96. Long Y, Lin XT, Zeng KL, Zhang L. Efficacy of intramuscular matrine in the treatment of chronic hepatitis B. *Hepatobiliary Pancreat Dis Int.* 2004;3(1):69-72.

97. Khan Z, Bhadouria P, Bisen PS. Nutritional and therapeutic potential of *Spirulina. Curr Pharm Biotechnol.* 2005;6(5):373-379.

98. Moura LP, Puga GM, Beck WR, et al. Exercise and *Spirulina* control non-alcoholic hepatic steatosis and lipid profile in diabetic Wistar rats. *Lipids Health Dis.* 2011;10(1):77.

99. Baicus C, Tanasescu C. Chronic viral hepatitis, the treatment with spir-uline for one month has no effect on the aminotransferases. *Rom J Intern Med.* 2002;40(1-4):89-94.

100. Ferreira-Hermosillo A, Torres-Duran PV, Juarez-Oropeza MA. Hepatoprotective effects of *Spirulina maxima* in patients with non-alco-holic fatty liver disease: a case series. *J Med Case Reports.* 2010;4:103.

101. Schütz K, Carle R, Schieber A. Taraxacum—a review on its phytochem-ical and pharmacological profile. *J Ethnopharmacol.* 2006;107(3):313-323.

102. Domitrovic R, Jakovac H, Romic Z, Rahelic D, Tadic Z. Antifibrotic activity of *Taraxacum officinale* root in carbon tetrachloride-induced liver damage in mice. *J Ethnopharmacol.* 2010;130(3):569-577.

103. Panchabhai TS, Kulkarni UP, Rege NN. Validation of therapeutic claims of *Tinospora cordifolia*: a review. *Phytother Res.* 2008;22(4):425-441.

104. Rivera-Espinoza Y, Muriel P. Pharmacological actions of curcumin in liver diseases or damage. *Liver Int.* 2009;29(10):1457-1466.

105. Darvesh AS, Aggarwal BB, Bishayee A. Curcumin and liver cancer: a review. *Curr Pharm Biotechnol.* 2011.

106. Rechtman MM, Har-Noy O, Bar-Yishay I, et al. Curcumin inhibits hepa-titis B virus via down-regulation of the metabolic coactivator PGC-1alpha. *FEBS Lett.* 2010;584(11):2485-2490.

107. Kheradpezhouh E, Panjehshahin MR, Miri R, et al. Curcumin protects rats against acetaminophen-induced hepatorenal damages and shows synergistic activity with N-acetyl cysteine. *Eur J Pharmacol.* 2010;628(1-3):274-281.

108. Chang HF, Lin YH, Chu CC, Wu SJ, Tsai YH, Chao JC. Protective effects of *Ginkgo biloba*, *Panax ginseng*, and *Schizandra chinensis* extract on liver injury in rats. *Am J Chin Med.* 2007;35(6):995-1009.

109. Singh AK, Jiang Y, Benlhabib E, Gupta S. Herbal mixtures consisting of puerarin and either polyenylphosphatidylcholine or curcumin provide comprehensive protection against alcohol-related disorders in P rats receiving free choice water and 15% ethanol in pure water. *J Med Food.* 2007;10(3):526-542.

110. Zuin M, Battezzati PM, Camisasca M, Riebenfeld D, Podda M. Effects of a preparation containing a standardized ginseng extract combined with trace elements and multivitamins against hepatotoxin-induced chronic liver disease in the elderly. *J Int Med Res.* 1987;15(5):276-281.

111. Tan YW, Yin YM, Yu XJ. Influence of *Salvia miltiorrhizae* and *Astragalus membranaceus* on hemodynamics and liver fibrosis indexes in liver cirrhotic patients with portal hypertension. *Zhongguo Zhong Xi Yi Jie He Za Zhi.* 2001;21(5):351-353.

Chapter

59 *Select Ayurvedic Remedies for Liver Disorders*

KEY POINTS

○ Ayurveda encompasses a comprehensive holistic approach, and the medicines are only one component.

○ Liv-52 is the most popular Ayurvedic herbal remedy for liver disorders.[1]

DIHAR

Dihar is an Ayurvedic formulation composed of 8 different herbs (ie, *Syzygium cumini, Momordica charantia, E officinalis, Gymnema sylvestre, Enicostemma littorale, A indica, T cordifolia,* and *C longa*). It has antihyperglycemic, antihyperlipidemic, and antioxidant properties in experimental animal models.[2] Several scientific studies have demonstrated beneficial effects of its components in liver dysfunction.

KAMALAHAR

Kamalahar contains *Tecoma undulata, Phyllanthus urinaria, Embelia ribes, T officinale, Nyctanthes arbor-tristis,* and *T arjuna.* Kamalahar given to patients with acute viral hepatitis results in a superior improvement in clinical symptoms and liver tests compared to placebo.[3]

Liv-52[4-9]

Liv-52 is perhaps the most popular Ayurvedic remedy for liver disorders today. It contains multiple herbs, including *Mandur bhasma*, Negro coffe (*Cassia occidentalis*), tamarisk or salt cedar (*Tamarix gallica*), capers (*C spinosa*), chicory (*C intybus*), black nightshade (*Solanum nigrum*), arjuna (*T arjuna*), and yarrow (*Achillea millefolium*).

Liv-52 is widely used for alcohol-related illness. It protects against experimental ethanol-induced fetotoxicity in rats. Results in alcoholic liver disease have been mixed. A double-blind placebo-controlled study found that Liv-52 improves symptoms, as well as jaundice, in patients with acute viral hepatitis.

A 6-month treatment with Liv-52 improves liver function tests in patients with liver cirrhosis.[9]

REFERENCES

1. Ghosh N, Ghosh R, Mandal V, Mandal SC. Recent advances in herbal medicine for treatment of liver diseases. *Pharm Biol.* 2011;49(9):970-988.

2. Patel SS, Shah RS, Goyal RK. Antihyperglycemic, antihyperlipidemic and antioxidant effects of Dihar, a polyherbal ayurvedic formulation in streptozotocin induced diabetic rats. *Indian J Exp Biol.* 2009;47(7):564-570.

3. Das DG. A double-blind clinical trial of kamalahar, an indigenous compound preparation, in acute viral hepatitis. *Indian J Gastroenterol.* 1993;12(4):126-128.

4. Gopumadhavan S, Jagadeesh S, Chauhan BL, Kulkarni RD. Protective effect of Liv-52 on alcohol-induced fetotoxicity. *Alcohol Clin Exp Res.* 1993;17(5):1089-1092.

5. Chauhan BL, Kulkarni RD. Alcohol hangover and Liv-52. *Eur J Clin Pharmacol.* 1991;40(2):187-188.

6. Kaláb M, Krechler T. The effect of the heptoprotective agent Liv-52 on liver damage. *Cas Lek Cesk.* 1997;136(24):758-760.

7. de Silva HA, Saparamadu PA, Thabrew MI, et al. Liv-52 in alcoholic liver disease: a prospective, controlled trial. *J Ethnopharmacol.* 2003;84(1):47-50.

8. Sama SK, Krishnamurthy L, Ramachandran K, Lal K. Efficacy of an indigenous compound preparation (Liv-52) in acute viral hepatitis—a double blind study. *Indian J Med Res.* 1976;64(5):738-742.

9. Huseini HF, Alavian SM, Heshmat R, Heydari MR, Abolmaali K. The efficacy of Liv-52 on liver cirrhotic patients: a randomized, double-blind, placebo-controlled first approach. *Phytomedicine.* 2005;12(9):619-624.

60 *Select Chinese Treatments for Liver Disorders*

KEY POINTS

○ Chinese herbal products containing ginseng, *Astragalus*, and *Mylabris* have a beneficial effect in hepatocellular cancer (HCC).[1]

○ Fuzheng Jiedu Tang (compound of herbs) is effective in clearing serum HBsAg, HBeAg, and HBV DNA.[2]

TREATMENTS

Because of overlap with other systems of medicine, some of the therapies mentioned may be in Chapter 58. Please see Table 60-1 for popular Chinese herbal remedies.[3]

Cardiotonic Pills

Cardiotonic pills are an oral, multicomponent herbal medicine that includes Danshen (*S miltiorrhiza*), *P notoginseng*, and *Dryobalanops aromatica Gaertn*. It has beneficial effects in alcohol-induced fatty liver in mice.[4]

CH-100

CH-100 is a Chinese herbal formulation of 19 different herbs used in liver disorders. It modifies the T-cell responses, especially in ethanol-fed rats.[5] Results of studies in patients with hepatitis C suggest a modest benefit at best.[6,7]

Chi-Shen

Chi-shen extract from *S miltiorrhiza* and *R Paeoniae* exerts antitumor effects on human HCC cells.

Dahuang zhechong

Dahuang zhechong herbal combination formula pills reduce immune-mediated liver fibrosis in rats.

Danning Pian

Chinese herbal medicine Danning Pian (composed of rhubarb, grant knotweed, dried green orange peel, and dried old orange peel) is beneficial for patients with NAFLD.[8]

Table 60-1. Select Chinese Herbal Remedies by Popularity[3]

Popularity	Drug/Regimen
Most popular herbal formula for chronic hepatitis	Long-dan-xie-gan-tang
Most popular single drug for chronic hepatitis	*S miltiorrhiza* (Dan-shen)
Most popular 2-drug regimen for liver disorders	Jia-wei-xia-yao-san, plus *S miltiorrhiza*
Most popular 3-drug regimen for liver disorders	Jia-wei-xia-yao-san, plus *S miltiorrhiza* and *Artemisia capillaris* (Yin-chen-hao)

A systematic review found that, compared to nonspecific treatment or placebo, the herbal compound Fuzheng Jiedu Tang is effective in clearing serum HBsAg, HBeAg and HBV DNA.[2] *P umbellatus* polysaccharide displays a positive effect on serum HBeAg and HBV DNA. *P amarus* has positive effects on serum HBeAg. *Phyllanthus* compound and kurorinone are similar in efficacy to interferon, as determined by the clearance of serums HBeAg and HBV DNA and the normalization of alanine aminotransferase.

Fuzheng Huayu Capsule

Fuzheng Huayu capsule is a multiherbal remedy, including cordyceps sinensis polysaccharide, amygdaloside, and gypenoside. Fuzheng Huayu treatment of patients with chronic hepatitis B results in improvement in biochemical liver tests as well as fibrosis.[2,9,10]

Jiedu Yanggan Gao

Jiedu Yanggan Gao is a multiherbal formula composed of *A capillaris*, *Taraxacum mongolicum*, *Plantago* seed, *Cephalanoplos segetum*, *Hedyotis diffusa*, *Flos chrysanthemi indici*, *Smilax glabra*, *A membranaceus*, *S miltiorrhiza*, *Fructus polygonii orientalis*, *R Paeoniae alba*, and *Polygonatum sibiricum*. Treatment of hepatitis B results in the normalization of liver enzymes and clearance of HBeAg and HBV DNA.[11]

Ninjin-Yoei-To (TJ-108)

Ninjin-yoei-to (Formula ginseng TJ-108) is used for hepatitis C. *Citrus unshiu* peel, *Schisandra* fruit, and *Polygala* root, which are specific to TJ-108, are the active components against HCV.

Polyporus umbellatus *(Chuling)*

Chuling plus mitomycin is effective against experimental liver cancer in mice.[12] Chuling administration has beneficial effects in patients with hepatitis B.[2]

Shengmai San

Shengmai San is composed of *P ginseng C A Meyer*, *S chinensis Baill*, and *Ophiopogon japonicus Ker-Gawl*. Shengmai San reduces hepatic lipids in rats fed a high-cholesterol diet.[13]

Sho-Saiko-To (TJ-9)[14,15]

Treatment of hepatitis B with herbal combination Sho-saiko-to (TJ-9) results in a decline of serum aspartate aminotransferase and alanine aminotransferase values.[15]

Songyou Yin

Herbal combination extract "Songyou Yin" (containing *S miltiorrhiza Bge-danshen* and 4 other herbs) inhibits tumor growth and prolongs survival in mice bearing human HCC.

Yanggan Aoping Mixture

Treatment of chronic persistent hepatitis with Yanggan Aoping mixture is effective in 61% of patients, whereas the response rate is 60% for chronic active hepatitis.[16]

Yin-Chen-Hao-Tang

Yin-Chen-Hao-Tang decoction from 3 different herbs (ie, *A capillaris Thunb* [*Compositae*], *Gardenia jasminoides Ellis* [*Rubiaceae*], and *R officinale Baill* [*Polygonaceae*]) is believed to protect the liver against various types of injury.[17] It ameliorates hepatic fibrosis in rats.[18]

Yo Jyo Hen Shi Ko

Yo Jyo Hen Shi Ko improves biochemical parameters in patients with nonalcoholic steatohepatitis.

Miscellaneous Chinese Therapies

The cultured broth of *G lucidum*, supplemented with *Radix Sophorae flavescentis*, protects mice from hepatitis B liver damage. Treatment with jiedu xiaozheng yin prior to surgery, and then fuzheng yiliu recipe postoperatively for HCC, results in decreased cancer recurrence.[19]

A controlled study of acute, subacute, and chronic severe hepatitis compared the effect of Western medicine alone or when combined with Chinese medicine based on the removing dampness and purgative principle.[20] Both the total effective rate and marked improvement rate were superior to controls.

Table 60-2 reviews some select Chinese medicine remedies in vogue these days.

References

1. Wu P, Dougoua JJ, Eyawo O, Mills EJ. Traditional Chinese medicines in the treatment of hepatocellular cancers: a systematic review and meta-analysis. *J Exp Clin Cancer Res.* 2009;28:112.

2. Liu JP, McIntosh H, Lin H. Chinese medicinal herbs for chronic hepatitis B. *Cochrane Database Syst Rev.* 2001;(1):CD001940.

3. Chen FP, Kung YY, Chen YC, et al. Frequency and pattern of Chinese herbal medicine prescriptions for chronic hepatitis in Taiwan. *J Ethnopharmacol.* 2008;117(1):84-91.

4. Horie Y, Han JY, Mori S, et al. Herbal cardiotonic pills prevent gut ischemia/reperfusion-induced hepatic microvascular dysfunction in rats fed ethanol chronically. *World J Gastroenterol.* 2005;11(4):511-515.

5. Batey R, Cao Q, Pang G, Clancy RL. Effects of CH-100, a chinese herbal medicine, on acute concanavalin A-mediated hepatitis in control and alcohol-fed rats. *Alcohol Clin Exp Res.* 2000;24(6):852-858. Erratum: 2002;26(9):1443.

6. Batey RG, Bensoussan A, Fan YY, Bollipo S, Hossain MA. Preliminary report of a randomized, double-blind placebo-controlled trial of a Chinese herbal medicine preparation CH-100 in the treatment of chronic hepatitis C. *J Gastroenterol Hepatol.* 1998;13(3):244-247.

7. Mollison L, Totten L, Flexman J, Beaman M, Batey R. Randomized double blind placebo-controlled trial of a Chinese herbal therapy (CH100) in chronic hepatitis C. *J Gastroenterol Hepatol.* 2006;21(7):1184-1188.

8. Fan JG; Shanghai Multicenter Clinical Cooperative Group of Danning Pian Trial. Evaluating the efficacy and safety of Danning Pian in the short-term treatment of patients with non-alcoholic fatty liver disease: a multicenter clinical trial. *Hepatobiliary Pancreat Dis Int.* 2004;3(3):375-380.

9. Liu P, Hu YY, Liu C, et al. Multicenter clinical study about the action of Fuzheng Huayu Capsule against liver fibrosis with chronic hepatitis B. *Zhong Xi Yi Jie He Xue Bao.* 2003;1(2):89-98,102.

10. Hu YY, Liu P, Liu C. Investigation on indication of fuzheng huayu capsule against hepatic fibrosis and its non-invasive efficacy evaluation parameters: data analysis of liver biopsy of 50 patients with chronic hepatitis B before and after treatment. *Zhongguo Zhong Xi Yi Jie He Za Zhi.* 2006;26(1):18-22.

Table 60-2. Miscellaneous Chinese Herbal Treatments for Liver Disorders Currently in Vogue

Drug/Author	Study Rationale/Setting	Comments
Potentilla anserine[21]	Triterpenoid saponin from the plant inhibits the expression of HBsAg, HBeAg, and HBV DNA	Inhibits duck HBV (DHBV) DNA replication
Oenanthe javanica[22]	Suppresses HBeAg and HBsAg in vitro	Reduces HBV DNA level
QHF formula containing Qingrejiedu, Huoxue-huayu, and Fuzheng-guben[23]	Effective in H(22) mouse (Balb/c) models with solid tumors and ascites tumors	Combination is better than the individual drugs in the formula
Astragali com-posita[24]	Effective in chronic per-sistent hepatitis and chronic active hepatitis	The seroconversion rates of HBeAg and HBV DNA is 28.0%
Xiaoshui decoction[25]	RCT (n = 61) in treating ascites patients with primary liver cancer	Addition of Xiaoshui decoction results in higher 1-year survival rate
Shenqi mix-ture[26]	RCT of Shenqi mixture combined with micro-wave coagulation versus microwave coagulation alone in primary hepa-tocellular carcinoma	Effective rate was significantly higher (75% versus 56%) in the treatment group along with prolonged survival
S miltiorrhiza plus *P umbel-latus*[27]	RCT (n = 90) compared the effect of *S miltiorrhi-za* plus *P umbellatus* to the individual drugs in hepatitis B	Combination group had a greater num-ber of HBeAg neg-ative subjects com-pared to the drugs

(continued)

Table 60-2 (continued). Miscellaneous Chinese Herbal Treatments for Liver Disorders Currently in Vogue

Drug/Author	Study Rationale/Setting	Comments
Kangxian Baogan decoction on liver fibrosis in patients with chronic hepatitis B[28]	An RCT (n = 81). Controls got conventional liver protecting treatment	Kangxian Baogan decoction group showed significantly better liver function tests and liver fibrosis
Da Ding Feng Zhu decoction[29]	RCT in patient with chronic hepatitis B; controls were treated with colchicine	Treatment group showed significantly lower levels of markers of fibrosis
Xuefu Zhuyu decoction (XZD)[30]	RCT of patients with chronic hepatitis B; controls got conventional treatment	Treatment resulted in significantly improved markers of liver fibrosis
Yi-Ganning granule is composed of *A membranaceus*, *A capillaris*, *Codonopsis pilosula*, etc[31]	A controlled study in chronic hepatitis B; controls received oleanolic acid granule	Yi-Ganning granule results in superior seronegative conversion rates of HBsAg and HBeAg
Cpd 861[32]	A randomized, double-blind, placebo-controlled trial in patients with HBV infection	Treatment reduces liver fibrosis and early cirrhosis compared to placebo

(continued)

Table 60-2 (continued). Miscellaneous Chinese Herbal
Treatments for Liver Disorders Currently in Vogue

Drug/Author	Study Rationale/Setting	Comments
Yo Jyo Hen Shi Ko[33]	Randomized, double-blind, placebo-controlled pilot study in patients with nonalcoholic steatohepatitis and abnormal transaminases	Patients in the Yo Jyo Hen Shi Ko group have a significant decline in alanine aminotransferase compared to baseline

11. Chen Z. Clinical study of 96 cases with chronic hepatitis B treated with jiedu yanggan gao by a double-blind method. *Zhong Xi Yi Jie He Za Zhi.* 1990;10(2):67,71-74.

12. You JS, Hau DM, Chen KT, Huang HF. Combined effects of chuling (*Polyporus umbellatus*) extract and mitomycin C on experimental liver cancer. *Am J Chin Med.* 1994;22(1):19-28.

13. Yao HT, Chang YW, Chen CT, Chiang MT, Chang L, Yeh TK. Shengmai San reduces hepatic lipids and lipid peroxidation in rats fed on a high-cholesterol diet. *J Ethnopharmacol.* 2008;116(1):49-57.

14. Yamashiki M, Nishimura A, Huang XX, Nobori T, Sakaguchi S, Suzuki H. Effects of the Japanese herbal medicine "Sho-saiko-to" (TJ-9) on interleukin-12 production in patients with HCV-positive liver cirrhosis. *Dev Immunol.* 1999;7(1):17-22.

15. Hirayama C, Okumura M, Tanikawa K, Yano M, Mizuta M, Ogawa N. A multicenter randomized controlled clinical trial of Shosaiko-to in chronic active hepatitis. *Gastroenterol Jpn.* 1989;24(6):715-719.

16. Yu RQ, Bi JJ, Wang QS. Clinical and experimental study on treatment of chronic hepatitis B with yanggan aoping mixture. *Zhongguo Zhong Xi Yi Jie He Za Zhi.* 1997;17(3):155-158.

17. Lee TY, Chang HH, Lo WC, Lin HC. Alleviation of hepatic oxidative stress by Chinese herbal medicine Yin-Chen-Hao-Tang in obese mice with steatosis. *Int J Mol Med.* 2010;25(6):837-844.

18. Tao Q, Sun MY, Feng Q. Syndrome identification of CCl4 induced liver fibrosis model rats based on syndrome detecting from recipe used. *Zhongguo Zhong Xi Yi Jie He Za Zhi.* 2009;29(3):246-250.

19. Chen LW, Lin J, Chen W, Zhang W. Effect of Chinese herbal medicine on patients with primary hepatic carcinoma in III stage during perioperational period: a report of 42 cases. *Zhongguo Zhong Xi Yi Jie He Za Zhi.* 2005;25(9):832-834.

20. Zhang JJ, Huang JQ. Clinical study on treatment of severe hepatitis with removing dampness and purgative method. *Zhongguo Zhong Xi Yi Jie He Za Zhi.* 2008;28(1):13-16.

21. Zhao YL, Cai GM, Hong X, Shan LM, Xiao XH. Anti-hepatitis B virus activities of triterpenoid saponin compound from *Potentilla anserine L. Phytomedicine.* 2008;15(4):253-258.

22. Han YQ, Huang ZM, Yang XB, Liu HZ, Wu GX. In vivo and in vitro anti-hepatitis B virus activity of total phenolics from *Oenanthe javanica. J Ethnopharmacol.* 2008;118(1):148-153.

23. Chen T, Li D, Fu YL, Hu W. Screening of QHF formula for effective ingredients from Chinese herbs and its anti-hepatic cell cancer effect in combination with chemotherapy. *Chin Med J (Engl).* 2008;121(4):363-368.

24. Liu KZ, Xu CH, Zhang MT. Clinical and experimental studies on effects of chronic hepatitis B treated with astragali composita. *Zhongguo Zhong Xi Yi Jie He Za Zhi.* 1996;16(7):394-397.

25. Wu D, Bao WG, Ding YH. Clinical and experimental study of xiaoshui decoction in the treatment of primary liver cancer caused ascites. *Zhongguo Zhong Xi Yi Jie He Za Zhi.* 2005;25(12):1066-1069.

26. Lin JJ, Jin CN, Zheng ML, Ouyang XN, Zeng JX, Dai XH. Clinical study on treatment of primary hepatocellular carcinoma by Shenqi mixture combined with microwave coagulation. *Chin J Integr Med.* 2005;11(2):104-110.

27. Xiong LL. Therapeutic effect of combined therapy of *Salvia miltiorrhizae* and *Polyporus umbellatus* polysaccharide in the treatment of chronic hepatitis B. *Zhongguo Zhong Xi Yi Jie He Za Zhi.* 1993;13(9):533-535,516-517.

28. Liang TJ, Zhang W, Zhang CQ. Clinical study on treatment of liver fibrosis in patients of hepatitis B by kangxian baogan decoction. *Zhongguo Zhong Xi Yi Jie He Za Zhi.* 2002;22(5):332-334.

29. Li W, Wang C, Zhang J. Effects of da ding feng zhu decoction in 30 cases of liver fibrosis. *J Tradit Chin Med.* 2003;23(4):251-254.

30. Ru QJ, Tang ZM, Zhang ZE, Zhu Q. Clinical observation on effect of xuefu zhuyu decoction in treating patients with liver fibrosis caused by chronic hepatitis B. *Zhongguo Zhong Xi Yi Jie He Za Zhi.* 2004;24:983-985.

31. Zhang BZ, Ding F, Tan LW. Clinical and experimental study on yi-gan-ning granule in treating chronic hepatitis B. *Zhongguo Zhong Xi Yi Jie He Za Zhi.* 1993;13(10):597-599,580.

32. Yin SS, Wang BE, Wang TL, Jia JD, Qian LX. The effect of Cpd 861 on chronic hepatitis B related fibrosis and early cirrhosis: a randomized, double blind, placebo controlled clinical trial. *Zhonghua Gan Zang Bing Za Zhi.* 2004;12(8):467-470.

33. Chande N, Laidlaw M, Adams P, Marotta P. Yo Jyo Hen Shi Ko (YHK) improves transaminases in nonalcoholic steatohepatitis (NASH): a randomized pilot study. *Dig Dis Sci.* 2006;51(7):1183-1189.

Nonherbal Treatments for Liver Disorders

Key Points

○ L-carnitine appears to be of benefit in hepatic encephalopathy, nonalcoholic steatohepatitis, and valproate poisoning.[1]

○ Vitamin E supplementation is effective in nonsteatohepatitis.[2]

○ Limited data indicate a benefit of S-adenosylmethionine in alcoholic liver disease and cholestatic disorders.[3]

○ Zinc may be of benefit in hepatic encephalopathy.[4]

Treatments

Acupuncture

Manual acupuncture and electroacupuncture promote clearance of HBsAg and HBeAg and positive turnover of anti-HBe.[5]

Alpha Lipoic Acid

Preadministration of alpha lipoic acid is hepatoprotective in several animal models of hepatotoxicity. Use of multiantioxidative treatments including alpha lipoic acid in chronic HCV patients has a beneficial effect on necroinflammatory variables.[6] Alpha lipoic acid therapy may be helpful in chronic alcohol-related liver disease.[7,8]

Antioxidants

Antioxidants vitamin E and vitamin C, and both combined, inhibit hepatic fibrosis in rats.[9] However, the role of vitamin supplementation in many such disorders is controversial in humans.[10] A 2011 systematic review concluded that there is no evidence to support or refute the use of antioxidants in liver diseases.[11]

The role of vitamin E alone is discussed separately later in this chapter.

Betaine

Betaine is found in plants and animals. It increases levels of S-adenosylmethionine. The human data have been disappointing. Betaine does not have an impact on NAFLD activity.[12]

Biotin[13]

Use of antioxidant therapy including biotin, with or without corticosteroids, does not improve 6-month survival in severe alcoholic hepatitis.

Clay

Phyllosilicate clay, also known as *hydrated sodium calcium aluminosilicate*, binds to aflatoxins in the GI tract and reduces their uptake. Urinary metabolites of aflatoxin are markedly reduced in animals fed aflatoxin plus hydrated sodium calcium aluminosilicate.

Choline

Polyunsaturated phosphatidylcholine treatment of patients with chronic hepatitis B and C, in combination with alpha-interferon, results in a higher response in hepatitis C patients, but not in hepatitis B patients.[14] Similar beneficial results are seen in patients with fulminant and subacute hepatic failure.[15]

Chlorophyll

Administration of chlorophyllin 3 times a day for 4 months results in a 55% reduction of median urinary levels of aflatoxin biomarker, compared to those taking placebo.[16]

Germanium

Germanium L-cysteine alpha-tocopherol complex is effective against radiation-induced toxicity. A 16-week treatment with propagermanium given to patients with chronic hepatitis B helps in the clearance of the hepatitis Be antigen.[17]

Lactoferrin

Results of studies in hepatitis C have been mixed. One study showed that oral bovine lactoferrin has no effect on virologic response or alanine aminotransferase levels.[18]

L-Carnitine[1,19-24]

L-carnitine treatment reduces steatosis in patients with chronic hepatitis C treated with alpha-interferon and ribavirin.[21] It improves liver function and histological injury of NAFLD.[22] Branched chain amino acids supplemented with L-acetylcarnitine are superior to branched chain amino acids treatment alone for treatment of patients in hepatic coma.[23] It is useful in patients with altered mental status following valproate overdose.[24]

Liver Extract

A mixture of liver extract and flavin adenin dinucleotide improves the histopathology seen in chronic liver injury.[25] Combination therapy with intravenous interferon-beta and the liver extract preparation and flavin adenine dinucleotide mixture is more effective than intravenous interferon-beta monotherapy for patients with chronic hepatitis C.[25]

Melatonin

Melatonin abnormalities occur in cirrhosis patients even without clinical encephalopathy.[26] Melatonin delays circadian rhythms when given in the morning and advances them when administered in the afternoon or early evening.[27] Melatonin administration at appropriately targeted times of day may modulate these disturbances and restore the biological clock toward baseline.

Phosphogliv

Phosphogliv is a Russian hepatoprotective drug. Phosphogliv improves symptoms and biochemical liver tests in patients with chronic viral hepatitis.[28]

S-Adenosylmethionine[3,29-34]

S-adenosylmethionine regulates hepatocyte growth, differentiation, and death.[29] Hepatic S-adenosylmethionine levels are decreased in alcohol liver disease, as well as viral cirrhosis.

A Cochrane database review concluded that there was not enough evidence to support or refute the use of S-adenosylmethionine for patients with alcoholic liver disease.[34] Meta-analysis suggested that S-adenosylmethionine is useful in patients with cholestatic liver diseases for the treatment of pruritus and jaundice. While it improves pruritus and bilirubin in females with cholestasis of pregnancy, it is not better than—and may actually be inferior to—ursodeoxycholic acid.

Selenium

Antitumorigenic effects of selenium compounds have been described in animals. Antioxidant therapy including selenium, alone or in combination with corticosteroids, does not improve 6-month survival rates in severe alcoholic hepatitis.[35] Increased consumption of wheat biofortified with selenium does not modify biomarkers of cancer risk or immune functions in healthy subjects. There is a lack of effect of antioxidant supplementation on hepatitis C. A Cochrane database systematic review reported that selenium seemed to show significant beneficial effect on GI cancer occurrence (RR = 0.59, 95% CI: 0.46 to 0.75).[36]

A recent systematic review concluded that there is no evidence to support or refute the promise of benefit from antioxidant supplements in patients with liver disease. On the other hand, antioxidant supplements may increase liver enzymes.[37]

Taurine

A taurine-supplemented diet has a beneficial effect on immune responses and performance in animals. There is a lack of literature to support its use in liver disorders.

Thymus

Interferon plus thymosin alpha-1 is superior to interferon alone for HBeAg positive chronic hepatitis B.[38] The role of thymosin in the treatment of hepatitis C remains to be established.[39,40]

A meta-analysis concluded that thymosin alpha-1 plus lamivudine may be superior to lamivudine alone for HBeAg-positive patients.[41]

Trace Elements

Iron and zinc content are lower in HCC than in controls. Copper content is lower in HCC than in surrounding tissues and cirrhotic controls.

While data are lacking, the use of zinc for alcoholic liver disease treatment has a therapeutic rationale.[42] Zinc supplementation prevents the increase of liver enzymes in chronic hepatitis C patients during combination therapy with pegylated interferon and ribavirin. Many, but not all, studies have shown zinc to be of benefit in hepatic encephalopathy.

Vitamin E

Vitamin E therapy, compared with placebo, results in a significantly higher rate of improvement in nonalcoholic steatohepatitis (43% versus 19%, p = 0.001).[2] This is associated with an improvement in liver biochemical tests and histology.

REFERENCES

1. Shores NJ, Keeffe EB. Is oral L-acyl-carnitine an effective therapy for hepatic encephalopathy? Review of the literature. *Dig Dis Sci.* 2008;53(9):2330-2333.

2. Sanyal AJ, Chalasani N, Kowdley KV, et al. Pioglitazone, vitamin E, or placebo for nonalcoholic steatohepatitis. *N Engl J Med.* 2010;362(18):1675-1685.

3. Cederbaum AI. Hepatoprotective effects of S-adenosyl-L-methionine against alcohol- and cytochrome P450 2E1-induced liver injury. *World J Gastroenterol.* 2010;16(11):1366-1376.

4. Takuma Y, Nouso K, Makino Y, Hayashi M, Takahashi H. Clinical trial: oral zinc in hepatic encephalopathy. *Aliment Pharmacol Ther.* 2010;32(9):1080-1090.

5. Chen J, Chen M, Zhao B, Wang Y. Effects of acupuncture on the immunological functions in hepatitis B virus carriers. *J Trad Chin Med.* 1999;19(4):268-272.

6. Melhem A, Stern M, Shibolet O, et al. Treatment of chronic hepatitis C virus infection via antioxidants: results of a phase I clinical trial. *J Clin Gastroenterol.* 2005;39(8):737-742.

7. Marshall AW, Graul RS, Morgan MY, Sherlock S. Treatment of alcohol-related liver disease with thioctic acid: a six month randomised double-blind trial. *Gut.* 1982;23(12):1088-1093.

8. Kravchuk IuA, Mekhtiev SN, Uspenskiï IuP, Grinevich VB, Koblov SV. Device laboratory and postmortem parallels in alcoholic hepatitis during combined therapy using thioctic (alpha-lipoic) acid. *Klin Med (Mosk).* 2004;82(6):55-57.

9. Soylu AR, Aydogdu N, Basaran UN, et al. Antioxidants vitamin E and C attenuate hepatic fibrosis in biliary-obstructed rats. *World J Gastroenterol.* 2006;12(42):6835-6841.

10. Di Sario A, Candelaresi C, Omenetti A, Benedetti A. Vitamin E in chronic liver diseases and liver fibrosis. *Vitam Horm.* 2007;76:551-573.

11. Bjelakovic G, Gluud LL, Nikolova D, Bjelakovic M, Nagorni A, Gluud C. Antioxidant supplements for liver diseases. *Cochrane Database Syst Rev.* 2011;(3):CD007749.

12. Abdelmalek MF, Sanderson SO, Angulo P, et al. Betaine for nonalcoholic fatty liver disease: results of a randomized placebo-controlled trial. *Hepatology.* 2009;50(6):1818-1826.

13. Fernandez-Mejia C. Pharmacological effects of biotin. *J Nutr Biochem.* 2005;16(7):424-427.

14. Niederau C, Strohmeyer G, Heintges T, Peter K, Göpfert E. Polyunsaturated phosphatidyl-choline and interferon alpha for treatment of chronic hepatitis B and C: a multi-center, randomized, double-blind, placebo-controlled trial. Leich Study Group. *Hepatogastroenterology.* 1998;45(21):797-804.

15. Singh NK, Prasad RC. A pilot study of polyunsaturated phosphatidyl choline in fulminant and subacute hepatic failure. *J Assoc Physicians India.* 1998;46(6):530-532.

16. Egner PA, Wang JB, Zhu YR, et al. Chlorophyllin intervention reduces aflatoxin-DNA adducts in individuals at high risk for liver cancer. *Proc Natl Acad Sci USA.* 2001;98(25):14601-14606.

17. Hirayama C, Suzuki H, Ito M, Okumura M, Oda T. Propagermanium: a nonspecific immune modulator for chronic hepatitis B. *J Gastroenterol.* 2003;38(6):525-532.

18. Ueno H, Sato T, Yamamoto S, et al. Randomized, double-blind, placebo-controlled trial of bovine lactoferrin in patients with chronic hepatitis C. *Cancer Sci.* 2006;97(10):1105-1110.

19. Anonymous. Acetyl-L-carnitine. Monograph. *Altern Med Rev.* 2010;15(1):76-83.

20. Ali SA, Faddah L, Abdel-Baky A, Bayoumi A. Protective effect of L-carnitine and coenzyme Q10 on CCl(4)-induced liver injury in rats. *Sci Pharm.* 2010;78(4):881-896.

21. Romano M, Vacante M, Cristaldi E, et al. L-carnitine treatment reduces steatosis in patients with chronic hepatitis C treated with alpha-interferon and ribavirin. *Dig Dis Sci.* 2008;53(4):1114-1121.

22. Malaguarnera M, Gargante MP, Russo C, et al. L-carnitine supplementation to diet: a new tool in treatment of nonalcoholic steatohepatitis—a randomized and controlled clinical trial. *Am J Gastroenterol.* 2010;105(6):1338-1345.

23. Malaguarnera M, Risino C, Cammalleri L, et al. Branched chain amino acids supplemented with L-acetylcarnitine versus BCAA treatment in hepatic coma: a randomized and controlled double blind study. *Eur J Gastroenterol Hepatol.* 2009;21(7):762-770.

24. Perrott J, Murphy NG, Zed PJ. L-carnitine for acute valproic acid overdose: a systematic review of published cases. *Ann Pharmacother.* 2010;44(7-8):1287-1293.

25. Yokochi S, Ishiwata Y, Saito H, Ebinuma H, Tsuchiya M, Ishii H. Stimulation of antiviral activities of interferon by a liver extract preparation. *Arzneimittelforschung.* 1997;47(8):968-974.

26. Velissaris D, Karamouzos V, Polychronopoulos P, Karanikolas M. Chronotypology and melatonin alterations in minimal hepatic encephalopathy. *J Circadian Rhythms.* 2009;7:6.

27. Lewy AJ, Ahmed S, Jackson JM, Sack RL. Melatonin shifts human circadian rhythms according to a phase-response curve. *Chronobiol Int.* 1992;9(5):380-392.

28. Archakov AI, Sel'tsovskiï AP, Lisov VI, et al. Phosphogliv: mechanism of therapeutic action and clinical efficacy. *Vopr Med Khim.* 2002;48(2):139-153.

29. Mato JM, Lu SC. Role of S-adenosyl-L-methionine in liver health and injury. *Hepatology.* 2007;45(5):1306-1312.

30. Purohit V, Abdelmalek MF, Barve S, et al. Role of S-adenosylmethionine, folate, and betaine in the treatment of alcoholic liver disease: summary of a symposium. *Am J Clin Nutr.* 2007;86(1):14-24.

31. Lu SC, Huang ZZ, Yang H, Mato JM, Avila MA, Tsukamoto H. Changes in methionine adenosyltransferase and S-adenosylmethionine homeostasis in alcoholic rat liver. *Am J Physiol Gastrointest Liver Physiol.* 2000;279(1):G178-G185.

32. Roncaglia N, Locatelli A, Arreghini A, et al. A randomised controlled trial of ursodeoxycholic acid and S-adenosyl-l-methionine in the treatment of gestational cholestasis. *BJOG.* 2004;111(1):17-21.

33. Mato JM, Cámara J, Fernández de Paz J, et al. S-adenosylmethionine in alcoholic liver cirrhosis: a randomized, placebo-controlled, double-blind, multicenter clinical trial. *J Hepatol.* 1999;30(6):1081-1089.

34. Rambaldi A, Gluud C. S-adenosyl-L-methionine for alcoholic liver diseases. *Cochrane Database Syst Rev.* 2006;(2):CD002235.

35. Stewart S, Prince M, Bassendine M, et al. A randomized trial of antioxidant therapy alone or with corticosteroids in acute alcoholic hepatitis. *J Hepatol.* 2007;47(2):277-283.

36. Bjelakovic G, Nikolova D, Simonetti RG, Gluud C. Antioxidant supplements for preventing gastrointestinal cancers. *Cochrane Database Syst Rev.* 2008;(3):CD004183.

37. Bjelakovic G, Gluud LL, Nikolova D, Bjelakovic M, Nagorni A, Gluud C. Meta-analysis: antioxidant supplements for liver diseases—the Cochrane Hepato-Biliary Group. *Aliment Pharmacol Ther.* 2010;32(3):356-367.

38. Mao HY, Shi TD. Treatment with interferon and thymosin alpha-1 versus interferon monotherapy for HBeAg positive chronic hepatitis B: a meta-analysis. *Zhonghua Gan Zang Bing Za Zhi.* 2011;19(1):29-33.

39. Raymond RS, Fallon MB, Abrams GA. Oral thymic extract for chronic hepatitis C in patients previously treated with interferon. A randomized, double-blind, placebo-controlled trial. *Ann Intern Med.* 1998;129(10):797-800.

40. Sherman KE. Thymosin alpha 1 for treatment of hepatitis C virus: promise and proof. *Ann N Y Acad Sci.* 2010;1194:136-140.

41. Zhang YY, Chen EQ, Yang J, Duan YR, Tang H. Treatment with lamivudine versus lamivudine and thymosin alpha-1 for e antigen-positive chronic hepatitis B patients: a meta-analysis. *Virol J.* 2009;6:63.

42. Barve A, Khan R, Marsano L, Ravindra KV, McClain C. Treatment of alcoholic liver disease. *Ann Hepatol.* 2008;7(1):5-15.

Chapter

62 *Prebiotics and Probiotics in Liver Health*

KEY POINTS

○ Patients with liver cirrhosis have varying degrees of imbalance of the intestinal flora.

○ Multiple studies have documented the benefit of probiotics in the treatment of hepatic encephalopathy.

○ A mixture of pre- and probiotics reduces the risk of postoperative infections in patients with liver transplantation.

Manipulation of intestinal bacteria has the potential to modulate liver dysfunction and heal hepatic disorders.[1-16] Pre- and probiotics protect against chemical-induced liver injury in animals.[4-6] Probiotic treatment results in lower aspartate aminotransferase and alanine aminotransferase activity in alcoholic liver disease.[7] Most, but not all, studies have shown beneficial effects of probiotics and synbiotics for hepatic encephalopathy.[8-15]

Multiple RCTs suggest that probiotics or synbiotics may be viable alternatives and/or adjuncts to lactulose for the management of hepatic encephalopathy.[16]

LIVER CIRRHOSIS

The role of probiotics in liver cirrhosis (without complications) remains to be established. Probiotics restore neutrophil phagocytic capacity in patients with liver cirrhosis and may play a role in reducing infectious complications. Treatment with *E coli Nissle* results in a trend toward lowering of the endotoxemia ($p = 0.07$) and improvement of liver functions in patients with liver cirrhosis ($p = 0.06$).[17]

NONALCOHOLIC FATTY LIVER DISEASE

Nonalcoholic steatohepatitis is associated with small intestinal diverticulosis and bacterial overgrowth.[18] Small bowel bacterial overgrowth is present in 50% of patients with nonalcoholic steatosis compared to only 22% of control subjects.[19] VSL#3 treatment results in improved biochemical tests in patients with NAFLD and alcoholic cirrhosis.[20]

A Cochrane database meta-analysis and systematic review concluded that lack of RCTs makes it impossible to support or refute the role for probiotics in NAFLD.[21] Since that report, emerging evidence has sparked a great deal of interest in the use of probiotics for NAFLD.[22]

Liver Cancer

A mixture of *L rhamnosus* and *P freudenreichii* blocks the intestinal absorption of aflatoxin B(1), which reduces urinary excretion of markers for aflatoxin exposure.

Preventing Infections After Liver Transplantation

Early enteral nutrition, supplemented with a mixture of lactic acid bacteria plus fibers, reduces bacterial infections with liver transplantation.[23]

REFERENCES

1. Gratz SW, Mykkanen H, El-Nezami HS. Probiotics and gut health: a special focus on liver diseases. *World J Gastroenterol.* 2010;16(4):403-410.

2. Babicska I, Rotkiewicz T, Otrocka-Domagała I. The effect of *Lactobacillus acidophilus* and *Bifidobacterium spp.* administration on the morphology of the gastrointestinal tract, liver and pancreas in piglets. *Pol J Vet Sci.* 2005;8(1):29-35.

3. Pawłowska J, Klewicka E, Czubkowski P, et al. Effect of *Lactobacillus casei* DN-114001 application on the activity of fecal enzymes in children after liver transplantation. *Transplant Proc.* 2007;39(10):3219-3221.

4. Xing HC, Li LJ, Xu KJ, et al. Protective role of supplement with foreign *Bifidobacterium* and *Lactobacillus* in experimental hepatic ischemia-reperfusion injury. *J Gastroenterol Hepatol.* 2006;21(4):647-656.

5. Mannaa F, Ahmed HH, Estefan SF, Sharaf HA, Eskander EF. *Saccharomyces cerevisiae* intervention for relieving flutamide-induced hepatotoxicity in male rats. *Pharmazie.* 2005;60(9):689-695.

6. Jeon TI, Hwang SG, Lim BO, Park DK. Extracts of *Phellinus linteus* grown on germinated brown rice suppress liver damage induced by carbon tetrachloride in rats. *Biotechnol Lett.* 2003;25(24):2093-2096.

7. Kirpich IA, Solovieva NV, Leikhter SN, et al. Probiotics restore bowel flora and improve liver enzymes in human alcohol-induced liver injury: a pilot study. *Alcohol.* 2008;42(8):675-682.

8. Jia L, Zhang MH. Comparison of probiotics and lactulose in the treatment of minimal hepatic encephalopathy in rats. *World J Gastroenterol.* 2005;11(6):908-911.

9.   Sharma P, Sharma BC, Puri V, Sarin SK. An open-label randomized controlled trial of lactulose and probiotics in the treatment of minimal hepatic encephalopathy. *Eur J Gastroenterol Hepatol.* 2008;20(6):506-511.

10.   Malaguarnera M, Greco F, Barone G, Gargante MP, Malaguarnera M, Toscano MA. *Bifidobacterium longum* with fructo-oligosaccharide (FOS) treatment in minimal hepatic encephalopathy: a randomized, double-blind, placebo-controlled study. *Dig Dis Sci.* 2007;52(11):3259-3265.

11.   Bajaj JS, Saeian K, Christensen KM, et al. Probiotic yogurt for the treatment of minimal hepatic encephalopathy. *Am J Gastroenterol.* 2008;103(7):1707-1715.

12.   Liu Q, Duan ZP, Ha DK, Bengmark S, Kurtovic J, Riordan SM. Synbiotic modulation of gut flora: effect on minimal hepatic encephalopathy in patients with cirrhosis. *Hepatology.* 2004;39(5):1441-1449.

13.   Loguercio C, Abbiati R, Rinaldi M, Romano A, Del Vecchio Blanco C, Coltorti M. Long-term effects of *Enterococcus faecium* SF68 versus lactulose in the treatment of patients with cirrhosis and grade 1-2 hepatic encephalopathy. *J Hepatol.* 1995;23(1):39-46.

14.   Malaguarnera M, Gargante MP, Malaguarnera G, et al. *Bifidobacterium* combined with fructo-oligosaccharide versus lactulose in the treatment of patients with hepatic encephalopathy. *Eur J Gastroenterol Hepatol.* 2010;22(2):199-206.

15.   Pereg D, Kotliroff A, Gadoth N, Hadary R, Lishner M, Kitay-Cohen Y. Probiotics for patients with compensated liver cirrhosis: a double-blind placebo-controlled study. *Nutrition.* 2011;27(2):177-181.

16.   Dhiman RK, Saraswat VA, Sharma BK, et al. Minimal hepatic encephalopathy: consensus statement of a working party of the Indian National Association for Study of the Liver. *J Gastroenterol Hepatol.* 2010;25(6): 1029-1041.

17.   Lata J, Novotný I, Príbramská V, et al. The effect of probiotics on gut flora, level of endotoxin and Child-Pugh score in cirrhotic patients: results of a double-blind randomized study. *Eur J Gastroenterol Hepatol.* 2007;19(12):1111-1113.

18.   Nazim M, Stamp G, Hodgson HJ. Non-alcoholic steatohepatitis associated with small intestinal diverticulosis and bacterial overgrowth. *Hepatogastroenterology.* 1989;36(5):349-351.

19.   Wigg AJ, Roberts-Thomson IC, Dymock RB, McCarthy PJ, Grose RH, Cummins AG. The role of small intestinal bacterial overgrowth, intestinal permeability, endotoxaemia, and tumour necrosis factor alpha in the pathogenesis of non-alcoholic steatohepatitis. *Gut.* 2001;48(2):206-211.

20.   Loguercio C, Federico A, Tuccillo C, et al. Beneficial effects of a probiotic VSL#3 on parameters of liver dysfunction in chronic liver diseases. *J Clin Gastroenterol.* 2005;39(6):540-543.

21.   Lirussi F, Mastropasqua E, Orando S, Orlando R. Probiotics for non-alcoholic fatty liver disease and/or steatohepatitis. *Cochrane Database Syst Rev.* 2007;(1):CD005165.

22. Iacono A, Raso GM, Canani RB, Calignano A, Meli R. Probiotics as an emerging therapeutic strategy to treat NAFLD: focus on molecular and biochemical mechanisms. *J Nutr Biochem.* 2011;22(8):699-711.

23. Rayes N, Seehofer D, Theruvath T, et al. Supply of pre- and probiotics reduces bacterial infection rates after liver transplantation—a randomized, double-blind trial. *Am J Transplant.* 2005;5(1):125-130.

BILIARY AND PANCREATIC DISORDERS

Chapter

63 *Biliary Disorders*

KEY POINTS

○ Acupuncture is widely used for biliary disorders.

○ Probiotics may alter the bile composition, and potentially the lithogenic potential, of bile.

While this section focuses on biliary disorders, I would suggest that the reader also review other sections under liver disorders as there is a significant overlap.

HERBAL THERAPIES

Muh-Shiang-Bin-Lang-Wan

Chinese medicinal herbs, Muh-Shiang-Bin-Lang-Wan, modulate the sphincter of Oddi function in rabbits through activation of muscarinic receptors.[1]

Yiqi-Yangyin Prescription

Yiqi-Yangyin prescription demonstrates a significant decline in bilirubin and calcium, while the concentration of bile acid is significantly increased in patients with cholelithiasis.[2]

Minocha A. *A Guide to Alternative Medicine and the Digestive System* (pp 381-392).
© 2013 Taylor & Francis Group.

Jinquiancao Gao

Animal experiments demonstrate a gallstone growth rate of 43% in the treatment group, compared to 79% in the control. A study of 120 patients with cholelithiasis for 2 months revealed that the clinical effective rate was 92.5%.[3]

ACUPUNCTURE[4]

Multiple studies have documented beneficial effects against gallstones and cholestasis.[5-12] Acupuncture results in a significant reduction of the rate, number, and size of gallstones in hamsters.[5] Treatment at acupoints Ganshu (GB 18) and Qimen (LI 14) inhibit lithogenesis induced by lithogenic diet in animals.[6]

Acupuncture results in a gallstone excretion rate of 86 to 91%.[10,11] Likewise, acupuncture also affects the sphincter of Oddi dysfunction.[13-15]

LASER

Laser irradiation improves gallbladder and the sphincter of Oddi physiology while restoring the normal balance of bile constituents in patients with biliary dyskinesia.[16]

WATER INJECTION

Water injection at the lines joining the Qimen (Liv 14), Riyue (GB 24), and Juque (Ren 14) points in patients with biliary colic results in a superior resolution of pain compared to controls.[17]

MULTIMODAL THERAPIES

An Hui Zhi Tong Decoction Plus Acupuncture

An Hui Zhi Tong decoction combined with acupuncture is beneficial in patients with biliary ascariasis complicated by infection.[18]

PROBIOTICS

Data are limited and disappointing.

REFERENCES

1. Kuo YI, Chiu JH, Lin JG, Hsieh CL, Wu CW. Chinese medicinal herbs Muh-Shiang Bin-Lang-Wan increases the motility of sphincter of Oddi in anesthetized rabbits through activation of M1 muscarinic receptors. *Life Sci.* 2003;74(4):533-542.

2. Wei DQ. Effect of yiqi-yangyin prescription on bile composition of cho-lelithiasis patients. *Zhong Xi Yi Jie He Za Zhi*. 1990;10(8):470-472,452.

3. Zhang GS, Li SZ. Clinical and experimental observations of jinqiancao gao on preventive and therapeutic effects in cholelithiasis. *Zhong Xi Yi Jie He Za Zhi*. 1989;9(7):396-397,387.

4. Xu X. Acupuncture in an outpatient clinic in China: a comparison with the use of acupuncture in North America. *South Med J*. 2001;94(8):813-816.

5. Ma C, Yang W. The preventing and treating effects of electro-acupunc-ture on cholelithiasis in golden hamster. *Zhen Ci Yan Jiu*. 1996;21(4):68-72.

6. Zhang S, Chen H, Gui J, Xu C, Zhu P, Cao Z. Clinical and experimental researches in the inhibition of bile pigment lithogenesis by cupuncture and moxibustion. *Zhen Ci Yan Jiu*. 1995;20(3):40-45.

7. Wu JQ, Liu T, Bai YL. Study on "massage to activate the meridian" apparatus in the treatment of cholecystolithiasis. *Zhong Xi Yi Jie He Za Zhi*. 1989;9(3):141-143,131.

8. Lin JG, Yang SH, Tsai CH. Acupuncture protection against experimental hyperbilirubinemia and cholangitis in rats. *Am J Chin Med*. 1995;23(2):131-137.

9. Yang SH, Lin JG, Tsai CH, Ma JJ. Protection by moxibustion against experimental hyperbilirubinemia and cholangitis in rats. *Am J Chin Med*. 1993;21(3-4):237-242.

10. Zhang Y, Zhang L, Yang H, Zhang H, Zhu Y. 1291 cases of cholelithiasis treated with electric shock on otoacupoints. *J Tradit Chin Med*. 1991;11(2):101-109.

11. Song MP. Clinical observation on frequency-changeable electroacu-puncture for treatment of cholelithiasis. *Zhongguo Zhen Jiu*. 2006;26(11):772-774.

12. Akimova LG. Laser puncture in the combined treatment of stenocardia with concomitant chronic cholecystitis. *Lik Sprava*. 1998;(3):135-137.

13. Kim MH. A brief commentary: electroacupuncture may relax the con-traction of sphincter of Oddi. *J Altern Complement Med*. 2001;7(Suppl 1):S119-S120.

14. Guelrud M, Rossiter A, Souney PF, Mendoza S, Mujica V. The effect of transcutaneous nerve stimulation on sphincter of Oddi pressure in patients with biliary dyskinesia. *Am J Gastroenterol*. 1991;86(5):581-585.

15. Lee SK, Kim MH, Kim HJ, et al. Electroacupuncture may relax the sphincter of Oddi in humans. *Gastrointest Endosc*. 2001;53(2):211-216.

16. Vorob'ev LP, Salova LM, Chubarov GV, Meshkov VM. The correction of functional disorders of the bile-secreting system by using laser radia-tion. *Vopr Kurortol Fizioter Lech Fiz Kult*. 1992;(4):25-31.

17. Jiang Y, Chen Y. Treatment of biliary colic by water injection in the region of Qimen, Riyue, and Juque points. *J Tradit Chin Med*. 1995;15(3):185-188.

18. Liangmin L. Clinical observation on combined use of herbal medicine and acupuncture for treatment of 50 cases of biliary ascariasis compli-cated by infection. *J Tradit Chin Med*. 1996;16(3):194-197.

Chapter

64 *Acute Pancreatitis*

KEY POINTS

○ Phytobotanicals show promise as an adjunct treatment in patients with acute pancreatitis.

○ The role of probiotics in acute pancreatitis is controversial.

○ Studies on the effect of antioxidants in acute pancreatitis have yielded conflicting results.

Limited evidence indicates that complimentary therapies may provide benefit in an adjunctive capacity.

ACUPUNCTURE[1-4]

Electroacupuncture at Zusanli (ST36) in rats reduces amylase and lipase levels in rat pancreatitis.[1] The efficacy of electroacupuncture is better if undertaken at an early stage of pancreatitis.[3] Paradoxically, pancreatitis may occur rarely as a complication of acupuncture.[4]

ANTIOXIDANTS

Exposure to antioxidants during acute pancreatitis ameliorates oxidative stress.[5] Results of clinical studies have been mixed.[6,7]

OTHER SUPPLEMENTS

Feeding zinc to rats with pancreatitis improves survival.[8] Enteral feeding supplemented with n-3 polyunsaturated fatty acids reduces hospital stay length in patients with acute pancreatitis.[9] Glutamine supplementation is also of benefit.

PROBIOTICS

Rarely, commensal gut flora like *Bifidobacterium* and *Veillonella* can turn pathogenic, which can lead to life-threatening conditions such as infected necrotizing pancreatitis in patients with gallstone pancreatitis.[10] Data on the efficacy of probiotics have provided conflicting results, perhaps due to study design as well as use of different probiotics in different doses.[11,12]

A meta-analysis concluded that use of pre- or probiotics or synbiotics has no effect on acute pancreatitis.[13]

PHYTOBOTANICALS

Please see Tables 64-1 and 64-2 for information.

REFERENCES

1. An HJ, Lee JH, Lee HJ, et al. Electroacupuncture protects against CCK-induced acute pancreatitis in rats. *Neuroimmunomodulation.* 2007;14(2):112-118.

2. Wang XY. Electroacupuncture for treatment of acute pancreatitis and its effect on the intestinal permeability of the patient. *Zhongguo Zhen Jiu.* 2007;27(6):421-423.

3. Luo YH, Zhong GW, Zhao SP, et al. Efficacy observation of electroacupuncture intervention on severe acute pancreatitis at early stage complicated with intestinal paralysis. *Zhongguo Zhen Jiu.* 2011;31(2):105-109.

4. Uhm MS, Kim YS, Suh SC, et al. Acute pancreatitis induced by traditional acupuncture therapy. *Eur J Gastroenterol Hepatol.* 2005;17(6):675-677.

5. Uden S, Schofield D, Miller PF, Day JP, Bottiglier T, Braganza JM. Antioxidant therapy for recurrent pancreatitis: biochemical profiles in a placebo-controlled trial. *Aliment Pharmacol Ther.* 1992;6(2):229-240.

6. Sateesh J, Bhardwaj P, Singh N, et al. Effect of antioxidant therapy on hospital stay and complications in patients with early acute pancreatitis: a randomised controlled trial. *Trop Gastroenterology.* 2009;30(4):210-216.

7. Siriwardena AK, Mason JM, Balachandra S, et al. Randomised, double blind, placebo controlled trial of intravenous antioxidant (n-acetylcysteine, selenium, vitamin C) therapy in severe acute pancreatitis. *Gut.* 2007;56(10):1439-1444.

8. Song MK, Adham NF. Role of zinc in treatment of experimental acute pancreatitis in mice. *Dig Dis Sci.* 1989;34(12):1905-1910.

9. Lasztity N, Hamvas J, Biro L, et al. Effect of enterally administered n-3 polyunsaturated fatty acids in acute pancreatitis—a prospective randomized clinical trial. *Clin Nutr.* 2005;24(2):198-205.

10. Verma R, Dhamija R, Ross SC, Batts DH, Loehrke ME. Symbiotic bacteria induced necrotizing pancreatitis. *JOP.* 2010;11(5):474-476.

11. Besselink MG, van Santvoort HC, Buskens E, et al. Probiotic prophylaxis in predicted severe acute pancreatitis: a randomised, double-blind, placebo-controlled trial. *Lancet.* 2008;371(9613):651-659.

12. Oláh A, Belágyi T, Pótó L, Romics L Jr, Bengmark S. Synbiotic control of inflammation and infection in severe acute pancreatitis: a prospective, randomized, double blind study. *Hepatogastroenterology.* 2007;54(74):590-594.

Table 64-1. Animal Studies of Phytobotanicals
Used in Acute Pancreatitis

Remedy	Model	Comment
G jasminoides Ellis[14]	In vitro	Protects cellular membranes
Acanthopanax[15]	In vivo	Improves biochemical tests and histopathology
Curcumin[16,17]	In vivo	Ameliorates pancreatitis
Emodin derived from R palmatum[18]	In vivo	Decreases pancreatic necrosis and serum amylase
Emodin plus Danshensu[19]	In vivo	Combination is superior to either agent individually
Resveratrol[20]	In vivo	Maintains intestinal barrier
Baicalin derived from skullcap[21]	In vivo	Improves survival
Tripterygium glycosides derived from Tripterygium wilfordii[22]	In vivo	Improves serum amylase and endotoxin levels without effect on mortality
G biloba[23]	In vivo	Improves histopathology
Ginseng, Korean red[24]	In vivo	Improves histopathology
Panax notoginoside derived from P notoginseng[25]	In vivo	Reduces histopathological pancreatic injury and serum amylase
Caulis piper Wallichii[26]	In vivo	Reduces pancreatic injury and improves survival
Chaiqin Chengqi decoction[27]	In vivo	Reduces severity of pancreatitis
Rhubarb[28]	In vivo	Improves survival
S miltiorrhiza (Danshen)[29]	In vivo	Decreases complications and mortality
Ligustrazine[30]	In vivo	Reduces mortality
Kakonein[30]	In vivo	Reduces mortality

Table 64-2. Human Studies of Phytobotanicals in Acute Pancreatitis

Remedy	Comment
Anisodamine from the root of *Anisodus tanguticus*[31]	Data are mixed
Curcumin[32]	Reduces oxidative stress in tropical pancreatitis
Tetrandrine extracted from *Stephania tetrandra*[33]	Reduces complications and mortality
Breviscapine, also known as *scutellarin*, extracted from *Erigeron breviscapus (Vant) Hand.-Mazz*[34]	Reduces mortality

13. Zhang MM, Cheng JQ, Lu YR, Yi ZH, Yang P, Wu XT. Use of pre-, pro- and synbiotics in patients with acute pancreatitis: a meta-analysis. *World J Gastroenterol.* 2010;16(31):3970-3978.

14. Jia YJ, Jiang MN, Pei DK, Ji XP, Yu GJ. The influence of *Gardenia jasminoides Ellis* in function of pancreatic celluar memberance on acute pancreatitis. *Chin J Surg Integr Tradit West Med.* 1996;2:176-178.

15. Zhang XP, Shi Y, Zhang L. Progress in the study of therapeutic effects of traditional Chinese medicine and extracts in treating severe acute pancreatitis. *JOP.* 2007;8(6):704-714.

16. Gukovsky I, Reyes CN, Vaquero EC, Gukovskaya AS, Pandol SJ. Curcumin ameliorates ethanol and nonethanol experimental pancreatitis. *Am J Physiol Gastrointest Liver Physiol.* 2003;284(1):G85-G95.

17. Chen KH, Chao D, Liu CF, Chen CF, Wang D. Curcumin attenuates airway hyperreactivity induced by ischemia-reperfusion of the pancreas in rats. *Transplant Proc.* 2010;42(3):744-747.

18. Gong Z, Yuan Y, Lou K, Tu S, Zhai Z, Xu J. Mechanisms of Chinese herb emodin and somatostatin analogs on pancreatic regeneration in acute pancreatitis in rats. *Pancreas.* 2002;25:154-160.

19. Wang G, Sun B, Zhu H, et al. Protective effects of emodin combined with danshensu on experimental severe acute pancreatitis. *Inflamm Res.* 2010;59(6):479-488.

20. Xin L, Ou YY, Wang Y, et al. Significance of determination of changes of serum IL-6 and TNF-alpha levels in rat models of severe acute pancreatitis (SAP) treated with resveratrol. *J Radioimmunol.* 2005;18:417-419.

21. Zhang XP, Zhang L, Yang P, et al. Protective effects of baicalin and octreotide on multiple organ injury in severe acute pancreatitis. *Dig Dis Sci.* 2008;53(2):581-591.

22. Jin C, Ni QX, Zhang QH, Xiang Y, Zhang N, Zhang YL. An experimental study on the immunoregulatory effect of an extract of *Tripterygium wilfordii Hook F* in rats with acute necrotizing pancreatitis. *Chin J Gen Surg.* 2000;15:283-285.

23. Xu LJ, Zhang P, Miao Y. The effects and mechanisms of *Ginkgo biloba* extract on apoptosis of pancreatic acinar cells in severe pancreatitis in rats. *Jiangsu Medical J.* 2003;29:502-504.

24. Joo KR, Shin HP, Cha JM, et al. Effect of Korean red ginseng on superoxide dismutase inhibitor-induced pancreatitis in rats: a histopathologic and immunohistochemical study. *Pancreas.* 2009;38(6):661-666.

25. Ge Z, Zhang DS, Hu YL, Wang Y. Experimental study on therapeutic effect of pngs and somatostatin for severe acute pancreatitis model in rats. *China J Mod Med.* 2002;12:17-19.

26. Xu BH, Zhao SD, Yang CM. Effect of Shi Nanteng extract on endotoxemia in rats with acute hemorrhagic necrotizing pancreatits. *Chin Crit Care Med.* 1998;10:611-613.

27. Li YH, Huang ZW, Xue P, et al. Effects of Chaiqin Chengqi Decoction on activation of nuclear factor-kappaB in pancreas of rats with acute necrotizing pancreatitis. *Zhong Xi Yi Jie He Xue Bao.* 2008;6(2):180-184.

28. Yang CY, Shen L, Xie ZG, Jiang X, Liang N, Chen ZH. Experimental studies of therapeutic effect of *Rheum officinale* on acute pancreatitis. *Zhong Yao Cai.* 2011;34(1):84-88.

29. Zhang XP, Li ZJ, Liu DR. Progress in research into the mechanism of *Radix Salviae miltiorrhizae* in treatment of acute pancreatitis. *Hepatobiliary Pancreat Dis Int.* 2006;5(4):501-504.

30. Zhang XP, Wang C, Wu DJ, Ma ML, Ou JM. Protective effects of ligustrazine, kakonein and *Panax notoginsenosides* on multiple organs in rats with severe acute pancreatitis. *Methods Find Exp Clin Pharmacol.* 2010;32(9):631-644.

31. Chen DZ, Wan SQ, Zhang XY. Prognostic factors and treatment of severe acute pancreatitis. *Zhonghua Nei Ke Za Zhi.* 1991;30(2):82-85,125.

32. Durgaprasad S, Pai CG, Vasanthkumar, Alvres JF, Namitha S. A pilot study of the antioxidant effect of curcumin in tropical pancreatitis. *Indian J Med Res.* 2005;122(4):315-318.

33. Leng DY, Yu J, Luo JY, et al. Clinical observation of Tet in treating severe acute pancreatitis 13 cases. *J Modern Physician.* 1997;2:59-60.

34. Huang DK. The effect of breviscapine in severe pancreatitis. *China Pract Med.* 2006;1:11-12.

Chapter

65 *Chronic Pancreatitis*

KEY POINTS

○ Lifestyle modifications, including diet, cooking, smoking, and alcohol intake, have the potential to play a big role in the management.

○ Curcumin, derived from turmeric, slows the progression of disease in animals.

○ Antioxidants help decrease pain and improve quality of life.

○ Data on the role of complementary and alternative medicine are limited.

STRICT AVOIDANCE OF ALCOHOL

Patients must stop drinking alcohol, even in cases where alcohol may not be suspected to be the etiology. Continued alcohol intake increases mortality risk.

SMOKING CESSATION

Smoking is a risk factor for chronic pancreatitis.[1] Smoking cessation helps retard the progression of disease and provide relief.

DIETARY MANIPULATION

Small, frequent, low-fat meals, especially in the form of medium chain triglycerides, help some patients. Encourage antioxidant-rich foods over the long term.[2] Cooking at high temperatures, frying food, etc destroys the bioavailability of vitamin C.

Role of Micronutrient Supplements

Micronutrients/antioxidants help in controlling pain. Methionine and vitamin C appear to be the most critical, followed by selenium as needed.[2,3] Antioxidant supplements improve the quality of life.[4] Zinc deficiency is common in patients with chronic pancreatitis, and the degree of deficiency is directly proportional to the exocrine and endocrine insufficiency.[5]

Table 65-1. Phytobotanical Treatments
for Chronic Pancreatitis

Herbal Remedy/ Extract	Study Model	Comment
Emodin[6]	Rats	Antifibrotic
Curcumin[7]	Animals	Retards progression of chronic pancreatitis
Chlorophyll[8]	Uncontrolled study in humans	Relieves pain in patients
Grapeseed[9]	Case series of 3 patients using commercially available IH636 grape seed proanthocyanidin extract (known as ActiVin [InterHealth Nutraceuticals Inc, Benicia, CA])	Addition of ActiVin results in pain relief.
Saiko-keishi-to (TJ-10)	Rats	Reduces acinar destruction and apoptotic index

Enzyme Supplements

Pancreatic enzyme supplements are a popular remedy for pain relief in chronic pancreatitis. However, the results from the studies have not been consistent. They are also used to treat steatorrhea due to exocrine enzyme deficiency.

MISCELLANEOUS

Since probiotics modulate inflammatory processes at both intestinal and extraintestinal levels, they may have a role in therapy. Acupuncture and transcutaneous electric nerve stimulation do not provide pain relief in chronic pancreatitis.

See Table 65-1 for phytobotanical treatment information.

REFERENCES

1. Andriulli A, Botteri E, Almasio PL, Vantini I, Uomo G, Maisonneuve P; ad hoc Committee of the Italian Association for the Study of the Pancreas. Smoking as a cofactor for causation of chronic pancreatitis: a meta-analysis. *Pancreas*. 2010;39(8):1205-1210.

2. Braganza JM, Lee SH, McCloy RF, et al. Chronic pancreatitis. *Lancet*. 2011;377:1184-1197.

3. Kirk GR, White JS, McKie L, et al. Combined antioxidant therapy reduces pain and improves quality of life in chronic pancreatitis. *J Gastrointest Surg*. 2006;10(4):499-503.

4. Shah NS, Makin AJ, Siriwarddena AK, et al. Quality of life assessment in patients with chronic pancreatitis receiving antioxidant therapy. *World J Gastroenterol*. 2010;16(32):4066-4071.

5. Girish BN, Rajesh G, Vaidyanathan K, et al. Zinc status in chronic pancreatitis and its relationship with exocrine and endocrine insufficiency. *JOP*. 2009;10(6):651-656.

6. Wang CH, Gao ZQ, Ye B, et al. Effect of emodin on pancreatic fibrosis in rats. *World J Gastroenterol*. 2007;13(3):378-382.

7. Talukdar R, Tandon RK. Pancreatic stellate cells: new target in the treatment of chronic pancreatitis. *J Gastroenterol Hepatol*. 2008;23(1):34-41.

8. Yoshida A, Yokono O, Oda T. Therapeutic effect of chlorophyll-a in the treatment of patients with chronic pancreatitis. *Gastroenterol Jpn*. 1980;15(1):49-61.

9. Banerjee B, Bagchi D. Beneficial effects of a novel IH636 grape seed proanthocyanidin extract in the treatment of chronic pancreatitis. *Digestion*. 2001;63(3):203-206.

HEALTHY NUTRITION POTPOURRI

Chapter

66 *Weight Loss Diet That Reduces Mortality Risk, Too!*

The war over body weight control consumes billions of dollars with numerous books and pundits promoting their own versions of anti-obesity and weight loss. The Atkins low-carbohydrate diet has been one of the most popular diet fads to hit the market in recent years.

CONCERN

Questions have been raised about the benefits versus the risks of a low-carbohydrate diet (ie, is the weight loss being achieved at the risk to overall health?). The concerns became heightened when Dr. Atkins himself died, due in part to heart-related illness.

AN AUTHORITATIVE ANSWER

The report of a study funded by the National Institute of Health and published in the *Annals of Internal Medicine* provides a definitive answer.[1]

Study Goals and Follow-Up

The authors assessed the effect of 2 types of low-carbohydrate diets—either animal-based (primarily animal fat and protein) or vegetable-based (predominantly vegetable sources of fat and protein)—based on scientifically validated food-frequency questionnaires done during follow-up of the study subjects.

Minocha A. *A Guide to Alternative Medicine and the Digestive System* (pp 393-402). © 2013 Taylor & Francis Group.

Study Subjects

The data from Nurses Health Study and Health Professionals follow-up study were included in analysis. A total of 85,168 women and 44,548 men without heart disease, cancer, or diabetes at baseline formed the database. Over the follow-up, there were 12,555 deaths.

Results

○ The low-carbohydrate diet is associated with a modest increase in overall mortality.

○ The animal-based low-carbohydrate diet results in higher all-cause mortality, cardiovascular mortality, and cancer mortality.

COMMENTS

A more recent prospective study of 43,000 Swedish women also concluded that regular use of a low-carbohydrate, high-protein diet is associated with a higher risk of cardiovascular disease.[2]

The short-term benefits of low-carbohydrate, high-protein diets for weight loss must be viewed in context of long-term harm resulting from an increased risk of cardiovascular diseases.[3] Vegetable-based low-carbohydrate diet consumption leads to lower all-cause mortality and cardiovascular mortality.

REFERENCES

1. Fung TT, van Dam RM, Hankinson SE, Stampfer M, Willett WC, Hu FB. Low-carbohydrate diets and all-cause and cause-specific mortality: two cohort studies. *Ann Intern Med.* 2010;153(5):289-298.

2. Lagiou P, Sandin S, Lof M, Trichopoulos D, Adami HO, Weiderpass E. Low carbohydrate-high protein diet and incidence of cardiovascular diseases in Swedish women: prospective cohort study. *BMJ.* 2012;344:e4026.

3. Floegel A. Low carbohydrate-high protein diets. *BMJ.* 2012;344:e3801

Chapter

67 Quinoa
One Complete Vegetarian Food

KEY POINTS

○ *Quinoa* is a fiber-richsource of nutrition and health benefits.[1-5]

○ *Quinoa* contains no gluten.

Quinoa (*Chenopodium quinoa*) is considered a pseudocereal or pseudograin. The high nutritional value of *quinoa* has been recognized in South America for thousands of years. It is considered a complete food.

While not a common household item, *quinoa* seed has a fluffy, creamy, slightly crunchy texture. Cooking tends to give it a distinct flavor. *Quinoa* flakes can be used as a breakfast cereal.

QUINOA CONTENTS

○ In addition to its fiber content, a high protein content of 15% makes it a very attractive protein source for vegetarians. Unlike other vegetarian sources, it contains all essential amino acids and is thus recognized as a complete protein source.

○ It is an excellent source of important minerals and vitamins, including magnesium and iron, omega fatty acids, and vitamin E.

○ *Quinoa* contains a variety of polyphenols, phytosterols, and flavonoids with possible nutraceutical benefits. Its physico-chemical properties, including solubility, water-holding capacity, gelation, emulsification, and foaming, allow for its use in a variety of ways.

○ Noteworthy for patients with celiac sprue and those interested in a gluten-free diet for other indications is that it contains no gluten.

Because of its nutritional features, *quinoa* has the potential to be used as a crop in NASA's Controlled Ecological Support Systems for use during long manned spaceflights (eg, to Mars).[6]

Full and complete nutrition can be accomplished with an appropriate selection of plant-based foods. *Quinoa* is unrivalled in its qualities and nutritional ingredients, and a 1993 NASA report declared that "while no single food can supply all the life sustaining nutrients, *quinoa* comes close as any other in the plant and animal kingdom."[6(p1)]

REFERENCES

1. Vega-Gálvez A, Miranda M, Vergara J, Uribe E, Puente L, Martínez EA. Nutrition facts and functional potential of *quinoa* (*Chenopodium quinoa Willd.*), an ancient Andean grain: a review. *J Sci Food Agric.* 2010;90(15):2541-2547.

2. Abugoch James LE. *Quinoa* (*Chenopodium quinoa Willd.*): composition, chemistry, nutritional, and functional properties. *Adv Food Nutr Res.* 2009;58:1-31.

3. Dixit AA, Azar KM, Gardner CD, Palaniappan LP. Incorporation of whole, ancient grains into a modern Asian Indian diet to reduce the burden of chronic disease. *Nutr Rev.* 2011;69(8):479-488.

4. Meneguetti QA, Brenzan MA, Batista MR, Bazotte RB, Silva DR, Garcia Cortez DA. Biological effects of hydrolyzed quinoa extract from seeds of *Chenopodium quinoa Willd.* *J Med Food.* 2011;14(6):653-657.

5. Paško P, Zagrodzki P, Bartoń H, Chłopicka J, Gorinstein S. Effect of quinoa seeds (*Chenopodium quinoa*) in diet on some biochemical parameters and essential elements in blood of high fructose-fed rats. *Plant Foods Hum Nutr.* 2010;65(4):333-338.

6. National Aeronautics and Space Administration [NASA]. *Quiona: An Emerging "New" Crop With Potential for CELSS.* NASA Technical Paper 3422. Washington, DC: NASA; 1993. Available at: http://ntrs.nasa.gov/archive/nasa/casi.ntrs.nasa.gov/19940015664_1994015664.pdf. Accessed August 14, 2012.

Chapter
68 *All Yogurts May Not Be Probiotic or Equal*

KEY POINTS

- ○ The live culture seal on yogurt containers is voluntary and its presence implies that the yogurt contains at least 100 million bacteria per gram at the time of manufacture.

○ Some brands subject yogurt to heat treatment in an attempt to boost the shelf life, resulting in killing the bacteria. This step gets rid of any potential benefits of these bacteria.

The knowledge that yogurt, with its probiotic bacteria, provides healthy nutrition has been passed on through generations. It was Dr. Metchnikoff[1] who, in the early 20th century, publicly espoused the benefits of yogurt for health. In fact, he attributed his own health and longevity to yogurt.

YOGURT CONSUMPTION IN THE UNITED STATES

An average American eats 4 to 6 pounds of yogurt per year. The commercial market for yogurt exceeds $2.2 billion in the United States, and the popularity of yogurt continues to grow. The texture of different yogurts is obviously different and depends on a variety of factors.[2]

YOGURT VERSUS MILK

A big advantage of yogurt over milk and its other products is that yogurt contains bacterial lactase. Yogurt may be better tolerated by those with a deficiency of the enzyme lactase, manifesting as lactose intolerance, although data are mixed. Yogurt is considered especially beneficial for gastrointestinal health.[2,3]

LIVE ACTIVE CULTURES

○ The application of heat treatment to yogurt results in killing the bacteria while extending the shelf life of the yogurt product. Most of the health-promoting beneficial effects of probiotic bacteria are thus lost.

○ A brand of yogurt containing live cultures has a logo or seal (in the form of "A C," which stands for active cultures) on the container. Thus, yogurt may be made by active cultures but may or may not have the bacteria depending upon the brand.

○ The seal is voluntary, and its presence implies that the yogurt contains at least 100 million bacteria per gram at the time of manufacture.

Standard yogurt contains *L bulgaricus* and *S thermophilus*, but their beneficial probiotic effects, especially in doses present in usual yogurt, is controversial and limited at best.

HEALTH-ORIENTED YOGURTS

Yogurt appears to fulfill the basic criteria for a probiotic.[4,5] Many immune-enhancing benefits have been ascribed.[6] Health-oriented yogurt brands tend to contain 1 or more bacteria in addition to the 2 outlined previously. Furthermore, the number of bacteria per serving is much higher so that enough bacteria can survive to the colon and exert their beneficial effects to the highest potential. Some of these are mentioned in the section discussing probiotic products available on market. The study of microbial interactions is increasingly using a combination of classic and genomic approaches.[7,8]

KEFIR

Conceptually similar to yogurt, Kefir is a fermented milk drink and usually contains multiple diverse species of probiotic. The number of probiotics may vary from 10 to as many as 30 species/strains. For example, Lifeway Organic Probiotic Kefir (plain; Lifeway Foods Inc, Morton Grove, IL) contains 12 probiotics.

WORDS OF CAUTION

❍ Many of the products from popular brands contain gelatin, which is derived from animal skin, bones, etc. Refrain from such products if you want strict vegetarian items based on religious, cultural, or health convictions. This may not always be mentioned on the label, so check out the company Web site.

❍ Some but not all yogurt products are gluten free.

❍ Choose plain yogurt over frozen or sweetened yogurts, as well as those with fruit, if your goal is the highest health benefit. You may add, if you wish, fresh fruit to the yogurt just before consumption.

❍ Yogurt without live cultures has a low likelihood of providing significant health benefits of probiotics.

REFERENCES

1. Weissmann G. It's complicated: inflammation from Metchnikoff to Meryl Streep. *FASEB J.* 2010;24(11):4129-4132.

2. Sodini I, Remeuf F, Haddad S, Corrieu G. The relative effect of milk base, starter, and process on yogurt texture: a review. *Crit Rev Food Sci Nutr.* 2004;44(2):113-137.

3. Adolfsson O, Meydani SN, Russell RM. Yogurt and gut function. *Am J Clin Nutr.* 2004;80(2):245-256.

4. Guarner F, Perdigon G, Corthier G, Salminen S, Koletzko B, Morelli L. Should yoghurt cultures be considered probiotic? *Br J Nutr.* 2005;93(6):783-786.

5. de Vrese M, Stegelmann A, Richter B, Fenselau S, Laue C, Schrezenmeir J. Probiotics—compensation for lactase insufficiency. *Am J Clin Nutr.* 2001;73(Suppl 2):421S-429S.

6. Meydani SN, Ha WK. Immunologic effects of yogurt. *Am J Clin Nutr.* 2000;71(4):861-872.

7. Sieuwerts S, de Bok FA, Hugenholtz J, van Hylckama Vlieg JE. Unraveling microbial interactions in food fermentations: from classical to genomics approaches. *Appl Environ Microbiol.* 2008;74(16):4997-5007.

8. Sieuwerts S, Molenaar D, van Hijum SA, et al. Mixed-culture transcriptome analysis reveals the molecular basis of mixed-culture growth in Streptococcus thermophilus and Lactobacillus bulgaricus. *Appl Environ Microbiol.* 2010;76(23):7775-7784.

Chapter
69

Fish Type and Risk of Mercury Toxicity
All Fish Are Not the Same

KEY POINTS

- ○ Fish is considered to be heart healthy.
- ○ An appropriate selection of fish allows for health benefits without increasing mercury toxicity.

BACKGROUND[1]

- ○ Fish contain high amounts of cardioprotective omega-3 fatty acids. Ingestion of fish (eg, 1 to 2 servings per week) reduces the risk of coronary death by 36%.
- ○ The mercury content of predatory fish is higher because they eat other fish containing mercury and indirectly attain higher levels than the fish at the lower end of the food chain.
- ○ The beneficial effect of fish intake can be demonstrated with as few as one fish serving per week, and greater intake provides increased protection.
- ○ Both wild and farmed fish are beneficial, although the wild variety may have more heart-healthy fatty acids than farmed.
- ○ The benefits of fish intake are tempered by the concern over mercury intake.

IDENTIFYING LOW VERSUS HIGH MERCURY FISH

Sardines, salmon, and shrimp have lower mercury content than the predatory sharks, tuna, swordfish, and orange roughy.[1]

FARMED FISH

Even more importantly, the farmed fish have the lowest mercury content while providing similar benefits. However, there is some evidence that changes in the fishing industry have produced widely eaten fish (eg, tilapia and catfish), which have fatty acid characteristics that are considered inflammatory by the health care community.[2] Sadly, it is the cheaper fish that are likely to be in this latter category. The differences may in part be due to what these farmed fish are fed.

RECOMMENDATIONS FOR FISH INTAKE

Individuals with a very high consumption of fish (5 or more servings per week) should limit their intake of types of fish with high mercury levels.

Nonpregnant persons may eat 1 predatory fish serving and 2 to 3 low mercury fish servings per week. Pregnant women should not eat more than 1 predatory fish serving per 2 weeks; however, they may eat other fish 2 to 3 times per week.

REFERENCES

1. Jeejeebhoy KN. Benefits and risks of a fish diet—should we be eating more or less? *Nat Clin Pract Gastroenterol Hepatol.* 2008;5(4):178-179.
2. Weaver KL, Ivester P, Chilton JA, et al. The content of favorable and unfavorable polyunsaturated fatty acids found in commonly eaten fish. *J Am Diet Assoc.* 2008;108(7):1178-1185.

Chapter

70

One Must-Have Healthy Spice/Herb in the Kitchen
Turmeric

KEY POINTS

- ❍ It has antimicrobial, anti-inflammatory, and antineoplastic properties.
- ❍ Human studies show that it is effective in ulcerative colitis.
- ❍ Preclinical data indicate its potential benefit in the treatment and prevention of cancer.

Turmeric, derived from the plant *C longa*, is a golden yellow spice that has been used in Indian and Chinese cultures since ancient times. Because of its numerous diverse clinical uses with no known adverse effects,[1] it has been labeled by many as the "spice of life."

It suppresses *H pylori* and protects against the development of experimental gastric ulcer in animals.[2] It is a chemosensitizer and radiosensitizer for cancer cells, while protecting human tissues.[3,4] It inhibits experimental colorectal carcinogenesis in mice.[5]

Its role in inflammatory bowel disease appears promising.[6] A randomized, multicenter, double-blind, placebo-controlled trial demonstrated that the relapse rate of ulcerative colitis in a curcumin group over 6 months was 5%, compared to 21% in the placebo group.[7] It demonstrates anticancer activity in liver cancer cells.[8]

Turmeric is a hepatoprotective agent.[9] It protects animals against chemical/ethanol-induced liver damage. It ameliorates the risk of fibrosis of fatty liver.[10] It suppresses viral hepatitis B, as well as C.[11,12] Oxy-Q (Farr Labs, Santa Monica, CA), which contains curcumin and quercetin, improves early outcomes in cadaveric renal transplantation[13] and may benefit liver transplant patients.

Curcumin with piperine inhibits lipid peroxidation in patients with tropical pancreatitis.[14] It inhibits the growth of pancreatic adenocarcinoma cells.[15]

REFERENCES

1. Epstein J, Sanderson IR, Macdonald TT. Curcumin as a therapeutic agent: the evidence from in vitro, animal and human studies. *Br J Nutr.* 2010;103(11):1545-1557.
2. Kim DC, Kim SH, Choi BH, et al. *Curcuma longa* extract protects against gastric ulcers by blocking H2 histamine receptors. *Biol Pharm Bull.* 2005;28(12):2220-2224.

3.   Ravindran J, Prasad S, Aggarwal BB. Curcumin and cancer cells: how many ways can curry kill tumor cells selectively? *AAPS J.* 2009;11(3):495-510.

4.   Goel A, Aggarwal BB. Curcumin, the golden spice from Indian saffron, is a chemosensitizer and radiosensitizer for tumors and chemoprotector and radioprotector for normal organs. *Nutr Cancer.* 2010;62(7):919-930.

5.   Patel BB, Majumdar AP. Synergistic role of curcumin with current therapeutics in colorectal cancer: minireview. *Nutr Cancer.* 2009;61(6):842-846.

6.   Hanai H, Sugimoto K. Curcumin has bright prospects for the treatment of inflammatory bowel disease. *Curr Pharm Des.* 2009;15(18):2087-2094.

7.   Hanai H, Iida T, Takeuchi K, et al. Curcumin maintenance therapy for ulcerative colitis: randomized, multicenter, double-blind, placebo-controlled trial. *Clin Gastroenterol Hepatol.* 2006;4(12):1502-1506.

8.   Darvesh AS, Aggarwal BB, Bishayee A. Curcumin and liver cancer: a review. *Curr Pharm Biotechnol.* 2012;13(1):218-228.

9.   Priya S, Sudhakaran PR. Curcumin-induced recovery from hepatic injury involves induction of apoptosis of activated hepatic stellate cells. *Indian J Biochem Biophys.* 2008;45(5):317-325.

10. Aggarwal BB. Targeting inflammation-induced obesity and metabolic diseases by curcumin and other nutraceuticals. *Annu Rev Nutr.* 2010;30:173-199.

11. Kim K, Kim KH, Kim HY, Cho HK, Sakamoto N, Cheong J. Curcumin inhibits hepatitis C virus replication via suppressing the Akt-SREBP-1 pathway. *FEBS Lett.* 2010;584(4):707-712.

12. Kim HJ, Yoo HS, Kim JC, et al. Antiviral effect of *Curcuma longa* Linn extract against hepatitis B virus replication. *J Ethnopharmacol.* 2009;124(2):189-196.

13. Shoskes D, Lapierre C, Cruz-Correa M, et al. Beneficial effects of the bioflavonoids curcumin and quercetin on early function in cadaveric renal transplantation: a randomized placebo controlled trial. *Transplantation.* 2005;80(11):1556-1559.

14. Durgaprasad S, Pai CG, Vasanthkumar, Alvres JF, Namitha S. A pilot study of the antioxidant effect of curcumin in tropical pancreatitis. *Indian J Med Res.* 2005;122(4):315-318.

15. Mach CM, Mathew L, Mosley SA, Kurzrock R, Smith JA. Determination of minimum effective dose and optimal dosing schedule for liposomal curcumin in a xenograft human pancreatic cancer model. *Anticancer Res.* 2009;29(6):1895-1899.

INDEX

Printed in the United States
by Baker & Taylor Publisher Services